BIOCHEMICAL SOCIETY SY.

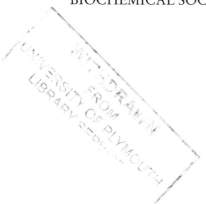

No. 61

FREE RADICALS AND OXIDATIVE STRESS:
ENVIRONMENT, DRUGS AND FOOD ADDITIVES

BIOCHEMICAL SOCIETY SYMPOSIUM No. 61
held at The University of Sussex, December 1994

Free Radicals and Oxidative Stress: Environment, Drugs And Food Additives

ORGANIZED AND EDITED BY

C. RICE-EVANS, B. HALLIWELL AND G. G. LUNT

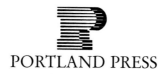

PORTLAND PRESS

Published by Portland Press, 59 Portland Place, London WIN 3AJ, U.K.
on behalf of The Biochemical Society
In North America orders should be sent to Ashgate Publishing Co.,
Old Post Road, Brookfield, VT 05036-9704, U.S.A.

ISBN I 85578 069 0   ISSN 0067-8694

British Library Cataloguing in Publication Data
A catalogue record for this book is available from the British Library

Typeset by Unicus Graphics Ltd, Horsham, Sussex
Printed in Great Britain by Henry Ling Ltd, Dorchester

Contents

Preface

It has been only in the past two decades that we have appreciated the 'paradox of aerobic life', to quote the title of the first chapter in this book. Oxygen is essential for human life, yet it is poisonous to all aerobic organisms. This is because some oxygen is metabolized to oxygen-derived free radicals and other reactive oxygen species which, in excess, can cause injury and have to be opposed by antioxidant defence systems, both endogenous and diet-derived. Ironically, moderate amounts of oxygen-derived free radicals and other free radical species (such as nitric oxide) are useful *in vivo*, so life is a balance.

This field of antioxidants, reactive oxygen species and reactive nitrogen species ramifies into all fields of biology and medicine, so it was appropriate to make it the subject of the Annual Symposium at the meeting of the Biochemical Society, held at the University of Sussex, Brighton, U.K. in December 1994. Experts from all over the world contributed to the symposium. This volume covers the basics of the chemistry of free radicals (including nitric oxide); the way in which side-effects of certain drugs and air pollutants can be mediated by free radicals; the mechanisms of action of antioxidants in foods, both as dietary phytochemicals and in food preservation; and the use of antioxidants in the treatment of human disease.

In the first section, the free radical that is currently most fashionable (nitric oxide) and its more toxic derivative (peroxynitrite) are described in relation to the balance of pro-oxidant versus protective reactions. This leads to the question of the role of nitric oxide and its derivatives in vascular injury and vascular protection. The biological importance of thiyl radicals and their role in the nitrosylation of protein and non-protein thiols gives rise to the proposal that 'free' thiols and protein thiols can act as potent antioxidants in radical-induced damage; however, the chemical reactivity of the resulting thiyl radicals must not be neglected. Since transition metal ion-catalysed reactions and their consequences have been at the root of much of the explosive growth in the free-radical field, both chemically and biologically, the chapter on the chemistry of lipid alkoxyl radicals and their role in metal-amplified lipid peroxidation is particularly appropriate. It helps to answer some of the many remaining questions pertaining to the non-enzymic mechanisms of lipid peroxidation.

The biological and biochemical effects of air pollutants are of great interest at present. Airborne soot and diesel exhaust particles are potential carcinogens and inducers of respiratory diseases. Sulphur dioxide continues to threaten plant life and episodes of elevated levels of ozone and nitrogen dioxide are becoming increasingly common in the world's major cities. The redox chemistry underlying the health-threatening effects resulting from air pollution is illustrated by the cooperation of catalytically active particles with sulphur dioxide, and the potential for oxidative damage by mixtures of ozone and nitrogen dioxide. Nowhere are the environmental effects of free radicals exemplified better than in the consideration of ultraviolet radiation and free-radical damage to the skin. Studies are described elucidating the functional role of the redox activation of the haem oxygenase gene by UVA as a general response to oxidative stress.

The section on antioxidants focuses on the highly topical issue of the constituents of higher plants as dietary antioxidants, especially the flavonoids and carotenoids, while approaches to protection against oxidative damage in pathological states and the accompanying chemistry are described in the context of therapeutic iron chelators. The criteria necessary to evaluate antioxidant activity are put into context, with methods that may be applied to establish antioxidant activity *in vitro* and how they would be relevant *in vivo*. Antioxidants in foods are important not only for the health of whoever eats the food, but also for the stability of the food itself. Therefore, the effect of processing on food antioxidants, as well as the mechanistic implications of the action of antioxidants and stabilizers in food packaging, are presented. The 'hot topic' of food irradiation is also discussed.

Drug-derived free radicals may contribute to the side-effects of certain drugs. This is reviewed in the context of activation by myeloperoxidase, and the kinetic basis for hypoxia-selective, bioreductive drugs which involves radicals from one-electron reduction of nitro compounds, aromatic N-oxides and quinones. The potential contribution of radicals to the side-effects of drugs in the treatment of rheumatoid arthritis is reviewed. In contrast, the drug tamoxifen may exert antioxidant properties *in vivo*, in addition to its better-established effects.

Most authors enthusiastically committed their thoughts to paper to create the present volume, which will make a significant contribution to the scientific literature available on this subject.

CATHERINE RICE-EVANS
BARRY HALLIWELL
August 1995

Abbreviations

AAPH	2,2'-azo*bis*(2-amidinopropane)-dihydrochloride
ABTS	2,2'-azino*bis*-(3-ethyl benzthiazoline-6-sulphonic acid)
ACH	acetohydroxamic acid
ALS	amyotrophic lateral sclerosis
AMVN	2,2'-azo*bis*(2,4-dimethylvaleronitrile)
AP site	apurinic/apyrimidinic site
BBB	blood–brain barrier
BHA	butylated hydroxyanisole
BHT	butylated hydroxytoluene
BPO	breath pentane output
CB-A	chain-breaking acceptor
CB-D	chain-breaking donor
CHD	coronary heart disease
COPS	cholesterol oxidation products
COSY	correlation spectroscopy
DEPMPO	5-diethoxyphosphoryl-5-methyl-1-pyrolline-*N*-oxide
DFO	desferrioxamine
DFT	desferrithiocin
DMPO	5,5-dimethyl-1-pyrolline-*N*-oxide
DMSO	dimethyl sulphoxide
DP	diesel soot particle
DTPA	diethylenetriamine penta-acetic acid
ECG	epicatechin gallate
EDTA	ethylene diamine tetra-acetic acid
EGCG	epigallocatechin gallate
ELF	epithelial lining fluid
EPR	electron paramagnetic resonance
ESR	electron spin resonance
FFA	flufenamic acid
GSH	glutathione
HBED	hydroxybenzyl ethylenediamine
HDL	high-density lipoprotein
HPLC	high-performance liquid chromatography
HPO	hydroxypyridone
KMB	ketomethylthiobutyrate
LDL	low-density lipoprotein
LOPS	lipid oxidation products
MFA	meclofenamic acid
MNP	2-methyl-2-nitrosopropane
MPO	myeloperoxidase
MRP	Maillard reaction product
NBT	Nitro-Blue tetrazolium
NMDA	*N*-methyl-D-aspartate
NMR	nuclear magnetic resonance

NO	nitric oxide
NOS	nitric oxide synthase
NSAID	non-steroidal anti-inflammatory drug
NTA	nitriloacetic acid
PB	phenylbutazone
PBN	α-phenyl-*tert*-butyl N-nitrone
PBS	phosphate-buffered saline
PMN	polymorphonuclear neutrophil
PP	polypropylene
PVC	poly(vinyl chloride)
RA	rheumatoid arthritis
ROS	reactive oxygen species
RT	respiratory tract
RTLF	respiratory tract lining fluid
SOD	superoxide dismutase
TAA	total antioxidant activity
TBA	thiobarbituric acid
TBARS	thiobarbituric acid reactive substance
TBPH	2,4,6-tri-*t*-butylphenol
TEAC	Trolox equivalent antioxidant activity
THF	tetrahydrofuran
VLDL	very-low-density lipoprotein

Biochem. Soc. Symp. **61**, 1–31
Printed in Great Britain

Oxidative stress: the paradox of aerobic life

Kelvin J.A. Davies

Department of Biochemistry & Molecular Biology, The Albany Medical College, Albany, NY 12208, U.S.A.

Abstract

The paradox of aerobic life, or the 'Oxygen Paradox', is that higher eukaryotic aerobic organisms cannot exist without oxygen, yet oxygen is inherently dangerous to their existence. This 'dark side' of oxygen relates directly to the fact that each oxygen atom has one unpaired electron in its outer valence shell, and molecular oxygen has two unpaired electrons. Thus atomic oxygen is a free radical and molecular oxygen is a (free) bi-radical. Concerted tetravalent reduction of oxygen by the mitochondrial electron-transport chain, to produce water, is considered to be a relatively safe process; however, the univalent reduction of oxygen generates reactive intermediates. The reductive environment of the cellular milieu provides ample opportunities for oxygen to undergo unscheduled univalent reduction. Thus the superoxide anion radical, hydrogen peroxide and the extremely reactive hydroxyl radical are common products of life in an aerobic environment, and these agents appear to be responsible for oxygen toxicity.

To survive in such an unfriendly oxygen environment, living organisms generate — or garner from their surroundings — a variety of water- and lipid-soluble antioxidant compounds. Additionally, a series of antioxidant enzymes, whose role is to intercept and inactivate reactive oxygen intermediates, is synthesized by all known aerobic organisms. Although extremely important, the antioxidant enzymes and compounds are not completely effective in preventing oxidative damage. To deal with the damage that does still occur, a series of damage removal/repair enzymes, for proteins, lipids and DNA, is synthesized. Finally, since oxidative stress levels may vary from time to time, organisms are able to adapt to such fluctuating stresses by inducing the synthesis of antioxidant enzymes and damage removal/repair enzymes.

In a perfect world the story would end here; unfortunately, biology is seldom so precise. The reality appears to be that, despite the valiant antioxidant and repair mechanisms described above, oxidative damage remains an inescapable outcome of aerobic existence. In recent years oxidative stress has been implicated in a wide variety of degenerative processes, diseases and syndromes, including the following:

mutagenesis, cell transformation and cancer; atherosclerosis, arteriosclerosis, heart attacks, strokes and ischaemia/reperfusion injury; chronic inflammatory diseases, such as rheumatoid arthritis, lupus erythematosus and psoriatic arthritis; acute inflammatory problems, such as wound healing; photo-oxidative stresses to the eye, such as cataract; central-nervous-system disorders, such as certain forms of familial amyotrophic lateral sclerosis, certain glutathione peroxidase-linked adolescent seizures, Parkinson's disease and Alzheimer's dementia; and a wide variety of age-related disorders, perhaps even including factors underlying the aging process itself. Some of these oxidation-linked diseases or disorders can be exacerbated, perhaps even initiated, by numerous environmental pro-oxidants and/or pro-oxidant drugs and foods. Alternatively, compounds found in certain foods may be able to significantly bolster biological resistance against oxidants. Currently, great interest centres on the possible protective value of a wide variety of plant-derived antioxidant compounds, particularly those from fruits and vegetables.

The radical nature of oxygen

Oxidative stress is an inevitable result of life in an oxygen-rich environment. For aerobic organisms oxygen is paradoxically both vital for existence and inherently dangerous. The Oxygen Paradox derives from the chemical nature of oxygen itself [1–5] which in atomic form (O) exists as a free radical, and in molecular form (O_2) is a bi-radical. The outer valence shell of atomic oxygen contains one unpaired electron. When two oxygen atoms combine to form molecular oxygen, the outer valence shell electrons do not spin-pair but remain as two unpaired electrons. A radical is defined as any atom or molecule with one or more unpaired electrons in an outer valence shell. Therefore, molecular oxygen is a true bi-radical.

The radical nature of molecular oxygen permits some very interesting oxidation/reduction chemistry [1–5]. In a non-enzymic, univalent, reduction pathway oxygen can undergo four successive one-electron reductions as shown in Fig. 1. Unlike the concerted four-electron (i.e. tetravalent) reduction of oxygen catalysed by cytochrome oxidase at the end of the mitochondrial electron transport chain, the non-enzymic univalent pathway for oxygen reduction results in the generation of several reactive intermediates. The first one-electron reduction of oxygen generates the superoxide anion radical ($O_2^{\cdot-}$) which is generally referred to simply as superoxide. Addition of a second electron and two protons (to $O_2^{\cdot-}$) generates the active species hydrogen peroxide (H_2O_2). A third electron addition produces the highly reactive hydroxyl radical ($^{\cdot}OH$) and releases a hydroxide ion (OH^-). A fourth electron addition harmlessly generates a water molecule.

It is interesting to note in Fig. 1 that both O_2 and $O_2^{\cdot-}$ are oxygen radicals (O_2 is a bi-radical, $O_2^{\cdot-}$ is a mono-radical) whereas H_2O_2, despite being a reactive oxygen species, is not a radical since all outer valence shell electrons are paired. The highly reactive hydroxyl radical is, of course, a true radical species. Also worth noting at this point is the fact that superoxide generation frequently occurs by hydrogen transfer (from a donor reductant) via a transient hydrodioxyl species ($HO_2^{\cdot}$). As shown in Fig. 2 the hydrodioxyl radical is a protonated superoxide

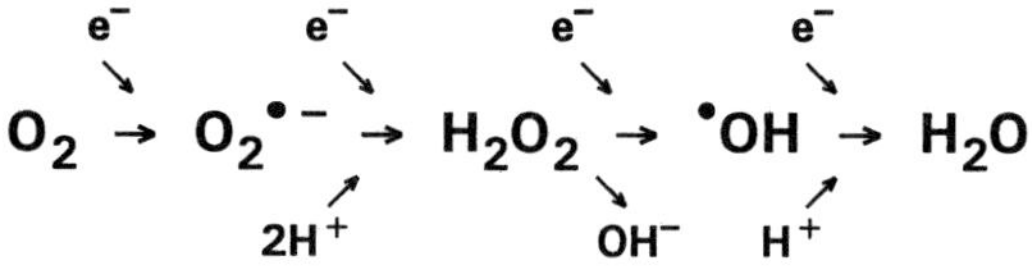

$$O_2 \xrightarrow{\quad e^- \quad} O_2^{\bullet -} \xrightarrow[2H^+]{\quad e^- \quad} H_2O_2 \xrightarrow[OH^-]{\quad e^- \quad} {}^{\bullet}OH \xrightarrow[H^+]{\quad e^- \quad} H_2O$$

$$O_2^{\bullet -} = \text{superoxide}$$
$$H_2O_2 = \text{hydrogen peroxide}$$
$${}^{\bullet}OH = \text{hydroxyl radical}$$

Fig. 1. The univalent pathway for oxygen reduction.

$$O_2 + RH \rightarrow HO_2^{\bullet} + R^{\bullet}$$

$$HO_2^{\bullet} \rightleftharpoons O_2^{\bullet -} + H^+ \quad (pKa = 4.8)$$

$$RH = \text{a hydrogen donor (reductant)}$$
$$HO_2^{\bullet} = \text{hydrodioxyl radical}$$
$$O_2^{\bullet -} = \text{superoxide}$$

Fig. 2. Hydrodioxyl radical and superoxide.

molecule and, at physiological pH, can rapidly dissociate to form $O_2^{\bullet -}$ and H^+. Since $HO_2^{\bullet}$ has a pK_a of 4.8 [1] it is possible that limited concentrations of this radical may be achieved in the acidic local environments of the outer surface of the inner mitochondrial membrane (where proton pumping generates a ΔpH) and within phagolysosomes of neutrophils, macrophages and monocytes.

Several oxygen species act as biological oxidants; but $O_2^{\bullet -}$ is actually a mild reductant [6]. The simple addition of a proton to $O_2^{\bullet -}$ (forming $HO_2^{\bullet}$) converts this mild reductant into a fairly active oxidizing agent. The redox potential of ${}^{\bullet}OH$ at approximately 1.77 V, however, clearly marks this radical as a highly oxidizing species [6]. Singlet molecular oxygen ($^1O_2$) is not produced by redox reactions but by absorption of electromagnetic energy which transiently inverts the spin of one of oxygen's two unpaired electrons, such that both spins attain an anti-parallel orientation [7]. Molecular oxygen or O_2 (also called ground state or triplet oxygen) is unable to accept two electrons directly (bivalent reduction) because the addition of a pair of anti-parallel electrons is restricted in the spins-parallel ground state. Singlet oxygen, however, with its anti-parallel valence electron spins has no such spin-restrictions on reactivity and is a very good two-electron oxidant for many biomolecules [1–7]. The absorption of large amounts of electromagnetic energy by O_2 to generate $^1O_2$ is largely restricted to photochemical events, however, and interest in singlet oxygen is, therefore, largely centred on environmental chemistry, plant biology and oxidant reactions in the tissues of the skin and the eye. Singlet oxygen is unstable and decays to the ground state with a lifetime of only 2–7 μs, emitting light as it decays [7].

Biological sources of reactive oxygen species

Over 95% of all the oxygen we breathe undergoes a concerted tetravalent reduction to produce water in a reaction catalysed by cytochrome oxidase (cytochrome c: oxygen oxidoreductase) of Complex IV in the mitochondrial electron transport chain $(O_2 + 4e^- + 4H^+ \rightarrow 2H_2O)$. Cytochrome oxidase is the terminal electron acceptor in the chain and must give up its reducing equivalents in order to allow continued electron transport; if electrons stop flowing through the chain the proton motive force dissipates, and ATP production cannot continue. Thus, the major role of oxygen for all aerobic organisms is simply to act as a sink or dumping ground for electrons.

Although the mitochondrial electron transport chain is a very efficient system the very nature of the alternating one-electron oxidation–reduction reactions it catalyses (generating a constantly alternating series of 'caged' radicals) predispose each electron carrier to side reactions with molecular oxygen. Thus, for example, as ubiquinone within the electron transport chain cycles between the quinone (fully oxidized) and semi-quinone (one-electron reduction product) and quinol (fully reduced by two electrons) states, there is a tendency for an electron to pass to oxygen directly (generating $O_2^{\cdot-}$) instead of to the next electron carrier in the chain. Several iron–sulphur clusters within the respiratory chain are also subject to such toxic, $O_2^{\cdot-}$-generating, side-reactions with oxygen. Thus it is commonly held that mitochondrial generation of $O_2^{\cdot-}$ represents the major intracellular source of oxygen radicals under physiological conditions [2]. With estimates of 1–2% of the total daily oxygen consumption going to mitochondrial $O_2^{\cdot-}$ generation, a 60 kg woman would produce some 160 to 320 mmol of superoxide each day from mitochondrial respiration alone (based on an O_2 consumption of $6.4 \, l \, kg^{-1} \, day^{-1}$) and an 80 kg man would produce some 215 to 430 mmol of $O_2^{\cdot-}$ per day.

Other potentially major sources of oxygen radical generation are phagocytic cells such as polymorphonuclear leucocytes (neutrophils), monocytes and macrophages. Such cells utilize an NADPH oxidase enzymic system to directly generate $O_2^{\cdot-}$ as part of their armoury against invading micro-organisms [8]. Under normal conditions most of the $O_2^{\cdot-}$ (and related species) generated by the NADPH oxidase should be accurately directed against micro-organisms enveloped within the phagocytic phagolysosome. Under conditions of chronic inflammation, however, surrounding tissues are directly exposed to high levels of $O_2^{\cdot-}$ and its metabolites. Such chronic inflammatory states are characteristic of many diseases such as rheumatoid arthritis, lupus erythematosus and psoriatic arthritis. Certain extreme acute inflammatory responses, such as those following extreme trauma, also appear to involve 'accidental' exposure of health tissues to bursts of $O_2^{\cdot-}$ generation. Various mammalian cell types express NADH- and/or NADPH-linked oxidases on their surfaces. Such oxidase complexes appear to function in a manner similar to phagocytic cell NADPH oxidases, and may generate a constant stream of $O_2^{\cdot-}$ to maintain a local environment that discourages bacterial/fungal infection; a sort of 'antiseptic superoxide tone'.

Autoxidation of biological molecules may account for a fairly significant source of oxygen radical production *in vivo*. Reduced carbon compounds are inherently susceptible to oxidation and this certainly includes the lipids, proteins, carbohydrates, DNA and RNA of which we are made. Historically, great interest has been focused on the autoxidation of membrane lipids and this approach enabled important advances in the food chemistry field, including the development of successful antioxidant compounds and packaging processes that enable foods to be stored for long periods without spoilage. Attention to lipid oxidation also paved the way for our understanding of the importance of the physiological antioxidant, vitamin E, that is lipid-soluble and partitions in all of our membranes [9]. Over the past 10 to 15 years new findings have revealed that cell proteins, carbohydrates and nucleic acids are also highly susceptible to autoxidation. Such agents as vitamin C (ascorbic acid), and uric acid, seem to provide significant protection against the effects of protein, carbohydrate and nucleic acid oxidation in the aqueous compartments of cells and organisms [10]. In reality, many of the protein, lipid, carbohydrate and nucleic acid oxidations that initially appear to be autoxidation reactions turn out to be metal-catalysed oxidations after more detailed investigations. The role of transition metals, such as iron and copper, in non-enzymic biological oxidations cannot be overestimated.

Fundamentals of oxidative stress

Oxidative stress may be considered as a state of increased turnover of biomolecules induced by elevated rates of non-enzymic oxidation. We usually think of the term oxidative stress as applied to cells, tissues, or organisms (including human beings) as an outcome of oxidative damage to biologically important molecules, such as proteins, lipids, carbohydrates and nucleic acids (DNA and RNA).

Proteins, lipids, carbohydrates and nucleic acids have all been studied for sensitivity to oxidative modification by a wide variety of free radicals and reactive oxygen species. Superoxide is not particularly reactive with lipids, carbohydrates, or nucleic acids, but does exhibit limited reactivity with certain proteins. The evidence to date indicates that $O_2^{\cdot-}$ will react with proteins that contain transition-metal prosthetic groups, such as haem moieties or iron–sulphur clusters [11,12]. Such transition-metal-mediated reactions result in damage to amino acids, usually those directly attached or proximal to the metal catalyst, and loss of protein/enzyme function. A good example of such reactions is the loss of aconitase activity that follows exposure of bacteria to $O_2^{\cdot-}$ [11].

One of the most important reactions of superoxide is actually with another superoxide molecule, as shown in Fig. 3. All of the reactions shown in Fig. 3 are dismutation reactions in which one molecule of $O_2^{\cdot-}$ or $HO_2^{\cdot}$ acts as the reductant and the other acts as the oxidant. Importantly, H_2O_2 and O_2 are the products of superoxide dismutation, whether one starts with $O_2^{\cdot-}$ or $HO_2^{\cdot}$. The rate constants for superoxide dismutation [1] do vary quite substantially, as shown in Fig. 3, depending on whether one starts with $O_2^{\cdot-}$ or $HO_2^{\cdot}$ and depending on whether the enzyme superoxide dismutase is used to catalyse the reaction. If one combines the information shown in Fig. 1 with that shown in Fig. 3, it will become clear that the second electron in the univalent pathway of Fig. 1 typically

Rate constant

Uncatalysed dismutation reactions

$$O_2^{\bullet-} + HO_2^{\bullet} + H^+ \rightarrow H_2O_2 + O_2 \qquad 8.5 \times 10^7 \text{ M}^{-1} \text{ sec}^{-1}$$

$$HO_2^{\bullet} + HO_2^{\bullet} + H^+ \rightarrow H_2O_2 + O_2 \qquad 7.6 \times 10^5 \text{ M}^{-1} \text{ sec}^{-1}$$

$$O_2^{\bullet-} + O_2^{\bullet-} + 2H^+ \rightarrow H_2O_2 + O_2 \qquad < 1 \times 10^2 \text{ M}^{-1} \text{ sec}^{-1}$$

Superoxide dismutase catalysed reaction

$$O_2^{\bullet-} + O_2^{\bullet-} + 2H^+ \rightarrow H_2O_2 + O_2 \qquad 1.9 \times 10^9 \text{ M}^{-1} \text{ sec}^{-1}$$

Fig. 3. The dismutation of superoxide.

1) $O_2^{\bullet-} + O_2^{\bullet-} + 2H^+ \rightarrow H_2O_2 + O_2$

2) $O_2^{\bullet-} + Fe^{3+} \rightarrow O_2 + Fe^{2+}$

3) $H_2O_2 + Fe^{2+} \rightarrow {}^{\bullet}OH + OH^- + Fe^{3+}$

Net: $O_2^{\bullet-} + H_2O_2 \rightarrow {}^{\bullet}OH + OH^- + O_2$

Fig. 4. Generation of hydroxyl radical.

is derived from $O_2^{\bullet-}$ (or $HO_2^{\bullet}$). Thus, whenever $O_2^{\bullet-}$ (or $HO_2^{\bullet}$) is generated there will always be a concomitant production of H_2O_2.

Hydrogen peroxide is clearly a major common intermediate, generated by multiple oxidation pathways. Hydrogen peroxide is an oxidant for many biological molecules, especially those containing sulphydryl groups, iron–sulphur clusters, reduced haem moieties and copper prosthetic groups [1–5]. Hydrogen peroxide can also readily react with transition-metal reductants/catalysts to generate the hydroxyl radical (${}^{\bullet}OH$), as shown in Fig. 4. Eqn. 3 in Fig. 4 shows that reduced iron (Fe^{2+}) is oxidized by H_2O_2 to generate ${}^{\bullet}OH$; this is basically the reaction described by Fenton in 1894 [13]. As also shown in Fig. 4, however, $O_2^{\bullet-}$ can act as the reductant to re-reduce Fe^{3+} to Fe^{2+}. This 'iron-catalysed Haber–Weiss reaction' was first proposed as one of several possible reaction schemes in 1934 [14] and has gained quite widespread support in recent years [15]. It should be noted that copper can substitute for iron as the transition metal in Fig. 4. The hydroxyl radical is the most reactive of all the oxygen radicals and will readily oxidize proteins, lipids, carbohydrates, DNA and RNA. In closely related reactions, proteins containing iron or copper prosthetic groups can react with H_2O_2 to produce high oxidation states of the bound metal. For example, haemoglobin can react with H_2O_2 to produce a ferryl-haemoglobin (Fe^{4+}) state [16]. Such high oxidation states can act as "OH', 'pseudo-'OH', or 'crypto-'OH' causing significant oxidative damage. The main difference is that true ${}^{\bullet}OH$ is a free radical which responds to Brownian motion in solution and reacts at nearly diffusion controlled rates. In contrast, agents like ferryl-haemoglobin have more limited mobility, and reactivity is hindered or determined by the position of the metal on the protein, and the access that a potential reactant may (or may not) have.

Other oxygen-based species also play major roles in the oxidative stresses to which we are subjected. One of the most common is hypochlorous acid or hypochlorite, which exists as a 50/50 ratio of $HOCl/OCl^-$ at physiological pH. $HOCl/OCl^-$ is generated by the enzyme myeloperoxidase in certain phagocytic cells such as neutrophils. It will be remembered from the previous section that phagocytes generate $O_2^{\cdot-}$ via a membrane NADPH oxidase system [8]. The $O_2^{\cdot-}$ so produced dismutates to H_2O_2 (as shown in Fig. 3) and neutrophils utilize myeloperoxidase to oxidize the abundant halide chloride to form hypochlorous acid/hypochlorite. Such cells then use the $HOCl/OCl^-$ to kill invading organisms such as bacteria [17]. $HOCl/OCl^-$ can directly oxidize proteins and increase their turnover [17–19] and it can generate secondary oxidants, such as chloroamines, that can migrate far from the site of production to cause multiple effects [17–19].

Various oxides of nitrogen are experienced as widespread environmental pollutants and some are actually generated intracellularly. Nitric oxide ($NO^{\cdot}$) and nitrogen dioxide ($NO_2^{\cdot}$) are common components of photochemical smog [20]. Nitric oxide, however, is also actively generated by the enzyme nitric oxide synthase in mammalian tissues, where it is used as a physiological vasodilating agent [21]. There is now serious concern [22–24] that $NO^{\cdot}$ may also be causing unwanted oxidative stress in our cells either directly, or through production of related species such as peroxynitrite ($ONOO^-$). Of course ozone (O_3) is another oxygen-based species that can cause significant oxidative stress [24,25]. In recent years there has been serious concern over the apparent loss of ozone from earth's upper atmosphere; the 'ozone hole'. At stratospheric levels ozone is extremely useful because it absorbs UV radiation and thereby protects animals and plant life on our planet from what would otherwise be dangerous, even life-threatening, exposure levels. In the lower atmosphere, however, ozone is decidedly undesirable because it is a powerful oxidizing agent [6,24,25]. Unfortunately ozone, like $NO^{\cdot}$ and $NO_2^{\cdot}$, is a common by-product of industrial combustion processes, and the internal combustion engine. Mankind's environmental ozone, nitric oxide and nitrogen dioxide exposures are man-made problems.

Antioxidant defences

So far I have painted a fairly dismal picture involving a cast of dangerous and damaging oxygen radicals, and other activated oxygen species, to which we are constantly exposed. Thankfully we are not defenceless against this onslaught. All aerobic organisms, including human beings, utilize a series of primary antioxidant defences in an attempt to protect against oxidant damage, and numerous damage removal and repair enzymes to remove and/or repair molecules that do get damaged [26]. This section will concentrate on the non-enzymic and enzymic primary antioxidant defences.

Antioxidant compounds

Our cells utilize a series of antioxidant compounds, many of which are reviewed in Table 1, to directly react with oxidizing agents and disarm them [9,10,26,27]. Such antioxidants are said to be 'scavengers' and their role

Table 1. Antioxidant compounds

Vitamin E
Caeruloplasmin
Vitamin C
Ferritin
β-Carotene
Selenium
Glutathione
Manganese
Ubiquinone
Zinc
Uric acid
Copper (?)
Iron (?)

is unavoidably suicidal. Thus, as has already been mentioned, vitamin E (α-tocopherol) is a major membrane-bound antioxidant, and vitamin C (ascorbic acid) is a major aqueous-phase antioxidant. The fact that these compounds are both human vitamins underscores their vital importance in maintaining health. Recently there has been significant *in vitro* evidence for a redox cycle in which vitamin C may re-reduce (i.e. regenerate) vitamin E [28]. If shown to be operative *in vivo* such a redox cycle would significantly alter our view of antioxidant functions.

Other lipid-soluble agents may also play important antioxidant roles *in vivo* (Table 1). These include β-carotene and ubiquinone [9,10,26,27]. A derivative of vitamin A (retinoic acid), β-carotene, has shown great promise as an antioxidant dietary supplement in several studies. Recently, however, a study from Finland has raised questions about the advisability of dietary β-carotene supplements [29]. Clearly more research is needed to resolve this important question and several major studies are, indeed, currently underway.

Other water-soluble antioxidant compounds (Table 1) include uric acid [30–32], glutathione and caeruloplasmin [33]. Uric acid, the end product of purine metabolism in humans, is particularly interesting because it may function both as a classic suicidal antioxidant and as a chelator of transition metals [30–32]. By binding iron and/or copper, uric acid may inhibit metal-catalysed oxidation reactions without itself becoming oxidized [32]. The very facility with which transition metals can act as oxidation/reduction catalysts, however, makes them ideal active-site constituents of many antioxidant enzymes. Thus, as discussed in greater detail below, various members of the superoxide dismutase family utilize copper, zinc, manganese, or iron as active-site catalysts [1,3,34,35]. Most glutathione peroxidases utilize selenium as the active-site catalyst [36], whereas catalases utilize iron [37]. Because of the absolute requirement of these metals for operation of the antioxidant enzymes, I suggest that selenium, manganese, zinc, copper and iron should be included in any list of requirements for antioxidant compounds (which is why they appear in Table 1). Diets deficient in these important metals result in serious oxidant disorders, in addition to other serious problems. So, for example, the selenium-deficient diets which can result from grasses and grains grown in selenium-poor New Zealand soils, have been shown to result in dangerously high levels of oxidative damage [4,10].

Interestingly those of us who live in the so-called 'developed' countries ingest larger quantities of antioxidant compounds and transition-metal chelators in virtually all processed foods. Thus a typical 'Western' diet contains significant quantities of the antioxidants butylated hydroxytoluene (BHT) and butylated hydroxyanisole (BHA) which are widely used as food preservatives in everything from potato chips (or crisps) to frozen lasagne! Also widely employed, and therefore ingested, is the transition-metal chelator EDTA. Significant tissue levels of BHT, BHA and EDTA are now to be found in humans (and many animals) from Western countries and these compounds presumably add a significant component to our antioxidant defences.

Antioxidant enzymes and proteins

Aerobic organisms also synthesize numerous antioxidant enzymes (reviewed in Fig. 5) in an attempt to minimize oxidative damage. Perhaps the best known of these enzymes is superoxide dismutase [1,3]. No single discovery was of greater significance to the development of the free-radical field than the discovery of the enzyme family of superoxide dismutases (SODs) [34]. The SODs catalyse the reaction $O_2^{\cdot-} + O_2^{\cdot-} \rightarrow H_2O_2 + O_2$ which readers will recognize from Figs. 3 and 4. As reported in Fig. 3 the rate constant of this important dismutation reaction is increased severalfold by SOD. All members of the SOD family utilize transition metals at their active sites [35]. Bacteria employ an Fe-SOD and an Mn-SOD, whereas mammals utilize distinct cytoplasmic and extracellular forms of Cu,Zn-SOD and a mitochondrial Mn-SOD that in evolutionary terms is closely related to the bacterial Mn-SOD [35]. Genetic deletion of SOD has been shown to be a lethal mutation in lower organisms [35], underpinning the essential importance of this enzyme family.

The product of SOD is H_2O_2, which is clearly toxic and must be rapidly removed. In mammalian cells this is accomplished by two enzyme families; the glutathione peroxidases and the catalases (Fig. 5). Both glutathione peroxidases

Glutathione Peroxidase:
$$H_2O_2 + GSH + GSH \rightarrow GS\text{-}SG + H_2O + H_2O$$

Glutathione Reductase:
$$GS\text{-}SG + NADPH + H^+ \rightarrow 2GSH + NADP^+$$

Catalase:
$$H_2O_2 + H_2O_2 \rightarrow H_2O + H_2O + O_2$$

DT Diaphorase:
$$Q + 2e^- + 2H^+ \rightarrow QH_2$$

GSH = reduced glutathione (L-γ-glutamyl-L-cysteinyl-glycine)
GS-SG = oxidized glutathione
Q = an oxidized quinone; QH_2 = a fully reduced quinol

Fig. 5. Mechanisms of antioxidant enzymes.

[36] and catalases [37] detoxify H_2O_2 by reducing it to water and oxygen. Glutathione peroxidases utilize the reducing power of glutathione (GSH), a tripeptide consisting of L-γ-glutamyl-L-cysteinyl-glycine, to detoxify H_2O_2 [36]. The sulphydryl moiety of the cysteine residue supplies the actual reducing equivalents required for glutathione peroxidase activity. Two molecules of GSH are oxidized, to form the disulphide-bonded compound GS–SG, in the reduction of a molecule of H_2O_2 (Fig. 5). The companion enzyme glutathione reductase utilizes NADPH to re-reduce one molecule of GS–SG to two molecules of GSH, thus permitting the continuous action of glutathione peroxidase (Fig. 5). So important are the roles of glutathione-utilizing enzymes to normal functions that most cells contain concentrations of GSH in excess of 5 mM [36].

Although the mechanism of action of catalase (Fig. 5) appears much simpler than that of glutathione peroxidase, appearances may be deceiving. There are reports in the literature for example that catalases may require NADH/NADPH for their continual operation [38], although there does not appear to be widespread acceptance of this concept. Certainly catalases are interesting enzymes, and they certainly do not follow classical Michaelis–Menten kinetics [37,38].

A good deal of interest has centred on the question of whether glutathione peroxidases or catalases are more important in detoxifying intracellular H_2O_2. In red blood cells Cohen and Hochstein [39,40] have reported that glutathione peroxidase is mostly responsible for removing the low levels of H_2O_2 generated by cellular metabolism and haemoglobin autoxidation, whereas catalase is important in dealing with the large H_2O_2 production rates induced by oxidizing drugs such as phenylhydrazine. Although well established, this view of red-blood-cell antioxidant functions has recently been questioned [41]. In other cell types there must be a very real question of the overall contribution of catalases to general scavenging. This is simply because, in most mammalian cell types, catalase is exclusively found within peroxisomes where it has a clear function of removing the H_2O_2 generated by β-oxidation of long-chain fatty acids [42]. Since catalase is not generally found in the cytoplasm of most mammalian cells, and since both H_2O_2 diffusion from the cytoplasm into peroxisomes seems rather unlikely, it seems probable that glutathione peroxidases largely deal with cytoplasmic H_2O_2 and catalases largely deal with peroxisomal H_2O_2.

Another important antioxidant enzyme is DT diaphorase, which is also called quinone reductase [43]. DT diaphorase is able to catalyse the direct bivalent reduction of many (dehydro)quinones to (dihydro)quinols, as shown in Fig. 5. By catalysing a direct two-electron reduction of substrate quinones, DT diaphorase avoids production of reactive semiquinone radical intermediates (such as $Q^{\cdot-}$ and $QH^{\cdot}$). DT diaphorase may play an important role in the detoxification of many quinonoid drugs and environmental agents by stabilizing the, relatively safe, quinol form, prior to conjugation and elimination by other enzyme systems.

Two non-enzymic proteins, ferritin [44] and ceruloplasmin [33], also appear to play important roles in transition-metal storage and antioxidant defence *in vivo* (and are included in Table 1). Transition metals such as iron and copper are involved in both metal-catalysed ('auto')oxidations, and reactions leading to hydroxyl radical production from superoxide, as discussed in detail in the previous two sections. Ferritin, which binds iron in mammalian cells, and ceruloplasmin, which binds copper in plasma, are thought by many to contribute a significant antioxidant capacity to bodily fluids [33,44].

Recently, despite the enormity of the task, significant progress has been made in detailed and quantitative analysis of the total antioxidant status of various bodily fluids [45].

Direct repair systems

Damage removal and/or repair systems may be classified as either direct or indirect [27,46,47] as shown in Fig. 6. Direct repair, about which we know only a little, has so far only been demonstrated for a few classes of oxidized molecules. One important direct repair process is the re-reduction of oxidized sulphydryl groups on proteins. Cysteine residues in proteins are highly susceptible to autoxidation and/or metal-catalysed oxidation. When two nearby cysteine residues within a protein oxidize they often form a disulphide bond, producing a more rigid protein. Disulphide bonds can also form between two proteins, promoting the formation of large supramolecular assemblies of inactivated enzymes and proteins; this is called intermolecular cross-linking. Both intramolecular disulphide cross-links and intermolecular disulphide cross-links can be reversed to some extent by disulphide reductases within cells [47]. Our understanding of such enzymic reactions is still at an early stage. Another important sulphydryl oxidation process is the oxidation of methionine residues to methionine sulphoxide, typically causing loss of enzyme/protein function. The enzyme methionine sulphoxide reductase can regenerate methionine residues within such oxidized proteins and restore function [48]. As with disulphide reductases, our understanding of methionine sulphoxide reductases is still in its infancy.

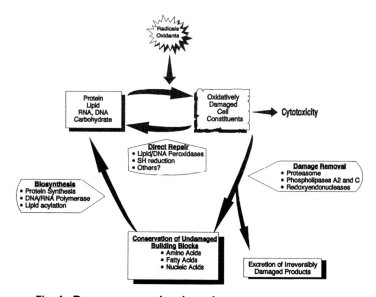

Fig. 6. Damage removal and repair systems.

Direct repair of DNA hydroperoxides by glutathione peroxidase has been reported from *in vitro* studies [49]. The extent to which DNA peroxides are actually formed *in vivo*, however, is not completely clear. Also not yet studied is the extent to which DNA peroxides may be directly repaired by glutathione peroxidases *in vivo*. Other, relatively straightforward, mechanisms of DNA repair are also being explored [50].

Damage removal and repair systems (indirect 'repair')

Although our knowledge of direct repair systems, as outlined above, is still rather rudimentary a great deal more is known about indirect repair systems (Fig. 6). Indirect repair involves two distinct steps [27,47]; first the damaged molecule (or the damaged part of a molecule) must be recognized and excised, removed, or degraded. Next, a replacement of the entire damaged molecule must be synthesized, or the excised portion of the damaged molecule must be made and inserted.

Degradation and replacement of oxidized proteins

Extensive studies have revealed that oxidized proteins are recognized by proteases and completely degraded (to amino acids); entirely new replacement protein molecules are then synthesized *de novo* [27,51–65]. It appears that oxidized amino acids within oxidatively modified proteins are eliminated, or used as carbon sources for ATP synthesis. Since an oxidatively modified protein may contain only two or three oxidized amino acids it appears probable that most of the amino acids from an oxidized and degraded protein are re-utilized for protein synthesis. Thus, during oxidative stress, many proteins synthesized as damage replacements are likely to contain a high percentage of recycled amino acids. During periods of particularly high oxidative stress the proteolytic capacity of cells may not be sufficient to cope with the number of oxidized protein molecules being generated. A similar problem may occur in aging, or with certain disease states, when proteolytic capacity may decline below a critical threshold of activity required to cope with normal oxidative stress levels [46]. Under such circumstances oxidized proteins may not undergo appropriate proteolytic digestion, and may, instead, cross-link with one another or form extensive hydrophobic bonds. Such aggregates of damaged proteins are detrimental to normal cell functions and lead to further problems. A summary of protein oxidative damage, recognition and degradation by proteases, or cross-linking and aggregation is presented in Fig. 7 and represents a pictorial synthesis of many detailed studies [57–65].

In bacteria such as *Escherichia coli* a series of proteolytic enzymes act cooperatively in the recognition and degradation of oxidatively modified soluble proteins [57,58]. A similar series of proteolytic enzymes appear to conduct the degradation of oxidatively modified soluble proteins in mammalian mitochondria [59]. In bacteria and in mitochondria, therefore, the proteolytic role shown for proteasome in Fig. 7 is actually played by a series of cooperative proteases. In the cytoplasm and nucleus of eukaryotic cells, however, oxidized soluble proteins largely appear to be recognized and degraded by the proteasome complex [60–65] as shown in Fig. 7. Proteasome is a 670 kDa multi-enzyme complex that appears

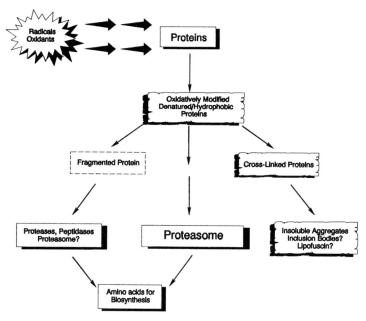

Fig. 7. Protein oxidation and the degradation of oxidatively modified proteins by proteasome in eukaryotic cells.

to be ubiquitously expressed in the cytoplasm and nuclei of all eukaryotic cells. More than 15 individual polypeptides, each present in multiple copies, with molecular masses ranging from 20000 Da to 35000 Da make up the proteasome complex; the exact composition varies with species and cell type. Each of the component proteasome polypeptides is encoded by a separate gene and many of these genes have now been cloned and sequenced [66]. The results of such cloning and sequencing studies reveal that proteasome is a completely non-classical protease complex. Indeed, the proteasome subunits have no discernable sequence identity with any known proteins, except for a small degree of sequence overlap with some of the heat shock proteins [66].

The core 670 kDa (20S) proteasome can combine with other, ubiquitin-conjugating and ATPase subunits to form a 1500 kDa (26S) proteolytic complex (sometimes called ubiquitin conjugate degrading enzyme or U.C.D.E.N.). This 1500 kDa form of proteasome is responsible for the ATP- and ubiquitin-dependent or stimulated proteolysis within eukaryotic cells, and probably plays an important role in antigen processing and cell differentiation [66]. The 1500 kDa proteasome form, however, appears not to recognize oxidized proteins [60]. It is in fact the 670 kDa 'core' proteasome complex that recognizes oxidatively modified proteins and selectively degrades them in an ATP- and ubiquitin-independent manner [60–65]. In this regard it is interesting that although reticulo-cytes contain both the 1500 kDa and the 670 kDa forms of proteasome, mature erythrocytes contain only the 670 kDa core proteasome [60]. Presumably the terminally differentiated erythrocyte can survive perfectly well without ATP/

ubiquitin-stimulated proteolysis, and has no need for antigen processing or further differentiation. The housekeeping function of recognizing and degrading oxidatively damaged proteins, however, conducted by the 670 kDa core proteasome, appears to be required throughout the entire life of the erythrocyte [27,47,60].

Recognition of oxidized soluble proteins in the cell cytoplasm and nucleus by proteasome appears to occur via binding to exposed hydrophobic patches on the damaged proteins [60–65]. Although the process of protein oxidation (which of course means oxidation of consistent amino acids) often involves changes that make some amino acid residues more hydrophilic, changes in charge relationships on a protein can cause significant unfolding or partial denaturation. Such partial denaturation exposes previously shielded stretches of primary sequence that are hydrophobic in nature. Exposed hydrophobic patches on the surface of oxidized proteins appear to act as recognition and binding sequences for the 670 kDa core proteasome [60–65].

Proteasome appears equally able to recognize and degrade damaged protein substrates generated by a wide variety of oxidant exposures. Thus, haemoglobin damaged by the indiscriminate hydroxyl radical is selectively degraded by proteasome at about the same efficiency as haemoglobin damaged by metal-catalysed oxidation with hydrogen peroxide at the haem moiety [60,61]. Similarly, Cu,Zn-SOD is recognized and degraded by proteasome equally well following either $^{\cdot}$OH exposure or specific copper-catalysed active-site inactivation by the enzymes product, H_2O_2 [60,61]. Again, the common link between the non-specific damage caused by $^{\cdot}$OH, and the site-specific oxidation caused by H_2O_2 reacting with a protein-bound transition-metal catalyst, is the partial denaturation and exposure of hydrophobic patches caused by both. Hydrophobic and bulky residues are the preferred substrates for proteolytic cleavage by the core proteasome [27,47,66]. Recently this laboratory has shown that treatment of epithelial cells in culture with an antisense oligonucleotide directed against the proteasome C-2 subunit gene, drastically diminishes C-2 expression, overall proteasome activity, and the ability of these mammalian cells to successfully degrade oxidatively modified proteins following an imposed oxidative stress [65].

Degradation and replacement/repair of oxidized membrane lipids

Lipid peroxidation was the first type of oxidative damage to be studied. Membrane phospholipids are continually subjected to oxidant challenges. The process of lipid peroxidation is comprised of a set of chain reactions which are initiated by the abstraction of a hydrogen atom (from carbon) in an unsaturated fatty acyl chain [67,68]. In an aerobic environment, oxygen will add to the fatty acid at the carbon-centred lipid radical (L$^{\cdot}$) to give rise to a lipid peroxyl radical (LOO$^{\cdot}$). Once initiated, LOO$^{\cdot}$ can further propagate the peroxidation chain reaction by abstracting a hydrogen atom from other vicinal unsaturated fatty acids [67,68]. The resulting lipid hydroperoxide (LOOH) can easily decompose into several reactive species including lipid alkoxyl radicals (LO$^{\cdot}$), aldehydes (e.g. malonyldialdehyde), alkanes, lipid epoxides and alcohols [67,68]. Cholesterol has also been shown to undergo oxidation, to give rise to a variety of epoxides and alcohols.

Peroxidized membranes become rigid, lose selective permeability and, under extreme conditions, can lose their integrity. Water-soluble lipid peroxidation products (most notably the aldehydes) have been shown to diffuse from membranes into other subcellular compartments [68–71]. Dialdehydes can act as cross-linking reagents, and are thought to play a role in the protein aggregation which forms the age pigment lipofuscin [72]. Several laboratories are investigating the possibility that lipid peroxidation products may form DNA adducts, thus giving rise to mutations and altered patterns of gene expression [71]. Others have noted inhibition of enzyme function by lipid peroxidation products. It is very clear that the process of lipid peroxidation, and its products, can be detrimental to cell viability. Cumulative effects of lipid peroxidation have been implicated as underlying mechanisms in numerous pathological conditions including athero-sclerosis, haemolytic anaemias, and ischaemia reperfusion injuries [68].

Lipid bilayers which have been oxidized become better substrates for phospholipase enzymes (Fig. 6). Phospholipase A_2 acts at the sn-2 position of the phospholipid glycerol backbone to generate a free fatty acid and a lysophospho-lipid. Phospholipase A_2 has been shown to preferentially hydrolyse fatty acids from oxidized liposomes [73]. Structural perturbations due to changes in membrane microviscosity, and the increased hydrophilic nature of oxidized lipids, may be responsible for the increased susceptibility to phospholipase A_2 action [70,74]. Removing fatty acid hydroperoxides from the membrane compartment will help prevent further propagation reactions. Additionally, it has been demonstrated that fatty acid hydroperoxides released into the cytosol are substrates for glutathione peroxidase. Glutathione peroxidase detoxifies fatty acid hydroperoxides by reducing them to their corresponding hydroxy fatty acids [74]. Lysophospholipids left in the membrane possess potential detergent properties which have been shown to disrupt membrane structure and function. Lysophospholipids can serve as substrates for re-acylation reactions (re-addition of fatty acids to the sn-2 position) to regenerate intact phospholipids [75,76].

Recent work suggests that it is possible to reduce fatty acid hydroperoxides (to their corresponding alcohols) without hydrolysis and release from the membrane compartment [49,77–79]. A member of the glutathione peroxidase family, phospholipid hydroperoxide glutathione peroxidase, which acts preferen-tially on phospholipid hydroperoxides, has been characterized by Ursini, Maiorino and their co-workers [77–80]. A glutathione transferase with activity towards lipid hydroperoxides has also been extracted from nuclei [49].

Peroxidized membranes and lipid oxidation products represent a constant threat to aerobic cells. It is now widely held that, in addition to preventing initiation of peroxidation (with compounds like vitamin E), cells have also developed a variety of mechanisms for maintaining membrane integrity and homoeostasis by repairing oxidatively damaged lipid components (Fig. 6).

Repair of oxidized DNA

RNAs and DNAs are also vulnerable to oxidative damage and, perhaps most importantly, DNA has been shown to incur oxidative damage *in vivo* [81–87]. Although DNA is a relatively simple biopolymer, made up of only four different nucleic acids, its integrity is vital to cell division and survival. Oxidative alterations to nucleic acid polymers has been shown to disrupt transcription, translation, and DNA replication, and to give rise to mutations and (ultimately) cell senescence or death [87–93]. Despite the precious nature of the genetic code, it too appears to be a target for oxidative damage. The amount of oxidative damage, even under normal physiological conditions, may be quite extensive, with estimates as high as one base modification per 130000 bases in nuclear DNA [86]. Damage to mitochondrial DNA is estimated to be even higher at one per 8000 bases. Fragments of oxidatively modified mitochondrial DNA have been implicated in cancer and aging [85].

Oxidants can elicit a wide variety of DNA damage products, several of which have been carefully characterized [87,94]. The types of DNA damage can be grouped into strand breaks (single and double), sister chromatid exchange, DNA–DNA and DNA–protein cross-links, and base modifications. All four DNA bases can be oxidatively modified; however, the pyrimidines (cytosine and, especially, thymidine) appear to be most susceptible [93]. Bases undergo ring saturation, ring opening, ring contraction and hydroxylation. These types of alteration usually result in a loss of aromaticity and planarity, which can cause local distortions in the double helix [93]. Depending on the type and extent of damage, the altered bases can be found either attached to, or dissociated from, the DNA molecule to generate apurinic/apyrimidinic (AP) sites [84,93,95].

Radical interactions with DNA appear to be fairly non-specific; hence, the phosphodiester backbone may also be oxidatively damaged. Damage to the sugar and phosphate moieties, which form the backbone, may result in strand breaks [87,94]. Depending on the site of radical attack, unusual 3′ and 5′ ends (i.e. non-3′-OH, non-5′-PO_4) can be generated. These abnormal ends are not substrates for DNA polymerases, and must be removed before any repair can occur [95].

Reports of glutathione transferases [95] and peroxidases using thymidine hydroperoxide as a substrate have been published (Fig. 6). DNA may also undergo oxidative demethylation [93,94]. DNA methylases may play an important role in restoring methylation patterns and maintaining epigenetic phenomena. Inhibition of poly(ADP-ribose) polymerase has been shown to exacerbate H_2O_2 genotoxicity, although the mechanism for this is not yet clear [92]. There is ample evidence that several prokaryotic and eukaryotic enzymes repair oxidatively damaged DNA by both direct [49,93,94], and excision–repair mechanisms [83,84,92–101] as shown in Fig. 6. Pilot studies using cell-free extracts *in vitro* indicated that some endo- and exo-nucleases preferentially cleave oxidized DNA. Bacterial mutants deficient in these putative DNA oxy-repair enzymes: *nth⁻* (endonuclease III), *xth⁻* (exonuclease III), and *nfo⁻* (endonuclease IV) were used to continue these studies *in vivo* [102]. It was found that strains deficient in exonuclease III (*xth⁻*) are hypersensitive to H_2O_2 [102]. Endonuclease IV deficiency (*nfo⁻*) also produced a hypersensitivity to organic hydroperoxides, and to oxidants generated by bleomycin [102]. When the *nfo* and *xth* mutations were combined, lethal oxidant effects are drastically increased.

The activity of these prokaryotic enzymes, with regard to oxidative DNA repair, has been extensively studied [96,99,102–104]. Endonuclease III has been shown to cleave at the 3′ side of AP sites [103]. Endonuclease III also appears to possess an N-glycosylase activity for thymine glycol and urea residues; two common products of oxidative damage to DNA. Exonuclease III possesses a 3' to 5' nucleolytic activity which may be responsible for removing the sugar fragments generated during oxidative strand breakage [94,103]. Exonuclease III is really a poor name for this enzyme which actually expresses 85% of the 5' AP endonucleolytic activity in *E. coli*. Endonuclease IV is also a 5' AP endonuclease.

Eukaryotic investigations are not as far along but several parallels with the results of prokaryotic studies have already been published [95,97,98,105]. Several glycosylases which act on DNA oxidation products have been characterized. A 3'-repair diesterase in yeast is apparently responsible for removing damaged 3' termini left by free radical reactions [95]. A mammalian endonuclease has been isolated based on its specificity for oxidatively modified DNA [97,98]. It bears remarkable similarities to the bacterial endonuclease III including molecular mass (~ 30 kDa), lack of bivalent cation requirement, and substrate specificity. The term 'redoxyendonucleases' (as used in Fig. 6) has been proposed for all nucleases which participate in repairing oxidatively damaged DNA [97].

There is mounting evidence that redoxyendonucleases function in higher eukaryotic cells (Fig. 6). DNA damage which appears in cells as a result of an acute oxidant challenge (including base damage and single-strand breaks) has been shown to diminish as a function of time [83]. These results suggest that a removal of lesions is being carried out by intracellular systems. Oxidatively damaged bases (8-hydroxydeoxyguanosine, thymine glycol and thymidine glycol) have been measured in animal urine [86]. Again this suggests that there is systematic excision and excretion of oxidized DNA *in vivo*. The vital importance of such DNA excision–repair processes was recently highlighted by the selection of DNA repair as the 'Molecule of the Year' for 1994 by Science magazine [106].

Inducible defence and repair systems

Thus far the picture of antioxidant defences and repair systems I have painted, although extensive, is a static one. In reality, however, both prokaryotes and eukaryotes are able to dramatically up-regulate their armoury of oxidant protections in response to an oxidative stress. Many researchers have utilized a fairly common cell-culture adaptive response protocol first used in heat-shock studies to study such phenomena. This approach involves first finding an oxidant concentration that is lethal to most of the cells. Next new cultures are exposed to much lower levels of the same oxidant (pretreatment exposures) for various periods of time before being exposed to the normally lethal concentration (the challenge dose). What has now been widely found is that, in cells from *E. coli* to human hepatocytes, pretreatment conditions can be found that will enable cells to survive the subsequent challenge dose. Such adaptive responses to oxidative stress have been shown to involve widespread alterations in gene expression [46,107–111].

In bacteria adaptation to hydrogen peroxide [109,112–128] has been shown to involve the *oxyR* regulon [114,115,119–126]. The *oxyR* gene encodes the OxyR protein that can bind to the nine or so target genes whose expression it regulates. In the reduced state the OxyR protein allows a basal level of transcription to occur. When oxidized, during the oxidative stress of H_2O_2 exposure for instance, the OxyR protein dramatically up-regulates transcription of its target genes, including a catalase, an alkyl-hydroperoxide reductase, a glutathione reductase, a non-specific DNA-binding protein, and the heat-shock protein DNAK. Each of these enzymes/proteins provides a clear advantage to oxidatively stressed cells. Recent work has revealed the existence of a second H_2O_2-inducible regulon, tentatively called the *oxoR* regulon, that appears to provide inducible protection in *E. coli* [107–109]. When *E. coli* are exposed to superoxide, instead of H_2O_2, the *soxRS* regulon provides inducible protection [96,99,127–134]. Genes induced by *soxRS* include a Mn-SOD, exonuclease IV, glucose-6-phosphate dehydrogenase, fumarase C, and an antisense RNA regulator.

Our understanding of eukaryotic adaptation to oxidative stress is not as advanced as the bacterial work. Limited studies have been performed with yeast, where it is clear that transcriptionally regulated adaptation to H_2O_2 exposure does occur [107,110,128,135–138]. Limited studies have also been performed in mammalian cell cultures. Mammalian H_2O_2 adaptation is a much slower, less extensive process than that seen for bacteria or yeast, but it does still occur [111,139–142]. Transcription of several genes has been shown to increase during mammalian responses to oxidative stress [143–153]. In this laboratory we have shown that HA-1, CHO, V79, C3H 10T1/2, and clone 9 liver cells all adapt to H_2O_2, although to varying degrees [111].

At the moment we are concentrating on H_2O_2 adaptation in the HA-1 cell line (a Chinese hamster ovary cell derivative) which relies on *de novo* protein synthesis for adaptation but does not appear to induce any of the classical anti-oxidant enzymes. A temporary growth arrest appears important for the successful H_2O_2 adaptation of HA-1 cells, and this growth-arrest includes expression of the *gadd153* and *gadd45* genes [144,152], as well as a novel growth-arrest-associated RNA transcript, called *adapt15*, that we are investigating [108]. A mammalian genetic library has been constructed that has sequences known to be induced by DNA damage [152]. Levels of transcripts which cross-hybridize with probes from this library have been shown to increase after H_2O_2 treatment, suggesting oxidative induction of DNA repair enzymes in mammals [144,152]. Haem oxygenase [145], DT diaphorase or quinone reductase [146], and a protein-tyrosine phosphatase [153] have all been shown to exhibit peroxide-inducible increases in expression, but the relative importance of any or all of these proteins to actual adaptation remains unclear. Obviously, the contribution of multiple proteins and enzymes to overall oxidative-stress adaptation remains an important area for future investigations.

Oxidative stress and disease states

Despite the antioxidant compounds, antioxidant enzymes, damage removal and repair enzymes, and inducible defences discussed in the previous sections many common diseases are thought to involve a significant oxidative-stress component. While a detailed review of disease states involving oxidative stress is beyond the scope of this chapter, an introduction to the topic is presented below.

Mutagenesis, cell transformation, and human cancers have all been linked with exposure to free radicals and other reactive oxygen species [29,154–156]. Encouragingly, at least some studies suggest that dietary antioxidants provide some protection against cancer [154–156], although recent work also advises caution [29].

Atherosclerosis, arteriosclerosis and ischaemia/reperfusion events are all thought to involve elements of oxidative stress. Thus, devastating events such as heart attacks and strokes now appear to involve free radicals. Oxidized low-density lipoproteins (LDLs) appear to play a major role in the formation of fatty lesions and fibrous plaques in the endothelial lining of blood vessels [157,158]. Such events are also associated with monocyte adherence and further LDL oxidation [159].

Atherosclerotic and arteriosclerotic blood vessels are, of course, the causes of heart attacks and strokes. Many heart attacks and strokes seem to involve an ischaemic period, during which blood flow and tissue oxygenation are minimal, followed by a reperfusion period, during which blood flow and oxygenation are re-established. Much research indicates that the ischaemic period is not the cause of irreversible tissue damage, provided that it is not too prolonged. Rather, it appears that events which occur during reperfusion, and reoxygenation, are the true causes of heart attack and stroke damage. An elegant hypothesis integrating all of these findings and explaining damage in terms of oxygen radical damage during reperfusion, was proposed by McCord [160] and has stimulated an enormous research effort. Although the original hypothesis has undergone some revisions, the basic idea that reperfusion involves an oxidative stress still seems tenable and is now supported by a good deal of experimental data [161].

Inflammatory diseases clearly involve significant exposure to oxidative stress. Acute inflammations, such as those associated with wound-healing, are probably relatively benign, but chronic inflammation is an altogether different matter. It is now quite clear that oxidative stresses involved in chronic inflammatory diseases are significant contributors to disease progression [19,162–167]. Diseases such as rheumatoid arthritis, lupus erythematosus and psoriatic arthritis involve chronic inflammation of joint tissues, with oxidant-associated gradual deterioration of joint structures [19,162–167].

Several diseases and disorders of the eye involve photo-oxidative stresses. One of the earliest diseases to be associated with photo-oxidative stress was cataract formation. The damage and cross-linking of lens proteins, particularly the crystallins, that characterize cataract are clearly a photo-oxidative event [168]. More recently studies have focused on the interaction of photo-oxidative damage and age-associated declines in protease and peptidase activities as causes for cataract [169–172]. In the young lens it is quite clear that photo-oxidative damage occurs but proteases like the proteasome complex, and peptidases such as leucine aminopeptidase, appear to remove damaged proteins and prevent cross-linking and cataract formation [169–172].

Several central-nervous-system diseases or syndromes are now thought to involve oxygen radicals. Most recently great excitement has been generated by the finding that amyotrophic lateral sclerosis (ALS) may involve a genetic defect in the gene encoding Cu,Zn-SOD [173–176]. While it now appears that only a percentage of those patients with the familial form of ALS exhibit SOD mutations, and the familial form of ALS accounts for less than 10% of all ALS cases, this still appears to be a case of an antioxidant genetic defect resulting in serious disease. Low glutathione peroxidase activity in red and white blood cells is associated with chronic seizures in children [177], and vitamin E deficiency can lead to lipid peroxidation, demyelination, and neuronal ceroid lipofuscinosis [178,179]. Similarly, abnormally low copper levels in the brain have been associated with diminished Cu,Zn-SOD activity, mental deterioration and even death [180]. Parkinson's disease [181–183] and Alzheimer's dementia [184–191] have both been associated with free radicals and oxidative stress, and the possibility that such associations may be causal in nature is now under very active investigation.

It will be noted that many of the diseases discussed above may be said to be 'age-associated disorders'. The concept that the aging process itself may actually be a free radical disease was advanced many years ago [192] and has recently received great attention [46,193,194]. Certainly aging is commonly associated with increased incidence of many degenerative diseases and disorders, an example being the age-associated decline in immune function that may be preventable by dietary (antioxidant) manipulation [195]. Whether aging is actually a free radical disease or a natural phenomenon may be more a question of semantics than of science, but it is, I suggest, abundantly clear that oxidative stress is at least a component of the aging process [46].

Environment, drugs and foods

The purpose of this volume is to emphasize the role of free radicals and oxidative stress as induced or affected by environmental factors, drugs and food additives. Each of these areas is now discussed in an introductory manner below.

Environmental sources of oxidative stress

The question of environmental exposure to singlet oxygen, as a photo-oxidative event, was covered in the first section ('The radical nature of oxygen') of this article. Similarly, the question of environmental production of, and exposure to, ozone and oxides of nitrogen such as $NO^{\cdot}$ and $NO_2^{\cdot}$ were discussed in the section entitled, 'Fundamentals of oxidative stress'.

Another major environmental source of oxygen radical exposure is through radiation. Many forms of electromagnetic radiation, including γ-rays and X-rays, are fairly common environmental 'pollutants'. Of major concern is the direct radiolysis of water that γ-rays and X-rays induce, since human beings are composed mostly of water and since water is 55 M in concentration. For most purposes this means that direct effects of radiation, on molecules such as DNA, are minimal in comparison with the indirect effects of radiation, mediated by the free radicals generated by radiolysis of water [196]. Radiolysis splits H_2O into $^{\cdot}OH$ and the solvated electron ($e^-_{aq.}$). Since our tissues contain oxygen, the $e^-_{aq.}$ so produced reduces oxygen to form $O_2^{\cdot-}$, which then dismutates to form H_2O_2. Thus radiation results in the generation of $^{\cdot}OH$, $O_2^{\cdot-}$ and H_2O_2 whose effects have already been reviewed in detail earlier in this introductory chapter.

Toxins released into the environment may affect oxidative metabolism. One compelling example is that of the industrial pollutant carbon tetrachloride. Although carbon tetrachloride itself is essentially harmless, it is oxidized by cytochrome *P*-450 enzymes, in the endoplasmic reticulum of the liver, to form the highly reactive trichloromethyl radical. Elegant and detailed investigations, spearheaded by Trevor Slater and Mario Dianzani over a period of decades, have given us a very intimate understanding of the free radical nature of carbon tetrachloride toxicity [197–199].

Studies are increasingly demonstrating the free radical (or non-radical oxidant) nature of an enormous variety of components found in cigarette, cigar and pipe smoke [3,5,10,24,25]. Radicals such as $NO^{\cdot}$, $NO_2^{\cdot}$, multiple carbon-centred radical species and O_3 are formed in vast quantities from the combustion of tobacco products. Also produced are multiple quinonoid compounds which may redox-cycle with mitochondrial or microsomal electron transport chains to generate oxygen radicals. The extent to which such tobacco-based radicals and other pro-oxidant species contribute to diseases in smokers, and those around them, is currently the subject of intense investigation.

Drugs and oxidative stress

Several medically useful drugs exhibit a variety of undesirable side-effects caused by generation of reactive oxygen species. One of the most widely studied of such free-radical-generating drugs is the anthracycline antibiotic doxorubicin, which is commercially (and clinically) known by the tradename Adriamycin. Ring B of Adriamycin's four-ring anthracycline structure is an unsubstituted quinone, that can readily redox cycle with appropriate electron donors. Detailed studies have shown that mitochondrial, microsomal (endoplasmic reticulum) and sarcosomal (sarcoplasmic reticulum) electron transport chains are good electron donors for Adriamycin [200–207]. Complex I is the mitochondrial site of Adriamycin one-electron reduction [203,205,206] to generate the semiquinone drug radical ($QH^{\cdot}$ or $Q^{\cdot-}$, depending on the local pH). The Adriamycin semiquinone radical next acts as a reductant for molecular oxygen, regenerating the native drug and producing superoxide [203,205,206]. Naturally the $O_2^{\cdot-}$ generated can participate in all the reactions detailed in Figs. 1–4.

Adriamycin can also undergo one-electron redox cycling with cytochrome *P*-450 species in the endoplasmic reticulum of the liver and the sarcoplasmic reticulum of cardiac muscle [201,202]. As with mitochondrial reduction above, a drug semiquinone radical ($QH^{\cdot}$ or $Q^{\cdot-}$) is the immediate product. Again, oxidation of the Adriamycin semiquinone radical by molecular oxygen generates $O_2^{\cdot-}$ and the native drug [201,202]. Both mitochondrial and cytochrome *P*-450-dependent redox cycling of Adriamycin are thought to account for most of the toxicity exhibited by this valuable anti-tumour agent [200–206] although non-oxidative inhibitory effects on mitochondrial electron transport are observed at high drug concentrations [207]. Cardiotoxicity is clearly the major form of damage seen with Adriamycin in clinical usage [200–207]. So severe is this toxicity that Adriamycin dosage treads a relatively fine line between anti-tumour effectiveness and cardiac death. A number of related drugs including daunorubicin, rubidazone, and aclacinomycin A are toxic for the same reasons detailed above for

Adriamycin [204]. Interestingly, an imino-substitution of Adriamycin's quinone ring, which produces 5-iminodaunorubicin, makes a drug that can no longer redox-cycle and is much less toxic [203,205,206]. Unfortunately, 5-iminodauno-rubicin has not been widely tested as an anti-tumour agent, and must currently be considered to be an 'orphan drug'.

Tylenol or acetaminophen (called paracetamol in the U.K.) has long been used as an effective, mild analgesic and antipyretic drug. Unfortunately, Parace-tamol can cause severe hepatic necrosis, and even death, when taken in very high doses [208]. Paracetamol poisoning clearly involves metabolism by cytochrome P-450 to generate the extremely reactive N-acetyl-p-benzoquinone imine [209]. Multiple toxic effects are exerted by the benzoquinone imine intermediate, including glutathione depletion [210,211], oxidation of protein thiols [212,213], oxidation of NADPH [213], depletion of ATP [213], and arylation/oxidation of the plasma membrane Ca^{2+}-ATPase, with a consequent rise in cytosolic calcium [213,214].

Naturally this section of my introduction to free radicals and oxidative stress, could expand to book-size if all possible drugs were included. For the purposes of this introduction it is enough to note that several widely available over-the-counter drugs (e.g. paracetamol) as well as an even larger number of prescription drugs (e.g. Adriamycin) can cause serious toxicity through the generation of free radicals. In some cases redox cycling by mitochondrial and cytochrome P-450 systems causes toxicity via superoxide generation, in other cases the drug may undergo an irreversible P-450-mediated oxidation to generate a powerful intracel-lular oxidant. It should also be noted in this section that several drugs appear to exert significant antioxidant effects that may underlie at least part of their clinical effectiveness. Examples of this category of 'antioxidant drugs' includes the corticosteroids, penicillamine, and many of the non-steroidal anti-inflammatory drugs (such as Piroxicam, Naproxen, and Ibuprofen) which are widely used in treating such chronic inflammatory diseases as rheumatoid arthritis, gout and lupus erythematosus [215,216].

Foods and oxidative stress

The past few years have seen an explosive interest from the general public in food additives. Significant attention has been paid to such additives as BHT, BHA and EDTA, with concern over possible mutagenic or carcinogenic effects. The reality, however, is that toxicity from such additives appears not to occur, whereas the carcinogens (formed by oxidation of foodstuffs) whose formation they inhibit are clearly undesirable [217,218].

A major growth area in the last few years has included detailed investigations of many naturally occurring antioxidant compounds for potential use as food additives or dietary supplements. Of course interest in, and use of, vitamin C, vitamin E and β-carotene by the general public has skyrocketed in recent years. These antioxidants are now widely available as dietary supplements and are also being incorporated into a large number of food products.

Newer 'natural' antioxidants are also being explored. Olive oils (particularly the first, or cold-pressed, variety) are widely considered to be healthy foods because they contain no cholesterol, have high levels of mono-unsaturated fatty acids (but low levels of saturates and polyunsaturates), and boast a wide variety of natural antioxidant compounds [219]. Considerable interest has also centred on the idea that moderate consumption of red wines may provide protection against heart attacks, possibly due to antioxidant properties of such wines. The concept that certain leaves, roots, or plant extracts may be useful as health aids is, of course, not new, and herbal or 'medicinal' teas have long been widely available. It has also been widely promulgated, and is now generally accepted, that diets rich in fruits and vegetables are associated with a diminished risk of cancer, heart attacks, strokes and other diseases [217]. There is, naturally, a strong desire to isolate, identify, and market the 'active-ingredients' in fruits and vegetables that promote such healthy lives.

Recently a considerable effort to extract potentially useful antioxidants from plants has begun. In addition to β-carotene, which has been of interest for a long time, other carotenoids such as β-cryptoxanthin, canthaxanthin, lutein, lycopene and bixin, are being studied and show early promise of significant antioxidant capacity [220–222]. Also under investigation (with promising initial results) are plant hydroxycinnamic acids such as ferulic acid, caffeic acid and p-coumaric acid [223–226].

Polyphenolic flavonoids are being extracted from fruits, vegetables, teas and wines, and studied as potentially useful antioxidants [223,227,228]. Research by Rice-Evans et al. [223] and others [227,228] indicates that both the classical antioxidant properties of the polyphenolic flavonoids (contributed by the hydrogen-donating capacity of their phenolic moieties) and their metal-chelating properties (effectively preventing transition metals from catalysing oxidation reactions) may be important elements in the overall effectiveness of such compounds against free radical oxidations [223]. Multiple polyphenolic flavonoids are currently being studied: these include the flavonols such as quercetin and rutin, the flavanols such as catechin and epicatechin, the anthocyanidins such as cyanidin and apigenidin, the flavones such as chrysin, and the flavanones such as taxifolin [223,227,228].

Many of the above plant antioxidants have demonstrated greater free radical-scavenging (hydrogen-donating) activity in vitro than urate, ascorbate, or glutathione. The flavonol quercetin and the flavanol catechin appear to exert particularly efficacious synergistic effects [223] and, since both are apparently absorbed by humans, may hold real promise for development as dietary supplements.

References

1. Fridovich, I. (1976) in Free Radicals in Biology, Vol. 1 (Pryor, W.A., ed.), pp. 239–277, Academic Press
2. Chance, B., Sies, H. and Boveris, A. (1979) Physiol. Rev. 59, 527–605
3. Pryor, W.A. (1986) Annu. Rev. Physiol. 48, 657–668
4. McCord, J.M. and Fridovich, I. (1988) Free Radical Biol. Med. 5, 363–370
5. Halliwell, B. and Cross, C.E. (1994) Environ. Health Perspect. 102 (Suppl. 10), 5–12
6. Koppenol, W.H. and Liebman, J.F. (1984) J. Phys. Chem. 88, 99–101

7. Frimmer, A.A. (ed.) (1985) Singlet Oxygen vols. 1–4, CRC Press, Boca Raton, FL

8. Babior, B.M. (1992) Adv. Enzymol. Relat. Areas Mol. Biol. **65**, 49–95

9. Kappus, H. and Diplock, A.T. (1992) Free Radical Biol. Med. **13**, 55–74

10. Rice-Evans, C. and Bruckdorfer, K.R. (1992) Mol. Aspects Med. **13**, 1–111

11. Gardner, P.R. and Fridovich, I. (1991) J. Biol. Chem. **266**, 19328–19333

12. Zhang, Y., Marcillat, O., Giulivi, C., Ernster, L. and Davies, K.J.A. (1990) J. Biol. Chem. **265**, 16330–16336

13. Fenton, H.J.H. (1894) J. Chem. Soc. (London) **65**, 899–910

14. Haber, F. and Weiss, J. (1934) Proc. R. Soc. London, Ser. A **147**, 332–351

15. McCord, J.M. and Day, E.D., Jr. (1978) FEBS Lett. **86**, 139–142

16. Giulivi, C. and Davies, K.J.A. (1990) J. Biol. Chem. **265**, 19453–19460

17. McKenna, S.M. and Davies, K.J.A. (1988) Biochem. J. **254**, 685–692

18. Davies, J.M.S., Horwitz, D.M. and Davies, K.J.A. (1993) Free Radical Biol. Med. **15**, 637–643

19. Davies, J.M.S., Horwitz, D.M. and Davies, K.J.A. (1994) Arthritis Rheum. **37**, 424–427

20. Kerr, J.A., Calvert, J.G. and Demerjian, K.L. (1976) in Free Radicals in Biology (Pryor, W.A., ed.), vol. 2, pp. 159–179, Academic Press, New York

21. Moncada, S., Palmer, R.M.J. and Higgs, E.A. (1991) Pharmacol. Rev. **43**, 109–143

22. Beckman, J.S., Beckman, T.W., Chen, J., Marshall, P.A. and Freeman, B.A. (1990) Proc. Natl. Acad. Sci. U.S.A. **87**, 1620–1624

23. Radi, R., Beckman, J.S., Bush, K.K.M. and Freeman, B.A. (1990) J. Biol. Chem. **266**, 4244–4250

24. Last, J.A., Sun, W.-M., and Witsch, H. (1994) Environ. Health Perspect. **102** (Suppl. 10), 179–184

25. Pryor, W.A. (1994) Free Radical Biol. Med. **17**, 451–465

26. Quintanilha, A.T., Packer, L., Davies, J.M.S., Racanelli, T.L. and Davies, K.J.A. (1982) Ann. N.Y. Acad. Sci. **393**, 32–47

27. Davies, K.J.A. (1986) Free Radical Biol. Med. **2**, 155–173

28. Packer, J.E., Slater, T.F. and Willson, R.L. (1979) Nature (London) **278**, 737–738

29. Heinonen, O.P., Albanes, D. and the members of the Alpha-Tocopherol, Beta-Carotene Cancer Prevention Study Group (1994) N. Engl. J. Med. **330**, 1029–1035

30. Ames, B.N., Cathcart, R., Schwiers, E. and Hochstein, P. (1981) Proc. Natl. Acad. Sci. U.S.A. **78**, 6858–6862

31. Sevanian, A., Davies, K.J.A. and Hochstein, P. (1985) Free Radical Biol. Med. **1**, 117–124

32. Davies, K.J.A., Sevanian, A., Muakkassah-Kelly, S.F. and Hochstein, P. (1986) Biochem. J. **235**, 747–754

33. Gutteridge, J.M.C., Richmond, R. and Halliwell, B. (1980) FEBS Lett. **112**, 269–272

34. McCord, J.M. and Fridovich, I. (1969) J. Biol. Chem. **244**, 6049–6055

35. Fridovich, I. (1989) J. Biol. Chem. **264**, 7761–7764

36. Flohé, L. (1982) in Free Radicals in Biology (Pryor, W.A., ed.), pp. 223–254,

Academic Press, New York

37. Halliwell, B. and Gutteridge, J.M.C. (1990) Arch. Biochem. Biophys. **200**, 1–8
38. Kirkman, H.N. and Gaetani, G.F. (1984) Proc. Natl. Acad. Sci. U.S.A. **81**, 4343–4347
39. Cohen, G. and Hochstein, P. (1963) Biochemistry **2**, 1420–1428
40. Cohen, G. and Hochstein, P. (1964) Biochemistry **3**, 895–900
41. Scott, M.D., Wagner, T.C. and Chiu, D.T.-Y. (1993) Biochim. Biophys. Acta **1181**, 163–168
42. del Río, L.A., Sandalio, L.M., Palma, J.M., Bueno, P. and Corpas, F.J. (1992) Free Radical Biol. Med. **13**, 557–580
43. Lind, C., Hochstein, P. and Ernster, L. (1982) Arch. Biochem. Biophys. **216**, 178–185
44. Balla, J., Jacob, H.S., Balla, J., Rosenberg, M., Nath, K.A., Apple, F., Eaton, J.W. and Vercellotti, G.M. (1992) J. Biol. Chem. **267**, 18148–18153 ·
45. Rice-Evans, C. and Miller, N.J. (1994) Methods Enzymol. **234**, 279–293
46. Pacifici, R.E. and Davies, K.J.A. (1991) Gerontology **37**, 166–180
47. Davies, K.J.A. (1993) Biochem. Soc. Trans. **21**, 346–353
48. Brot, N. and Weissbach, H. (1991) Biofactors **3**, 91–96
49. Ketterer, B. and Meyer, D.J. (1989) Mutat. Res. **214**, 33–40
50. Demple, B. and Harrison, L. (1994) Annu. Rev. Biochem. **63**, 915–948
51. Davies, K.J.A. and Goldberg, A.L. (1987) J. Biol. Chem. **262**, 8220–8226
52. Davies, K.J.A. and Goldberg, A.L. (1987) J. Biol. Chem. **262**, 8227–8234
53. Davies, K.J.A. (1987) J. Biol. Chem. **262**, 9895–9901
54. Davies, K.J.A., Delsignore, M.E. and Lin, S.W. (1987) J. Biol. Chem. **262**, 9902–9907
55. Davies, K.J.A. and Delsignore, M.E. (1987) J. Biol. Chem. **262**, 9908–9913
56. Davies, K.J.A., Lin, S.W. and Pacifici, R.E. (1987) J. Biol. Chem. **262**, 9914–9920
57. Davies, K.J.A. and Lin, S.W. (1988) Free Radical Biol. Med. **5**, 215–223
58. Davies, K.J.A. and Lin, S.W. (1988) Free Radical Biol. Med. **5**, 225–236
59. Marcillat, O., Zhang, Y., Lin, S.W. and Davies, K.J.A. (1988) Biochem. J. **254**, 677–683
60. Pacifici, R.E., Salo, D.C., Lin, S.W. and Davies, K.J.A. (1989) Free Radical Biol. Med. **7**, 521–536
61. Salo, D.C., Pacifici, R.E. and Davies, K.J.A. (1990) J. Biol. Chem. **265**, 12751–12757
62. Giulivi, C. and Davies, K.J.A. (1993) J. Biol. Chem. **268**, 8752–8759
63. Pacifici, R.E., Kono, Y. and Davies, K.J.A. (1993) J. Biol. Chem. **268**, 15405–15411
64. Giulivi, C., Pacifici, R.E. and Davies, K.J.A. (1994) Arch. Biochem. Biophys. **311**, 329–341
65. Grune, T., Reinheckel, T., Joshi, M. and Davies, K.J.A. (1995) J. Biol. Chem. **270**, 2344–2351
66. Rivett, A.J. (1993) Biochem. J. **291**, 1–10
67. Mead, J.F. (1976) in Free Radicals in Biology (Pryor, W.A., ed.), pp. 51–68, Academic Press, New York
68. Sevanian, A. and Hochstein, P. (1985) Annu. Rev. Nutr. **5**, 365–390
69. Comporti, M. (1985) **53**, 599–623

70. Sevanian, A., Wratten, M.L., McLeod, L.L. and Kim, E. (1988) Biochim. Biophys. Acta **961**, 316–327
71. Vaca, C.E., Wilhelm, J. and Harms-Ringdahl, M. (1988) Mutat. Res. **195**, 137–149
72. Davies, K.J.A. (1988) in Lipofuscin-1987: State of the Art. (Zs.-Nagy, I., ed.), pp. 109–133, Elsevier, Amsterdam
73. Sevanian, A. and Kim, E. (1985) Free Radical Biol. Med. **1**, 263–271
74. Van Kuijk, F.J.G.M., Sevanian, A., Handelman, G.J. and Dratz, E.A. (1987) Trends Biochem. Sci. **12**, 31–34
75. Lubin, B.H., Shohet, S.B. and Nathan, D.G. (1972) J. Clin. Invest. **51**, 338–344
76. Zimmerman, W.F. and Keys, S. (1988) Exp. Eye Res. **47**, 247–260
77. Thomas, J.P., Maiorino, M., Ursini, F. and Girotti, A.W. (1990) J. Biol. Chem. **265**, 454–461
78. Ursini, F., Maiorino, M., Valente, M., Ferri, L. and Gregolin, C. (1982) Biochim. Biophys. Acta **710**, 197–211
79. Zhang, L., Maiorino, M., Roveri, A. and Ursini, F. (1989) Biochim. Biophys. Acta **1006**, 140–143
80. Maiorino, M., Chu, F.F., Ursini, F., Davies, K.J.A., Doroshow, J.H. and Esworthy, R.S. (1991) J. Biol. Chem. **266**, 7728–7732
81. Adelman, R., Saul, R.L. and Ames, B.N. (1988) Proc. Natl. Acad. Sci. U.S.A. **85**, 2706–2708
82. Fridovich, I. (1978) Science **201**, 875–880
83. Kasai, H., Crain, P.F., Kuchino, Y., Nishimura, S., Ootsuyama, A. and Tanooka, H. (1986) Carcinogenesis **7**, 1849–1851
84. Povirk, L.F. and Steighner, R.J. (1989) Mutat. Res. **214**, 13–22
85. Richter, C. (1988) FEBS Lett. **241**, 1–5
86. Richter, C., Park, J.W. and Ames, B.N. (1988) Proc. Natl. Acad. Sci. U.S.A. **85**, 6465–6467
87. Simic, M.G., Bergtold, D.S. and Karam, L.R. (1989) Mutat. Res. **214**, 3–12
88. Ames, B.N. (1989) Mutat. Res. **214**, 41–46
89. Harman, D. (1956) J. Gerontol. **11**, 298–300
90. Harman, D. (1981) Proc. Natl. Acad. Sci. U.S.A. **78**, 7124–7128
91. Schraufstätter, I., Hyslop, P.A., Jackson, J.H. and Cochrane, C.G. (1988) J. Clin. Invest. **82**, 1040–1050
92. Spector, A., Kleiman, N.J., Huang, R.C. and Wang, R.R. (1989) Exp. Eye Res. **49**, 685–698
93. Tice, R.R. and Setlow, R.B. (1985) in Handbook of the Biology of Aging, 2nd edn. (Finch, C.E. and Schneider, R., eds.), pp. 173–224, Van Nostrand Reinhold Company, New York
94. Teebor, G.W., Boorstein, R.J. and Cadet, J. (1988) Int. J. Radiat. Biol. **54**, 131–150
95. Johnson, A.W. and Demple, B. (1988) J. Biol. Chem. **263**, 18017–18022
96. Chan, E. and Weiss, B. (1987) Proc. Natl. Acad. Sci. U.S.A. **84**, 3189–3193
97. Doetsch, P.W., Helland, D.E. and Haseltine, W.A. (1986) Biochemistry **25**, 2212–2220
98. Doetsch, P.W., Henner, W.D., Cunningham. R.P., Toney, J.H. and Helland, D.E. (1987) Mol. Cell. Biol. **7**, 26–32

99. Greenberg, J.T. and Demple, B. (1989) J. Bacteriol. **171**, 3933–3939

100. Levin, J.D., Johnson, A.W. and Demple, B. (1988) J. Biol. Chem. **263**, 8066–8071

101. Wallace, S. (1988) Environ. Mol. Mutagen. **12**, 431–477

102. Cunningham, R.P., Saporito, S.M., Spitzer, S.G. and Weiss, B. (1986) J. Bacteriol. **168**, 1120–1127

103. Demple, B., Johnson, A. and Fung, P. (1986) Proc. Natl. Acad. Sci. U.S.A. **83**, 7731–7735

104. Kow, Y.W. and Wallace, S.S. (1985) Proc. Natl. Acad. Sci. U.S.A. **82**, 8354–8358

105. Helland, D.E., Doetsch. P.W. and Haseltine, W.A. (1986) Mol. Cell. Biol. **6**, 1983–1990

106. Koshland, D.E., Jr. (1994) Science **266**, 1925–1929

107. Crawford, D.R., Edbauer-Nechamen, C., Lowry, C.V., Salmon, S.L., Kim, Y.K., Davies, J.M.S. and Davies, K.J.A. (1994) Methods Enzymol. **234**, 175–217

108. Crawford, D.R. and Davies, K.J.A. (1994) Environ. Health Perspect. **102** (Suppl. 10), 25–28

109. Davies, K.J.A. and Lin, S.W. (1994) in Free Radicals in the Environment, Medicine, and Toxicology (Nohl, H., Esterbauer, H. and Rice-Evans, C., eds.), pp. 563–578, Richelieu Press, London

110. Davies, J.M.S., Lowry, C.V. and Davies, K.J.A. (1995) Arch. Biochem. Biophys. **317**, 1–6

111. Wiese, A.G., Pacifici, R.E. and Davies, K.J.A. (1995) Arch. Biochem. Biophys **318**, 1–10

112. Demple, B. and Halbrook, J. (1983) Nature (London) **304**, 466–468

113. Richter, H.E. and Loewen, P.C. (1981) Biochem. Biophys. Res. Commun. **100**, 1039–1046

114. Christman, M.F., Morgan, R.W., Jacobson, F.S. and Ames, B.N. (1985) Cell **41**, 753–762

115. Morgan, R.W., Christman, M.F., Jacobson, F.S., Storz, G. and Ames, B.N. (1986) Proc. Natl. Acad. Sci. U.S.A. **83**, 8059–8063

116. Jenkins, D.E., Schultz, J.E. and Matin, A. (1988) J. Bacteriol. **170**, 3910–3914

117. Goerlich, O., Quillardet, P. and Hofnung, M. (1989) J. Bacteriol. **171**, 6141–6147

118. Farr, S.B. and Kogoma, T. (1991) Microbiol. Rev. **55**, 561–585

119. Christman, M.F., Storz, G. and Ames, B.N. (1989) Proc. Natl. Acad. Sci. U.S.A. **86**, 3484–3488

120. Tao, K., Makino, K., Yonei, S., Nakata, A. and Shinagawa, H. (1989) Mol. Gen. Genet. **218**, 371–376

121. Tartaglia, L.A., Storz, G. and Ames, B.N. (1989) J. Mol. Biol. **210**, 709–719

122. Storz, G., Tartaglia, L.A. and Ames, B.N. (1990) Science **248**, 189–194

123. Storz, G., Tartaglia, L.A., Farr, S.B. and Ames, B.N. (1990) Trends Genet. **6**, 363–368

124. Tartaglia, L.A., Gimeno, C.J., Storz, G. and Ames, B.N. (1992) J. Biol. Chem. **267**, 2038–2045

125. Kullik, I. and Storz, G. (1994) Redox Report **1**, 23–29

126. Toledano, M.B., Kulik, I., Trinh, F., Baird, P.T., Schneider, T.D. and Storz, G. (1994) Cell **78**, 897–909

127. Demple, B. (1991) Annu. Rev. Genet. **25**, 315–337
128. Davies, K.J.A., Wiese, A.G., Pacifici, R.E. and Davies, J.M.S. (1993) in Free Radicals: From Basic Science to Medicine (Poli, G., Albano, E. and Dianzani, M.U., eds.), pp. 18–30, Birkhuser-Verlag, Basel
129. Greenberg, J.T., Monach, P.A., Chou, J.H., Josephy, D.P. and Demple, B. (1990) Proc. Natl. Acad. Sci. U.S.A. **87**, 6181–6185
130. Tsaneva, I.R. and Weiss, B. (1990) J. Bacteriol. **172**, 4197–4205
131. Wu, J. and Weiss, B. (1991) J. Bacteriol. **173**, 2864–2871
132. Greenberg, J.T., Chou, J.H., Monach, P.A. and Demple, B. (1991) J. Bacteriol. **173**, 4433–4439
133. Farr, S.B., Natvig, D.O. and Kogoma, T. (1985) J. Bacteriol. **164**, 1309–1316
134. Kogoma, T., Farr, S.B., Joyce, K.M. and Natvig, D.O. (1988) Proc. Natl. Acad. Sci. U.S.A. **85**, 4799–4803
135. Collinson, L.P. and Dawes, I.W. (1992) J. Gen. Microbiol. **138**, 329–335
136. Flatter-O'Brien, J., Collinson, L.P. and Dawes, I.W. (1993) J. Gen. Microbiol. **139**, 501–507
137. Jamieson, D.J. (1992) J. Bacteriol. **174**, 6678–6681
138. Kuge, S. and Jones, N. (1994) EMBO J. **13**, 655–664
139. Spitz, D.R., Dewey, W.C. and Li, G.C. (1987) J. Cell. Physiol. **131**, 364–373
140. Laval, F. (1988) Mutat. Res. **201**, 73–79
141. Gupta, S.S. and Bhattacharjee, S.B. (1988) Int. J. Radiat. Biol. **53**, 935–942
142. Lu, D., Maulik, N., Moraru, I.I., Kreutzer, D.L. and Das, D.K. (1993) Am. J. Physiol. **264**, C715–C722
143. Crawford, D., Zbinden, I., Amstad, P. and Cerutti, P. (1988) Oncogene **3**, 27–32
144. Fornace, A.J., Alamo, I., Jr. and Hollander, M.C. (1988) Proc. Natl. Acad. Sci. U.S.A. **85**, 8800–8804
145. Keyse, S.M. and Tyrrell, R.M. (1989) Proc. Natl. Acad. Sci. U.S.A. **86**, 99–103
146. Rushmore, T.H., King, R.G., Paulson, K.E. and Pickett, C.G. (1990) Proc. Natl. Acad. Sci. U.S.A. **87**, 3826–3830
147. Salo, D.C., Donovan, C.M. and Davies, K.J.A. (1991) Free Radical Biol. Med. **11**, 239–246
148. Shull, S., Heintz, N.H., Periasamy, M., Manohar, M., Janssen, Y.M.W., Marsh, J.P. and Mossman, B.T. (1991) J. Biol. Chem. **266**, 24398–24403
149. Stevens, J.B. and Autor, A.P. (1977) J. Biol. Chem. **10**, 3509–3514
150. White, C.W., Ghezzi, P., McMahon, S., Dinarello, C.A. and Repine, J.E. (1989) J. Appl. Physiol. **66**, 1003–1007
151. Devary, Y., Gottlieb, R.A., Lau, L.F. and Karin, M. (1991) Mol. Cell Biol. **11**, 2804–2811
152. Fornace, A.J., Nebert, D.W., Hollander, M.C., Luethy, J.D., Papathanasiou, M., Fargnoli, J. and Holbrook, N.J. (1989) Mol. Cell Biol. **9**, 4196–4203
153. Keyse, S.M. and Emslie, E.A. (1992) Nature (London) **359**, 644–647
154. Daoud, A.H. and Griffin, A.C. (1980) Cancer Lett. **9**, 299–304
155. Ames, B.N., Shigenaga, M.K. and Hagen, T.M. (1993) Proc. Natl. Acad. Sci. U.S.A. **90**, 7915–7922
156. Block, G., Patterson, B. and Subar, A. (1992) Nutr. Cancer **18**, 1–29
157. Krieger, M. (1992) Trends Biochem. Sci. **17**, 141–146

158. Steinberg, D., Parthasarathy, S., Carew, T.E., Khoo, J.C. and Witztum, J.L. (1989) N. Engl. J. Med. **320**, 915–924

159. Ross, R. (1981) Arteriosclerosis **1**, 293–311

160. McCord, J.M. (1985) N. Engl. J. Med. **312**, 159–163

161. Kloner, R.A., Przyklenk, K. and Whitaker, P. (1989) Circulation **80**, 1115–1127

162. Stevens, C.R., Benboubetra, M., Harrison, R., Sahinoglu, T., Smith, E.C. and Blake, D.R. (1991) Ann. Rheum. Dis. **50**, 760–762

163. Situnayake, R.D., Thurnham, D.I., Kootathep, S., Chirico, S., Lunec, J., Davis, M. and McConkey, B. (1991) Ann. Rheum. Dis. **50**, 81–86

164. Blake, D.R., Merry, P., Unsworth, J., Kidd, B.L., Outhwaite, J.M., Ballard, R., Morris, C.J., Gray, L. and Lunec, J. (1989) Lancet **i**, 289–293

165. Chidwick, K., Winyard, P.G., Zhang, Z. Farrell, A.J. and Blake, D.R. (1991) Ann. Rheum. Dis. **50**, 915–916

166. Lunec, J., Halloran, S.P., White, A.G. and Dormandy, T.L. (1981) J. Rheumatol. **8**, 233–245

167. Fairburn, K., Kus, M.L., Winyard, P.G. and Blake, D.R. (1994) in Free Radicals in the Environment, Medicine and Toxicology (Nohl, H., Esterbeuer, H. and Rice-Evans, C.A., eds.), pp. 469–492, Richelieu Press, London

168. Varma, S.D., Chand, D., Sharma, Y.R., Kuck, J.F., Jr. and Richards, R.D. (1984) Curr. Eye Res. **3**, 35–57

169. Taylor, A., Daims, M.A., Lee, J. and Surgenor, T. (1982) Curr. Eye Res. **2**, 47–56

170. Taylor, A. and Davies, K.J.A. (1987) Free Radical Biol. Med. **3**, 371–377

171. Davies, K.J.A. (1989) in Antioxidants in Therapy and Preventive Medicine (Emerit, I., Packer, L. and Auclair, C., eds.), pp. 503–511, Plenum Press, London

172. Murakami, K., Jahngen, J.H., Lin, S.H., Davies, K.J.A. and Taylor, A. (1990) Free Radical Biol. Med. **8**, 217–222

173. Rosen, D.R., Siddique, T., Patterson, D. et al. (1993) Nature (London) **362**, 59–62

174. Deng, H.-X., Hentati, A., Tainer, J.A. et al. (1993) Science **261**, 1047–1051

175. Gurney, M.E., Pu, H., Chiu, A.Y. et al. (1994) Science **264**, 1772–1775

176. Rothstein, J.D., Bristol, L.A., Hosler, B., Brown, Jr., R.H. and Kuncl, R.W. (1994) Proc. Natl. Acad. Sci. U.S.A. **91**, 4155–4159

177. Weber, G.F., Maertens, P., Meng, X.Z. and Pippenger, C.E. (1991) Lancet **337**, 1443–1444

178. Saito, Y., Yokoyama, T. and Kamoshita, S. (1982) Acta Neuropathol. **58**, 187–192

179. Marklund, S.L., Santavuori, P. and Westermarck, T. (1981) Clin. Chim. Acta **116**, 191–198

180. Hochstein, P., Kumar, K.S. and Forman, H.J. (1980) Ann. N.Y. Acad. Sci. **355**, 240–248

181. Barbeau, A. (1984) Can. J. Neurol. Sci. **11**, 24–28

182. Youdim, M.B.H., Ben-Shachar, D. and Riederer, P. (1989) Acta Neurol. Scand. **126**, 47–54

183. Gee, P. and Davison, A.J. (1989) Free Radical Biol. Med. **6**, 271–284

184. Neve, R.L., Finch, E.A. and Dawes, L.R. (1988) Neuron **1**, 669–677

185. Glenner, G.G. (1988) Cell **52**, 307–308

186. Johnson, S.A., McNeill, T., Cordell, B. and Finch, C.E. (1990) Science **248**, 854–857

187. Selkoe, D.J. (1991) Neuron **6**, 487–498

188. Mattson, M.P., Barger, S.W., Cheng, B., Lieberburg, I., Smith Swintosky, V.L. and Rydel, R.E. (1993) Trends Neurosci. **16**, 409–414

189. Mattson, M.P., Cheng, B., Davis, D., Bryant, K., Lieberburg, I. and Rydel, R.E. (1992) J. Neurosci. **12**, 376–389

190. Hensley, K., Carney, J.M., Mattson, M.P., Aksenova, M., Harris, M., Wu, J.F., Floyd, R.A. and Butterfield, D.A. (1994) Proc. Natl. Acad. Sci. U.S.A. **91**, 3270–3274

191. Behl, C., Davis, J.B., Lesley, R. and Schubert, D. (1994) **77**, 817–827

192. Harman, D. (1956) J. Gerontol. **11**, 298–300

193. Harman, D. (1992) Mutat. Res. **275**, 257–266

194. Harman, D. (1994) Ann. N.Y. Acad. Sci. **717**, 1–15

195. Weindruch, R., Gottesman, S.R. and Walford, R.L. (1982) Proc. Natl. Acad. Sci. U.S.A. **79**, 898–902

196. Butler, J., Hoey, B.M. and Swallow, A.J. (1989) Annu. Rep. (Series C) R. Soc. Chem. 49–93

197. Tomasi, A., Albano, E., Dianzani, M.U., Slater, T.F. and Vannini, V. (1983) FEBS Lett. **160**, 191–194

198. Albano, E., Bellomo, G., Carini, R., Biasi, F., Poli, G. and Dianzani, M.U. (1985) FEBS Lett. **192**, 184–188

199. Poli, G., Albano, E. and Dianzani, M.U. (1987) Chem. Phys. Lipids **45**, 117–142

200. Thayer, W.S. (1977) Chem.-Biol. Interact. **19**, 265–278

201. Goodman, J. and Hochstein, P. (1977) Biochem. Biophys. Res. Commun. **77**, 797–803

202. Bachur, N.R., Gordon, S.L. and Gee, M.V. (1977) Mol. Pharmacol. **13**, 901–910

203. Davies, K.J.A., Doroshow, J.H. and Hochstein, P. (1983) FEBS Lett. **153**, 227–230

204. Doroshow, J.H. and Davies, K.J.A. (1983) Biochem. Pharmacol. **32**, 2935–2939

205. Davies, K.J.A. and Doroshow, J.H. (1986) J. Biol. Chem. **261**, 3060–3067

206. Doroshow, J.H. and Davies, K.J.A. (1986) J. Biol. Chem. **261**, 3068–3074

207. Marcillat, O., Zhang, Y. and Davies, K.J.A. (1989) Biochem. J. **259**, 181–189

208. Black, M. (1984) Annu. Rev. Med. **35**, 577–593

209. Dahlin, D.C., Minwa, G.T., Lu, A.Y.H. and Nelson, S.D. (1984) Proc. Natl. Acad. Sci. U.S.A. **81**, 1327–1331

210. Rosen, G.M., Rauckman, E.J., Ellington, S.P., Dahlin, D.C., Christie, J.L. and Nelson, S.D. (1984) Mol. Pharmacol. **25**, 151–157

211. Albano, E., Rundgren, M., Harvison, P.J., Nelson, S.D. and Moldéus, P. (1985) Mol. Pharmacol. **28**, 306–311

212. Streeter, A.J., Dahlin, D.C., Nelson, S.D. and Baille, T.A. (1984) Chem. Biol. Interact. **48**, 348–366

213. Anderson, B.S., Rundgren, M., Porubek, D., Nicotera, P., Nelson, S.D. and Moldéus, P. (1989) Adv. Biosci. **76**, 5–11

214. Moore, M., Thor, H., Moore, G., Nelson, S., Moldéus, P. and Orrenius, S. (1985) J. Biol. Chem. **260**, 13035–13040

215. Fehér, J., Csomós, G. and Vereckei, A. (1987) Free Radical Reactions in Medicine, pp. 1–199, Springer-Verlag, Berlin
216. Greenwald, R.A. (1981) J. Rheumatol. **8** (Suppl. 7), 9–13
217. Ames, B.N. (1983) Science **221**, 1256–1264
218. Kubow, S. (1992) Free Radical Biol. Med. **12**, 63–82
219. Ursini, F. (1989) in Molecular Mechanisms of Aging: The Role of Dietary Lipids. pp. 1–94, CCIAA, Lucca, Italy
220. Krinsky, N.J. (1989) Free Radical Biol. Med. **7**, 617–635
221. Burton, G.W. and Ingold, K.U. (1984) Science **224**, 569–573
222. Bendich, A. and Olson, J.A. (1989) FASEB J. **3**, 1927–1932
223. Rice-Evans, C., Miller, N., Bolwell, P., Bramley, P. and Pridham, J. (1995) Free Radical Res. **22**, 375–383
224. Herrman, K. (1989) Crit. Rev. Food Sci. Nutr. **28**, 315–347
225. Graf, E. (1992) Free Radical Biol. Med. **13**, 435–448
226. Scott, B.C., Butler, J., Halliwell, B., and Aruoma, O.I. (1993) Free Radical Res. Commun. **19**, 241–253
227. Afanas'ev, I.B., Dorozhko, A.I., Brodskii, A.V., Kostyuk, A. and Potapovich, A.I. (1989) Biochem. Pharmacol. **38**, 1763–1769
228. Hanasko, Y., Ogawa, S. and Fukui, S. (1994) Free Radical Biol. Med. **16**, 845–850

Biochem. Soc. Symp. **61**, 33–45
Printed in Great Britain

Nitric oxide and reactive oxygen species in vascular injury

Homero Rubbo, Margaret Tarpey and Bruce A. Freeman*

Department of Anesthesiology, The University of Alabama at Birmingham, Birmingham, AL 35233, U.S.A.

Abstract

Nitric oxide ('NO), a free radical species produced by several mammalian cell types, plays a role in regulation of vascular, neurological and immunological signal transduction and function. The role of 'NO in cytotoxic events is acquiring increased significance. The high rate of production and broad distribution of sites of production of 'NO, combined with its facile direct and indirect reactions with metalloproteins, thiols and various oxygen radical species, assures that 'NO will play a central role in regulating vascular, physiological and cellular homoeostasis, as well as critical intravascular free radical and oxidant reactions. At the same time, there are contradictions as to whether 'NO mediates or limits free-radical-mediated tissue injury, and uncertainty regarding its mechanisms of action. 'NO has been portrayed as a pathogenic mediator during ischaemia–reperfusion, and inflammatory and septic tissue injury. In contrast, cell-, metal- and oxidant-induced lipoprotein oxidation events, as well as hepatic, cerebrovascular, pulmonary and myocardial inflammatory and ischaemia-reperfusion injury studies, show convincingly that stimulation of endogenous 'NO production or exogenous administration of 'NO-donating molecules can serve a protective role by inhibition of often oxidant-related mechanisms. The final outcome of toxic versus tissue-protective reactions of 'NO will depend on several factors, including sites and relative concentrations of individual reactive species and their diffusion distances. The following sections address these issues and conclude with a proposal as to how 'NO serves as a central regulator of oxidant reactions and diverse free radical-related disease processes.

Pro-oxidant versus tissue-protective reactions of nitric oxide

Nitric oxide in vascular physiology

Nitric oxide ('NO, nitric oxide, nitrogen monoxide) is an endogenously synthesized free radical first characterized as a non-eicosanoid component of

*To whom correspondence should be addressed.

endothelial-derived relaxation factor, EDRF [1]. Nitric oxide is synthesized by the oxidation of L-arginine to L-citrulline by nitric oxide synthases (NOSs), with both constitutive (cNOS) and inducible (iNOS) forms of NOS reported [2]. Nitric oxide has proven to be a ubiquitous signal transduction molecule and a potent mediator of tissue injury because of its low molecular mass, volatility, lipophilicity, free radical nature and diverse reactivities. Owing to its chemical nature, ˙NO is an active participant in tissue free radical reactions, readily reacting with partially reduced oxygen species [i.e. superoxide anion (O_2˙⁻) and organic-derived free radicals]. Nitric oxide has a relatively low reactivity for a free radical species, resulting in a long biological half-life ($t_{1/2} = 5$–30 s); however, Kelm and Schrader [3] have reported the half-life of ˙NO *in vivo* to be considerably shorter (~ 0.1 s). Nitric oxide and oxygen closely resemble each other in diffusivity, with ˙NO slightly less lipophilic, resulting in a greater apparent rate of ˙NO diffusion in protein and lower apparent rate of ˙NO diffusivity in lipid, both relative to oxygen [4].

The high rate of production and broad distribution of sites of production of ˙NO, combined with its facile direct and indirect reactions with metalloproteins, thiols and various oxygen radical species, assures that ˙NO will play a central role in regulating vascular physiological and cellular homoeostasis as well as critical intravascular free radical and oxidant reactions. It thus becomes evident that reactive species and their reactions with each other play important roles in diverse pathogenic as well as tissue-protective aspects of vascular disease. From this, the following questions arise. What role does ˙NO and its myriad of secondary oxygen radical reactions play in the pathology of atherosclerosis and other vascular disease or injury processes such as ischaemia–reperfusion phenomena? Does ˙NO always act as a pro-oxidant, via its reaction with O_2˙⁻? Can ˙NO sometimes be tissue-protective during vascular disease/injury processes (all of which are already established to include enhanced rates of production of reactive oxygen species and oxidant injury in their pathogenesis)?

Reactivity and cellular targets of nitric oxide

The toxicity of ˙NO in cell-mediated immune reactions was initially attributed to direct ˙NO reaction with thiol- and iron–sulphur-containing mitochondrial enzymes [5] and the inhibition of DNA synthesis via inactivation of the non-haem iron enzyme ribonucleotide reductase [6]. Since tissue ˙NO concentrations are generally low (< 1 μM), it is important to note concepts derived from studies *in vitro* may not lend insight into events *in vivo*. In fact, ˙NO reactivity with haem-, iron–sulphur- and thiol-containing proteins often require very high concentrations of ˙NO, which may not be achievable in biological systems.

A critical reaction that ˙NO undergoes in oxygenated biological media is a direct bimolecular reaction with superoxide anion (O_2˙⁻), yielding peroxynitrite (ONOO⁻) at almost diffusion-limited rates (6.7×10^9 $M^{-1} \cdot s^{-1}$) [7]. Thus, ONOO⁻ formation represents a major potential pathway of ˙NO reactivity which depends on tissue rates of both ˙NO and O_2˙⁻ production. Peroxynitrite has a half-life of < 1 s under physiological conditions, due to proton-catalysed decomposition and target molecule reactions [8]. To date, it has been shown using pure preparations of ONOO− that this species is a potent oxidant capable of directly oxidizing protein and non-protein sulphydryls [9,10]. This process is mediated by both one- and two-electron transfer reactions, representing a major pathway of biological ONOO⁻ reactivity. Thiols readily react with other oxidants as well, including ˙OH, H_2O_2, $O_2^{\cdot -}$ and nitrogen dioxide (˙NO_2) [9,11]. While ˙NO_2 and ONOO⁻ react efficiently with thiols, ˙NO does not at neutral pH. Low yields of S-nitrosylated thiol products are also generated following ONOO⁻ reaction with sulphydryl compounds. The formation of peroxynitrous acid (ONOOH) from ONOO⁻ yields a species with unique ˙OH⁻-like reactions (i.e. stimulation of membrane lipid peroxidation) via metal-independent mechanisms [8,12]. Peroxynitrite is also capable of reaction with metal centres to yield a species with the reactivity of nitronium cation (NO_2^+), an oxidizing and nitrating intermediate [13].

It is apparent that ONOO⁻ can serve as a mediator in oxidative actions originally attributed to ˙NO or other oxygen-derived species. Nitric oxide will potentiate $O_2^{\cdot -}$-mediated tissue damage and leads to ONOO⁻ formation, which can represent a major pathway of ˙NO reactivity. Peroxynitrite is now being revealed to be a key contributing reactive species in pathological events associated with stimulation of tissue production of ˙NO, i.e. systemic hypotension, inhibition of intermediary metabolism, ischaemia–reperfusion injury, immune complex-stimulated pulmonary oedema, cytokine-induced oxidant lung injury and inflammatory cell-mediated pathogen killing/host injury [14–17]. While many studies of ONOO⁻ reactivity have, to date, necessarily utilized pure preparations of ONOO⁻, it is clear that the concurrent presence of other reactive species such as $O_2^{\cdot -}$ and ˙NO will dramatically affect the reaction pathways of ONOO⁻. Thus, as we translate insights from *in vitro* studies into mechanisms of disease, model systems must be designed to better reflect biological conditions.

Protective effects of nitric oxide

Despite the evidence that the co-generation of $O_2^{\cdot -}$ and ˙NO often leads to cytotoxic events via direct toxic reactions, as well as from the generation of secondary products such as ONOO⁻, there are a growing number of observations indicating that ˙NO can sometimes serve a protective role in pathological events associated with excess production and reactions of partially reduced oxygen species. Numerous studies of cell or metal-induced lipoprotein oxidation reactions, as well as hepatic, cerebrovascular, splanchnic, pulmonary and myocardial inflammatory and ischaemia–reperfusion injury studies have recently shown that stimulation of endogenous ˙NO production or exogenous administration of ˙NO often inhibits oxidant-related mechanisms and blunts the ultimate expression of tissue injury at both molecular and functional levels [18–31]. In some of these models, inhibition of ˙NO synthesis enhanced injury, again emphasizing the salutary role often observed for ˙NO in oxidant injury-related processes.

Nitric oxide–oxygen radical interactions in atherosclerosis

Mechanisms of low-density lipoprotein (LDL) oxidation

Recent evidence now compellingly reveals that reactive oxygen species are central mediators of the initiation and progression of both the structural and functional lesions characteristic of atherosclerosis. In fact, oxidation of LDL, a critical event in the initiation of atheroma formation, is associated with enhanced cellular production of $O_2{}^{\cdot-}$ [32]. LDL is normally incorporated by cells via receptor-mediated endocytosis [33]. Oxidation of LDL by $O_2{}^{\cdot-}$ or other reactive species reduces the affinity of LDL for this uptake mechanism. Consequently, macrophages and other cell types incorporate oxidized LDL via an acetylated-LDL or 'scavenger' receptor, leading to the formation of lipid-engorged foam cells. Oxidized lipoproteins can also promote direct vascular injury through the formation of lipid hydroperoxides within the LDL particle [34]. This event then initiates radical chain oxidation reactions of unsaturated LDL lipids, yielding additional anionic modified lipoprotein species with increased affinity for lipoprotein scavenger receptors.

While the *in vivo* mechanism of LDL oxidation remains controversial, information from several *in vitro* systems show that reactive species known to be present in the vascular compartment [$O_2{}^{\cdot-}$, $\cdot OH$, $ONOO^-$, peroxyl radical ($LOO^\cdot$) generators, copper ion, haem proteins and phospholipases] can readily contribute to oxidative mechanisms. Cell types including monocytes/macrophages, endothelial cells, smooth muscle cells and platelets have all been proposed to serve as sources of these reactive species. The observation that LDL may be oxidatively modified by incubation with soybean lipoxygenase and phospholipase A_2 [35], coupled with data showing that lipoxygenase inhibitors prevent LDL oxidation by endothelial cells or macrophages, suggest that cellular lipoxygenases are critically involved in oxidative modification of LDL. The presence of increased 15-lipoxygenase mRNA and protein mass in macrophage-rich atherosclerotic lesions of humans and Watanabe heritable hyperlipidaemic rabbits also supports this contention [36].

Peroxidation of lipoprotein lipids, no matter how the mechanism of initiation occurs, proceeds via free radical-mediated chain propagation reactions. These reactions serve to modify several properties of LDL, including electrophoretic mobility, fatty acid peroxide and thiobarbituric acid-reactive material content, the extent of apoprotein amino acid oxidation, polypeptide chain scission of apolipoprotein B and ultimately, the increased uptake, degradation and accumulation of modified LDL by macrophages [34]. The oxidation of LDL can be enhanced by transition metals such as iron or copper, via promotion of propagation reactions through the transition metal-mediated decomposition of endogenous lipoprotein lipid hydroperoxides to $LOO^\cdot$ and alkoxyl radical species ($LO^\cdot$). Existing 'seeded' lipoprotein and vascular cell lipid hydroperoxides (LOOH) play a key role in these oxidative processes and their consequences, by giving rise to a variety of reactive radical species [i.e. lipid peroxyl ($LOO^\cdot$) or alkoxyl ($LO^\cdot$) radicals] and secondary breakdown products (i.e. reactive aldehydes) which will react with primary amines to yield fluorescent Schiff's base products [37]. This resultant oxidized lipoprotein product is the more anionic species which becomes a ligand recognized by macrophage scavenger receptor(s).

Nitric oxide in lipid and lipoprotein oxidation

Nitric oxide has been observed to play a critical role in regulating lipid and lipoprotein oxidation induced by reactive oxygen and nitrogen species ($O_2{}^{\cdot-}$,

H_2O_2, 'OH and ONOO⁻) and activated reticuloendothelial cells [24,38,39]. Nitric oxide can act as a vitamin E-like inhibitor of radical chain propagation reactions via radical–radical reaction with cytotoxic species such as LOO' or LO' (at the same time yielding unstable nitrogen-containing species as products) [38,39]. In fact, 'NO reacts with LO' and LOO' at near diffusion-limited rates (for LOO', $k = 1.3 \times 10^9 \, M^{-1} \cdot s^{-1}$) [40]. The reaction of 'NO with $O_2^{\cdot-}$ (yielding the potent oxidant ONOO⁻) and reaction with LO' and LOO' to inhibit lipid oxidation suggests that 'NO can both enhance and inhibit lipoprotein oxidation in the vessel wall. The pro-oxidant versus antioxidant outcome of these reactions which are sensitive to 'NO regulation are critically dependent on relative concentrations of individual reactive species [38,39].

Accumulating evidence supports the view that the salutary effects of 'NO are diminished in atherosclerotic vessels due to its reactions with oxygen free radicals. The removal of 'NO from the vascular compartment by its rapid reactions with these free radical species will concomitantly lower its steady-state concentration, thus increasing platelet and inflammatory cell adhesion to the vessel wall and impairing endothelial-dependent mechanisms of relaxation. In this manner, the loss of 'NO bioactivity may promote atherogenic processes.

Nitric oxide has been reported to have contrasting effects on LDL oxidation, for which no mechanistic explanation has been advanced (Fig. 1). For both macrophage and endothelial cell model systems, increased 'NO production or addition of 'NO donors or cytokine-mediated stimulation of the inducible macrophage NOS have been shown to inhibit cell and $O_2^{\cdot-}$-mediated lipoprotein oxidation [24]. In contrast, the simultaneous production of 'NO and $O_2^{\cdot-}$ by 1,3-morpholinosydnonimine hydrochloride (SIN-1) has been shown to oxidize LDL to a potentially atherogenic form via formation of ONOO⁻ [41,42]. We have also observed that direct addition of synthetic ONOO⁻ readily oxidizes β-very-

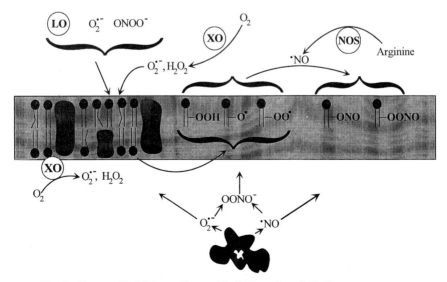

Fig. 1. Free radical interactions with LDL and endothelium.

low-density lipoprotein, as detected by the formation of conjugated dienes and thiobarbituric acid-reactive substances [43]. Graham *et al.* [44] have also shown that ONOO⁻ depletes LDL of native antioxidants and converts the LDL into a form readily recognized by macrophage scavenger receptors.

A stable product of ONOO⁻ reaction with proteins is the addition of a nitro group to the *ortho* position of tyrosine, which can then be used as a 'fingerprint' for ONOO⁻ reaction in tissues. Monoclonal and polyclonal antibodies to nitro-tyrosine formation show immunoreactivity in fatty streaks of coronary arteries of young autopsy subjects. In older patients, nitrotyrosine immuno-reactivity is found in close association with foam cells, vascular endothelium and in the neointima of advanced atherosclerotic lesions. These results show that ONOO⁻-dependent reactions occurred during both early and chronic stages of atherosclerotic disease [45]. Nitrotyrosine immunoreactivity may therefore be an effective marker for oxidative vascular injury due to ONOO⁻, as well as indicating the formation and location of highly immunogenic and potentially pro-inflammatory protein oxidation products.

Nitric oxide and vasomotor responses

Nitric oxide displays numerous vascular actions beyond modulation of vessel tone. As already noted, this reactive species inhibits platelet aggregation, as well as platelet and leucocyte adhesion to the vessel wall [19]. Nitric oxide inhibits smooth-muscle proliferation and acts as a potent antioxidant towards lipids. The diversion of ˙NO from these anti-atherogenic, anti-thrombotic regulatory actions has important implications for atherogenic processes.

Considerable evidence has accumulated in recent years suggesting that the alterations in vascular reactivity associated with atherosclerosis are related to changes in endothelial-cell-dependent (EC-dependent) mechanisms of relaxation. Acetylcholine and other endothelial-cell agonists normally promote the relaxation of isolated vascular ring segments via stimulating the production of ˙NO. Nitric oxide diffuses to underlying vascular smooth-muscle cells where it activates soluble guanylate cyclase and induces vessel relaxation via cyclic GMP-dependent mechanisms. *In vitro* bioassay of arteries from atherosclerotic patients [46] and hypercholesterolaemic animals [47,48] demonstrates that ˙NO-mediated vessel relaxation is severely impaired. Numerous mechanisms have been suggested for this impaired response, including substrate (L-arginine) depletion [47], changes in endothelial cell receptor-coupling mechanisms [49], and abrogation of the vaso-active action of ˙NO following its reactions with $O_2^{˙-}$, LOO˙ and LO˙. Several studies have shown that incubation of vessels with L-arginine restores EC-dependent relaxation [47,50]. Similarly, L-arginine may provide some protection against graft atherosclerosis in cardiac transplant recipients via ˙NO-mediated inhibition of intimal cell proliferation [51] and may attenuate the adhesion of monocytes to the endothelial-cell surface in a dietary model of experimental atherosclerosis [52]. In contrast, other data suggest that ˙NO production is actually enhanced in hypercholesterolaemic vessels [53].

Superoxide dismutase (SOD), an endogenous scavenger of $O_2^{˙-}$, has been used experimentally to limit cellular $O_2^{˙-}$ concentrations (thus ONOO⁻ formation from ˙NO) in an attempt to restore normal ˙NO-mediated vessel responses.

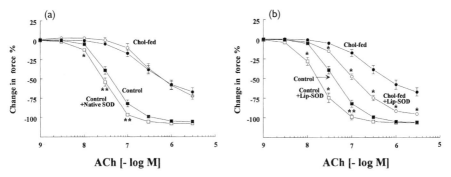

Fig. 2. Cumulative dose–response curves for acetylcholine (ACh) in femoral artery rings from cholesterol-fed rabbits (Chol-fed). (a) Separate groups of vessels from control (squares; $n = 21$) and cholesterol-fed (circles; $n = 15$) rabbits were incubated with bovine CuZn SOD (200 units/ml) before addition of ACh. Native SOD failed to improve EC-dependent relaxation in segments from Chol-fed animals. (b) Control (□) ($n = 20$) and Chol-fed rabbits (○) ($n = 30$) were treated with Lip-SOD for 5 days prior to study. Liposomal-SOD enhanced ACh-induced relaxation in both groups. The DEC$_{50}$ (effective concentration for 50% relaxation) for ACh-induced relaxation as well as the change in maximal relaxation was greater in the Chol-fed group. Data are presented as the mean $\pm$ S.E.M. (*$P < 0.01$; **$P < 0.05$). Adapted from (White, 1994) with permission.

Exogenous administration of native SOD showed little protective effect towards the impaired relaxation response of vessel ring segments from cholesterol-fed rabbits (Fig. 2). Native SOD, which is relatively membrane-impermeable due to its net negative charge at pH 7.4, is electrostatically repelled from cell membranes. Alternate means to target the delivery of SOD to potential intracellular sites of free radical injury have been developed. We have shown [43] that intravenous injection of liposome-entrapped SOD (Lip-SOD) restores ˙NO-mediated relaxation responses in cholesterol-fed rabbits (Fig. 2). A 2–3-fold increase in intracellular SOD enzymic activity was associated with Lip-SOD treatment in these animals. Additionally, poly(ethylene glycol)-derivatized SOD (PEG-SOD) has been used to enhance vascular endothelial antioxidant enzyme levels in hypercholesterolaemic rabbits, yielding similar improvement in ˙NO-mediated relaxation [54]. Treatment of vessels with oxypurinol, an inhibitor of xanthine oxidase, also facilitates ˙NO-dependent relaxation in this model [55]. These different approaches to restoration of EC-dependent relaxation all involve reducing steady-state concentrations of oxygen radical species, suggesting that $O_2^{\cdot-}$-mediated injury (and possibly the formation of oxidized lipid species) resulted in a functional modification of ˙NO.

Nitric oxide–oxygen radical interactions in reperfusion injury

It has been widely accepted in recent years that enhanced rates of production of reactive oxygen species ($O_2^{\cdot-}$, H_2O_2, ˙OH) occur following both focal and global myocardial ischaemia–reperfusion, as well as during the reperfusion associated with thrombolytic therapy and other forms of interventional recanalization for the treatment of ischaemic syndromes. There have been extensive studies in both animal models and humans to support the view that the excess production of reactive oxygen species contributes to loss of myocardial function and/or tissue necrosis, based on direct measurement of free-radical-reaction by-products as well as from the protective effects lent by exogenous administration of antioxidant enzymes and free radical scavengers.

It has recently been observed that enhanced tissue production of ˙NO occurs following reperfusion of both ischaemic brain cortex and myocardium and that inhibitors of ˙NO synthesis will protect from myocardial reoxygenation injury. Both cNOS and iNOS have been reported in human myocardial tissue, first noted after biopsy of right ventricular tissue from patients with dilated cardiomyopathy. Vascular endothelium, as well as other myocardial cells (endocardial endothelium, fibroblasts and vascular smooth cells) are competent to produce ˙NO, with greater extents of ˙NO production expected during events which expose myocardial and vascular tissues to elevated levels of inflammatory stimuli. This includes vessel injury induced by balloon angioplasty, exposure of myocytes to macrophage-derived soluble inflammatory mediators and macrophage accumulation at sites of vascularized allograft rejection. From *in vitro* studies, it is also apparent that some cell types, such as smooth-muscle cells, are capable of generating much greater levels of ˙NO than vascular endothelium, and thus must be considered to contribute a more direct role in myocardial ˙NO reactions than previously thought. From this, it has been concluded that (a) the free radical injury occurring consequent to reperfusion of ischaemic myocardium came predominantly from the potent oxidizing species formed by the reaction of $O_2^{˙-}$ with ˙NO, and (b) that treatment of tissues with inhibitors of ˙NO synthesis can induce mild tissue ischaemia, thus 'preconditioning' myocardium for a second more injurious ischaemic assault.

Some reports have observed that the earliest anomaly in reperfusion injury is an endothelial dysfunction manifested by a loss of ˙NO-dependent vasorelaxation, due to formation of and reaction with oxygen radical species, principally $O_2^{˙-}$ [56]. The stimulation of endogenous ˙NO synthesis or addition of exogenous ˙NO-donating molecules will thus be therapeutic in platelet-mediated ischaemic syndromes such as unstable angina and coronary thrombosis. The protective effects observed for ˙NO with *in vivo* models of reperfusion injury, when administered as a bolus of nitrosothiol or other ˙NO donors, are often ascribed to ˙NO inhibition of inflammatory cell margination and function [21,22,28,29]. In addition, there is a rapid fall in ˙NO levels upon reperfusion, thus augmenting ˙NO-mediated signal transduction pathways at the level of cyclic GMP provides a useful pharmacological approach for normalizing vascular function and blood flow in the critical early stages following tissue ischaemia [56].

The dual role of ˙NO in ischaemia–reperfusion injury is postulated to include an initial increased ˙NO production, which will be tissue-protective by inducing collateral perfusion, but after a time ˙NO formation ceases because of lowered oxygen tension, with oxygen serving a critical role in oxidative deamination of arginine to yield ˙NO. Upon reoxygenation, ˙NO production again recovers, but now, due to the increased presence of other oxygen free radicals, formation of peroxynitrite can occur, thus potentially contributing to further tissue damage.

In brain ischaemia–reperfusion phenomena, ˙NO has been reported to serve a protective role by inducing vasodilation and reducing neutrophil/platelet adhesion and aggregation, thus leading to increased blood flow, tissue perfusion and attenuation of the ischaemic insult. Nitric oxide may also protect from ischaemic-induced brain injury by ˙NO-mediated down-modulation of N-methyl-D-aspartate (NMDA) receptors, thus diminishing NMDA-induced neurotoxicity [23,31,57]. Excess central nervous system ˙NO production during ischaemia–reperfusion will also lead to pathological responses, via activation of NMDA receptor-induced ˙NO synthesis [58]. It is postulated that ˙NO exerts neurotoxic actions primarily through combination with $O_2^{˙-}$ to yield ONOO˙ and its secondary reactive species [59], although a cause and effect relationship has yet to be established. Nonetheless, the presence of critical concentrations of ˙NO may exert cytoprotective effects by counterbalancing or offsetting its cytotoxic effects [23,38].

Conclusions

In biological systems where co-generation of multiple reactive species occurs, ˙NO will exacerbate oxidant injury via production of the potent oxidant ONOO⁻ and can also exert tissue-protective roles. While ˙NO will exert apparent antioxidant effects by terminating radical chain propagation reactions of alkoxyl and peroxyl radicals, it is important to note that (a) when the ratio of the relative rates of $O_2^{˙-}$ to ˙NO production in test systems is less than 1:1, ˙NO serves as a pro-oxidant, via formation of the potent oxidant ONOO⁻, and (b) the products of ˙NO termination of lipid radical species are unstable and may mediate a different spectrum of as yet undefined target molecule and pathological reactions. Thus, ˙NO regulates critical lipid and lipoprotein oxidation events, by contributing to the formation of potent secondary oxidants from $O_2^{˙-}$, catalysing the redirection of $O_2^{˙-}$- and H_2O_2-mediated cytotoxic reactions to other oxidative pathways, serving as an antioxidant via different mechanisms:

(1) Nitric oxide can act as an inhibitor of radical chain propagation reactions via radical–radical reaction with LOO˙ and LO˙, with the formation of nitrogen-containing lipid adducts. These novel lipid oxidation adducts are, in part, organic peroxynitrites and would be expected to occur *in vivo* when diverse inflammatory and pathological processes give rise to similar combinations of reactive species.

(2) Because ˙NO can serve as an iron ligand to form iron–nitrosyl complexes, it has been proposed that ˙NO will modulate the pro-oxidant effects of iron and other transition metals, thereby limiting their role in the Haber–Weiss-catalysed formation of ˙OH and iron-dependent electron transfer reactions. However, the rate of ˙NO reaction with ferrous iron ($2 \times 10^7 \, M^{-1} \cdot s^{-1}$) is significantly lower than for ˙NO reaction with either $O_2^{˙-}$ or LO˙ and LOO˙ radical species. It should be noted that with transition metals, ˙NO can exert pro-oxidant effects as well, by reducing ferric iron complexes.

(3) Nitric oxide is a potent endogenous vasodilator, playing a major role in modulating vascular tone. Endothelial release of ˙NO stimulates soluble guanylate

cyclase in the underlying vascular smooth-muscle cells, thereby elevating intracellular levels of cyclic GMP and inducing relaxation of the vascular smooth muscle. Nitric oxide also inhibits interaction of the vessel wall with circulating blood elements (i.e. platelets and neutrophils). The effect of ˙NO in inhibiting platelet adhesion and aggregation to the vessel wall is associated with increases in the level of platelet cyclic GMP.

(4) Nitric oxide reaction with $O_2^{˙-}$ may in some cases also serve to protect $O_2^{˙-}$-sensitive target molecules. This 'diversionary reaction' of ˙NO, which kinetically can outcompete SODs, forces $O_2^{˙-}$ through $ONOO^-$ oxidation and decomposition pathways. At the same time, this will limit the accumulation of H_2O_2 and decrease the formation of secondary reactive species derived from H_2O_2 reaction with transition metals. This 'superoxide diverting' reaction pathway of ˙NO may promote the extracellular decomposition or less toxic alternative reactions of $ONOO^-$, while at the same time limiting the accumulation and reactions of H_2O_2, toxic to tissues in its own right.

The reaction between ˙NO and $O_2^{˙-}$ in the vasculature also has the combined effect of eliminating a putative antioxidant (˙NO) while at the same time generating a more potent oxidant than $O_2^{˙-}$ ($ONOO^-$). Since the rate constant for ˙NO reaction with $LOO˙$ is greater than that for α-tocopherol reaction with $LOO˙$ and considering that the sometimes $>1\,\mu M$ tissue concentrations of ˙NO can concentrate in membranes, ˙NO could act more readily than (or in concert with) the lipophilic antioxidants α-tocopherol, lycopene, retinyl derivatives and β-carotene as an adjunct antioxidant defence against oxygen radical and lipoxygenase-derived oxidized lipid species. The relative rates of production, sites of production and steady-state concentrations of reactive species, antioxidants and tissue mediators will critically influence the observed apparent toxic or protective effects of ˙NO in biological systems. The cellular and anatomical sites of production of $O_2^{˙-}$ and ˙NO, and the dominant operative mechanisms of oxidant damage in tissues at the time of $O_2^{˙-}$ and ˙NO production will also profoundly influence expression of the differential oxidant injury-enhancing and protective effects of ˙NO. Development of a better understanding of the physiological roles of ˙NO, coupled with detailed insight into ˙NO regulation of oxygen radical-dependent reactions and the chemistry of ˙NO and $ONOO^-$, should yield a more rational basis for the present and future therapeutic use of inhaled ˙NO gas mixtures, ˙NO donors and inhibitors of NOSs. The recent observations of (a) the extremely fast and direct reactivity of ˙NO with oxidizing lipids as well as $O_2^{˙-}$, (b) the tenuous balance between $O_2^{˙-}$, oxidized lipoproteins and ˙NO in regulating endothelial-dependent relaxation, (c) the potent inhibitory effects of ˙NO towards platelet function and neutrophil margination on the vessel wall, and (d) the diversity of pro-atherogenic oxidizing events which occur in the vascular compartment all strongly support a central role for ˙NO in regulating vascular pathogenic processes.

References

1. Furchgott, R.F. and Zawadski, J.B. (1980) Nature (London) **288**, 373–376
2. Marsden, P.A., Schappert, K.T., Chen, H.S., Flowers, M., Sundell, C.L., Wilcox, J.N., Lamas, N. and Michel, T. (1992) FEBS Lett. **307**, 287–293

3. Kelm, M. and Schrader, J. (1990) Circ. Res. **66**, 1561–1575
4. Vanderkooi, J.M., Wright, W.W. and Erecinska, M. (1994) Biochim. Biophys. Acta **1207**, 249–254
5. Hibbs, J.B., Taintor, R.R., Vavrin, Z. and Rachlin, E.M. (1988) Biochem. Biophys. Res. Commun. **157**, 87–94
6. Lepoivre, M., Flaman, J., Bobe, P., Lemaire, G. and Henry, Y. (1994) J. Biol. Chem. **269**, 21891–21897
7. Huie, R.E. and Padmaja, S. (1993) Free Radical Res. Commun. **18**, 195–199
8. Beckman, J.S., Beckman, T.W., Chen, J., Marshall, P.A. and Freeman, B.A. (1990) Proc. Natl. Acad. Sci. U.S.A. **87**, 1620–1624
9. Radi, R., Beckman, J.S., Bush, K. and Freeman, B.A. (1991) J. Biol. Chem. **266**, 4244–4250
10. Rubbo, H., Denicola, A. and Radi, R. (1994) Arch. Biochem. Biophys. **308**, 96–102
11. Radi, R., Bush, K., Cosgrove, T. and Freeman, B.A. (1991) Arch. Biochem. Biophys. **286**, 117–125
12. Radi, R., Beckman, J.S., Bush, K. and Freeman, B.A. (1991) Arch. Biochem. Biophys. **288**, 481–487
13. Ischiropoulos, H., Zhu, L., Chen, J., Tsai, M., Martin, J., Smith, C. and Beckman, J.S. (1992) Arch. Biochem. Biophys. **298**, 431–437
14. Denicola, A., Rubbo, H., Rodriguez, D. and Radi, R. (1993) Arch. Biochem. Biophys. **304**, 279–286
15. Radi, R., Rodriguez, M., Castro, L. and Telleri, R. (1994) Arch. Biochem. Biophys. **308**, 89–95
16. Castro, L., Rodriguez, M. and Radi, R. (1994) J. Biol. Chem. **269**, 29409–29415
17. Mulligan, M.S., Hevel, J.M., Marletta, M.A. and Ward, P.A. (1991) Proc. Natl. Acad. Sci. U.S.A. **88**, 6338–6342
18. Guo, J.P., Siegfried, M.R. and Lefer, A.M. (1994) Methods Exp. Clin. Pharmacol. **16**, 347–354
19. Yao, S., Ober, J., Krishnaswami, A., Ferguson, J., Anderson, H., Golino, P., Buja, L. and Willerson, J.T. (1992) Circulation **86**, 1302–1309
20. Clancy, R.M., Leszczynska, J. and Abramson, S.B. (1992) J. Clin. Invest. **90**, 1116–1121
21. Siegfried, M.R., Carey, C., Ma, X. and Lefer, A.M. (1992) Am. J. Physiol. **263**, H771–H777
22. Lefer, D.J., Nakanishi, K. and Vinten-Johansen, J. (1993) J. Cardiovasc. Pharmacol. **22** (Suppl. 7), S34–S43
23. Wink, D.A., Hanbauer, I., Krishna, M.C., DeGraff, W., Gamson, J. and Mitchell, J.B. (1993) Proc. Natl. Acad. Sci. U.S.A. **90**, 9813–9817
24. Hogg, N., Kalyanaraman, B., Joseph, J., Struck, A. and Parthasarathy, S. (1993) FEBS Lett. **334**, 170–174
25. Malo-Ranta, U., Yla-Herttuala, S., Metsa-Ketela, T., Jaakkola, O., Moilanen, E., Vuorinen, P. and Nikkari, T. (1994) FEBS Lett. **337**, 179–183
26. Jessup, W. and Dean, R.T. (1993) Atherosclerosis **101**, 145–155
27. Payne, D. and Kubes, P. (1993) Am. J. Physiol. **265**, G189–G195
28. Kubes, P., Suzuki, M. and Granger, D.N. (1991) Proc. Natl. Acad. Sci. U.S.A. **88**, 4651–4655

29. Kurose, I., Wolf, R., Grisham, M.B. and Granger, D.N. (1994) Circ. Res. **74**, 376–382

30. Kavanagh, B.P., Mouchawar, A., Goldsmith, J. and Pearl, R.G. (1994) J. Appl. Physiol. **76**, 1324–1329

31. Choi, D.W. (1993) Proc. Natl. Acad. Sci. U.S.A. **90**, 9741–9743

32. Steinbrecher, U.P. (1988) Biochim. Biophys. Acta **959**, 20–30

33. Schwartz, C.J., Valente, A.J., Sprague, E.A., Kelley, J.L. and Nerem, R.M. (1991) Clin. Cardiol. **14**, I1–I16

34. Steinberg, D., Parthasarathy, S., Carew, T.E., Khoo, J.C. and Witztum, J.L. (1989) N. Engl. J. Med. **320**, 915–924

35. Sparrow, C.P., Parthasarathy, S. and Steinberg, D. (1988) J. Lipid. Res. **29**, 745–753

36. Yla-Herttuala, S., Rosenfeld, M.E., Parthasarathy, S. et al. (1991) J. Clin. Invest. **87**, 1146–1152

37. Fruebis, J., Parthasarathy, S. and Steinberg, D. (1992) Proc. Natl. Acad. Sci. U.S.A. **89**, 10588–10592

38. Rubbo, H., Radi, R., Trujillo, M., Telleri, R., Kalyanaraman, B., Barnes, S., Kirk, M. and Freeman, B.A. (1994) J. Biol. Chem. **269**, 26066–26075

39. Rubbo, H., Parthasarathy, S., Kalyanaraman, B., Barnes, S., Kirk, M. and Freeman, B.A. (1995) Arch. Biochem. Biophys., in the press

40. Padmaja, S. and Huie, R.E. (1993) Biochem. Biophys. Res. Commun. **195**, 539–544

41. Hogg, N., Darley-Usmar, V., Graham, A. and Moncada, S. (1993) Biochem. Soc. Trans. **21**, 358–361

42. Darley-Usmar, V.M., Hogg, N., O'Leary, V.J., Wilson, M.T. and Moncada, S. (1992) Free Radical Res. Commun. **17**, 9–20

43. White, R., Brock, T., Chang, L., Crapo, J., Briscoe, P., Ku, D., Bradley, W., Gianturco, S., Gore, J., Freeman, B.A. and Tarpey, M.M. (1994) Proc. Natl. Acad. Sci. U.S.A. **91**, 1044–1048

44. Graham, A., Hogg, N., Kalyanaraman, B., O'Leary, V., Darley-Usmar, V. and Moncada, S. (1993) FEBS Lett. **330**, 181–185

45. Beckman, J.S., Ye, Y.Z., Anderson, P.G., Chen, J., Accavitti, M.A., Tarpey, M.M. and White, R. (1994) Biol. Chem. Hoppe-Seyler **375**, 81–88

46. Forstermann, U., Mugge, A., Alheid, U., Haverich, A. and Frolich, J.C. (1988) Circ. Res. **62**, 185–190

47. Shimokawa, H., Kim, P. and VanHoutte, P.M. (1988) Circ. Res. **63**, 604–612

48. Harrison, D.G., Freiman, P.C., Armstrong, M., Marcus, M. and Heistad, D.D. (1987) Circ. Res. **61** (Suppl. II), II-74–II-80

49. Cohen, R.A., Zitnay, K., Haudenschild, C. and Cunningham, L.D. (1988) Circ. Res. **63**, 903–910

50. Cooke, J.P., Andon, N.A., Girerd, X., Hirsch, A. and Creager, M.A. (1991) Circulation **83**, 1057–1062

51. Drexler, H., Fischell, T.A., Pinto, F.J., Chenzbraun, A., Botas, J., Cooke, J.P. and Alderman, E.L. (1994) Circulation **89**, 1615–1623

52. Tsao, P.S., McEvoy, L.M., Drexler, H., Butcher, E.C. and Cooke, J.P. (1994) Circulation **89**, 2176–2182

53. Minor, R.L., Myers, P., Guerra, R., Bates, J.N. and Harrison, D.G. (1990) J. Clin.

Invest. **86**, 2109–2116

54. Mugge, A., Elwell, J.H., Peterson, T.E., Hofmeyer, T.G., Heistad, D.D. and Harrison, D.G. (1991) Circ. Res. **69**, 1293–1300

55. Ohara, Y., Peterson, T.E. and Harrison, D.G. (1991) J. Clin. Invest. **91**, 2546–2551

56. Pinsky, D., Naka, Y., Chowdhury, N., Liao, H., Oz, M., Michler, R., Kubaszewiski, E., Malinski, T. and Stern, D. (1994) Proc. Natl. Acad. Sci. U.S.A. **91**, 12086–12090

57. Lipton, S., Choi, Y., Pan, Z., Lei, S., Chen, H., Sucher, N., Loscalzo, J., Singel, D. and Stamler, J. (1993) Nature (London) **364**, 626–632

58. Dawson, V., Dawson, T., London, E. and Snyder, S. (1991) Proc. Natl. Acad. Sci. U.S.A. **88**, 6368–6371

59. Beckman, J.S. (1991) J. Dev. Physiol. **15**, 53–59

Biochem. Soc. Symp. **61**, 47–53
Printed in Great Britain

Ultraviolet radiation and free radical damage to skin

Rex M. Tyrrell

Swiss Institute for Experimental Cancer Research, CH-1066 Epalinges, Switzerland

Abstract

Solar UVB (290–320 nm) and particularly UVA (320–380 nm) radiations have a capacity to generate reactive chemical species, including free radicals, in cells. These intermediates have been shown to be involved in various biological effects in cultured human skin cells (e.g. cell death) and skin (e.g. erythema). Endogenous glutathione is a critical molecule in protection against the cytotoxic effects of both wavelength ranges. Although there is evidence from cellular studies for the involvement of an oxidative component of UVC/UVB radiations in activation of several genes, the doses used are generally extremely cytotoxic and could cause aberrant signalling. Genes activated by sublethal doses of UVA radiations (e.g. haem oxygenase 1 and the CL100 phosphatase) are clearly redox regulated. The strong induction of haem oxygenase 1 in human fibroblasts has been implicated in an adaptive response to oxidative membrane damage that involves increased synthesis of the iron storage protein, ferritin.

Introduction

Chronic exposure to sunlight is the major cause of skin cancer in man and a major factor in the ageing of human skin. Epidemiological evidence now clearly links UV exposure to human melanoma and there is provocative evidence from studies using a fish model that the oxidative UVA component could be involved [1]. However, for the most part, the evidence for the involvement of free radicals and oxidative processes in the chronic effects of sunlight on skin is based on animal (usually rodent) experiments involving topical application or dietary supplementation with antioxidants. In contrast, there is evidence from various experimental approaches for the involvement of oxidative processes in the acute effects of UV on cultured mammalian cells and human skin cells in particular and the main purpose of this overview is to draw together some of the evidence in this area before briefly summarizing our own data related to free radical-mediated gene activation.

Penetration of UV through skin

Solar UV radiation incident at the surface of the earth is composed of UVB (290–320 nm) and UVA (320–380 nm) radiation. UVB radiation is essentially defined by the short wavelength cut-off for solar radiation reaching the surface of the earth and this precise cut-off is largely determined by the thickness of the ozone column. Decreased ozone will lead to increased UVB and this effect is particularly dramatic at the shorter wavelengths. In humans the major targets for UV are the skin and the eyes, and it is important to emphasize that the transmission of UV through these tissues increases with increase in wavelength. In practice this means that, in normal skin, the proportion of UVB penetrating through to the basal layer of the epidermis (at an average of 70 μm from the skin's surface) is of the order of 1–10% (according to wavelength) while approximately 20% of a mid-UVA wavelength (365 nm) can penetrate as far. Indeed, significant levels of UVA radiation penetrate beyond the dermis and into subcutaneous tissue and will undoubtedly be 'seen' by blood components. So, while many of the biological effects of UV diminish dramatically with increase in wavelength, this is compensated for to some extent by tissue penetration. Furthermore, more of the solar UV energy incident on the skin is in the UVA region than in the UVB region. These factors clearly influence the levels, magnitude and effectiveness of UV received by the epidermal (keratinocytes and melanocytes) and dermal (fibroblasts) layers of skin.

UV and the generation of active species including free radicals

Both UVA and UVB radiations interact with several biomolecules to generate free radicals and other active intermediates (reviewed in [2]). Sufficient levels of hydrogen peroxide are almost certainly generated by UV in cells to cause generation of hydroxyl radical in the ferrous ion-catalysed Fenton reaction. The ferric ion produced in this reaction may be continuously reduced by superoxide anion and this is generated not only during normal oxidative metabolism but also as a result of the absorption of UV radiation by molecules such as NADH and NADPH. Another important intermediate is singlet oxygen which is generated as a result of the interaction of UV with endogenous photosensitizer molecules that include flavins and porphyrins. These are classical photodynamic agents which undergo reactions (defined as type II) in which the porphyrin chromophore is excited to a triplet state and transfers energy or an electron to oxygen to generate active oxygen intermediates. Porphyrins are probably the most important endogenous photosensitizers in cells and, since they exhibit a Soret band absorption with a peak around 405 nm, it is assumed that the longer UVA wavelengths are primarily responsible for generation of singlet oxygen in cells. A good example of a powerful sensitizer is protoporphyrin IX (the immediate precursor to haem) which is found in the mitochondria and whose levels may be elevated under certain conditions. Nevertheless, it should be mentioned that the major UV chromophore in skin is usually melanin which has a broad absorption spectra which ranges through the UVB, UVA and visible ranges. Although melanin is generally considered to be protective by virtue of its UV-absorbing properties, its degradation can lead to the appearance of melanin free radicals whose biological consequences have not yet been fully evaluated.

Evidence that certain biological effects of UV involve free radical species and active oxygen intermediates

Most of the evidence that UV generates active intermediates in skin cells is indirect and is based on either observed oxygen effects or experiments designed to study the modifying effects of endogenous or exogenous antioxidants (free radical scavengers).

Oxygen effects

There are only a few reports (e.g. [3]) of dose-modifying effects of aerobic versus anaerobic irradiation with UVB in cultured cells. However, there are numerous examples of oxygen effects on the biological action of UVA radiation. These include induction of damage to macromolecules such as DNA (e.g. strand breaks and DNA–protein cross-links) and proteins (including many enzymes), as well as a strong oxygen-dependence for inactivation of populations of both cultured bacterial cells [4,5] and mammalian cells [6]. However, even whole organ effects such as UVA-induced erythema in human skin appear to depend on the presence of oxygen. Such observations provide firm evidence that active species are generated by UVA in the presence of molecular oxygen.

Endogenous antioxidants

In addition to antioxidant vitamins, cells cultured from human skin and other organs contain high (3–5 mM) levels of reduced glutathione, a ubiquitous sulphydryl tripeptide with strong reducing properties. Depletion of cellular glutathione levels using the highly specific γ-glutamyl synthetase inhibitor, buthionine S,R-sulphoximine, strongly sensitizes cells to the lethal action of both UVB and UVA radiations [7,8]. These observations clearly implicate active intermediates in cytotoxicity caused by both wavelength regions. It is also important to note that glutathione levels in both dermis and epidermis are rapidly depleted as a result of UVA irradiation [9], a clear indicator of oxidative stress. UVA also depletes glutathione in cultured dermal fibroblasts [10], but epidermal keratinocytes appear to be relatively resistant to UVA depletion (L. Laurent-Applegate and R.M.Tyrrell, unpublished work). It is worthy of note that glutathione depletion of newborn rodents leads to a strong disposition to cataract [11].

Inhibition of antioxidant enzymes, including superoxide dismutase, catalase and glutathione peroxidase, does not appear to have significant effects on the

UVA sensitivity of cultured human fibroblasts [12] but simultaneous inhibition of a combination of enzymes has not been tried. Similarly, addition of antioxidant vitamins does not normally increase protection of cell cultures against UVB or UVA irradiation, although there is a single report that UVA-sensitive cells cultured from actinic reticuloid patients can be protected by Trolox-C, a water-soluble derivative of vitamin E [13]. In one report, α-tocopherol has been shown to protect against UV-induced cytotoxicity but not DNA damage [14]. A brief summary of the possible evidence of a photoprotective role for vitamin E in animal cells and tissues [15] includes evidence that vitamin E protects lens epithelial tissue from the oxidizing component of UV radiation. Furthermore, there is evidence that UVB-induced erythema and sunburn in the skin of mice can be prevented by topical application of α-tocopherol acetate [16].

Modulation of UV effects by exogenously added agents

In addition to antioxidant vitamins, which have occasionally shown protective effects (see above), other antioxidants or free-radical scavengers may be used to test the involvement of radical intermediates in UV effects. Indeed, the antioxidant drug N-acetylcysteine has been increasingly used after it was shown that it can prevent the UVC-activated signal transduction pathway involving membrane-bound tyrosine kinases [17]. This is almost the only evidence for an oxidative component of UVC radiation in a biological system and it is possible that the high doses of UVC employed rapidly disrupt cellular function and increase oxidative processes which cause aberrant signalling. As discussed above, there is evidence for an oxidative component of UVB radiation but most experiments using chemical modulating agents have involved longer UVA wavelengths. Classical hydroxyl-radical scavengers such as dimethyl sulphoxide (DMSO) and mannitol have little effect on the cytotoxic action of UVA [12] but, in the same study, significant sensitization to the lethal effects of UVA radiation on human fibroblasts was obtained by irradiating them in deuterium oxide, an agent which enhances singlet oxygen lifetime. Interestingly, singlet oxygen has also been implicated as the effector species in the UVA activation of the haem oxygenase (HO)-1 gene (see next section).

UV activation of gene expression and cellular defence

Numerous genes are activated by non-solar UVC radiation and to the extent that these studies have been extrapolated to the UVB region a similar set of genes is involved. Clearly, UVB activates the AP-1/ras signalling pathway and this is linked to activation of many genes including collagenase [18] and c-fos [19], a critical component of the AP-1 transcription factor complex. UVB also activates the c-jun gene [20] and leads to enhanced production of the corresponding protein that constitutes another component of the AP-1 transcription factor. Activation of c-fos and c-jun also occurs in rodent skin after treatment with solar-simulated UV [21]. Both UVC and UVB radiations enhance levels of the p53 tumour-suppressor protein in skin [22,23], a phenomenon which is believed to reflect increased p53 protein lifetime [24] rather than modulation of messenger RNA levels.

Activation of gene expression by UVC and UVB radiation often requires very high doses and there is little evidence that these phenomena are actually related to enhanced cellular defence, either in terms of altered DNA repair or elevated antioxidant activity. Based on studies with ionizing radiation, the p53 protein has been postulated to act in a cell-cycle checkpoint pathway which would allow time for enhanced DNA repair [25]. Interestingly, UVA radiation also enhances p53 protein levels in skin, but, for reasons yet to be clarified, this phenomenon is restricted to the basal layer of the epidermis [22].

In my laboratory, we have been particularly concerned with elucidating the functional role of the activation of the HO-1 gene by UVA and other oxidants. The activation which results in a strong enhancement of the corresponding enzymic activity appears to be a general response to oxidative stress in mammalian cells and occurs to high levels in cultured human skin fibroblasts.

Several lines of evidence, in addition to activation of the gene by oxidants such as hydrogen peroxide, are consistent with the conclusion that this gene is redox-regulated. Perhaps most significant is the observation that both basal levels of expression and the extent of transcriptional activation are strongly influenced by cellular glutathione levels [10]. More recently we have observed that anti-oxidants such as N-acetylcysteine suppress activation of the gene [26]. Further-more, there is evidence that both iron and singlet oxygen are critical to the activation response [27,28].

The normal role of HO in tissue is the breakdown of haem proteins (and particularly haemoglobin) to generate biliverdin which is then normally converted into bilirubin. Although these breakdown products are considered important antioxidants in plasma [29], they are unlikely to play a crucial role in cells where the actual levels generated are low. Rather we have proposed a model in which the final result of UVA activation of the HO-1 gene is increased levels of ferritin. This protein appears to play a critical role in cellular antioxidant defence by keeping the levels of free intracellular iron, a catalyst in many oxidative reactions (see above), to a minimum. We now have strong experimental support for this model [30,31] which is summarized below.

Low fluences of UVA radiation lead to a dramatic increase in HO-1 transcription rate and specific HO-1 mRNA accumulation [32] which is followed several hours later by the predicted several-fold increase in HO enzymic activity. Corresponding to this increase in activity, there is a sharp increase in haem catabolism which will lead to release of chelatable iron. As expected from the known role of iron in stimulating ferritin translation via its interaction with iron responsive factor, this increase in HO activity is followed by a two-fold increase in ferritin levels [30]. We have now observed a UVA-inducible protective response against oxidative damage to membranes, consistent with a lowering of the pro-oxidant state of the cell as a result of increased scavenging of free intracellular iron [31]. Both the increase in ferritin levels and the newly observed adaptive response appear to be mediated via the transient stimulation of HO activity that results from oxidative stress, since these processes are prevented by antisense oligo-nucleotides targeted to the start site of the HO-1 gene. We have also isolated cDNA for the constitutively expressed HO-2 gene (A. Noël, unpublished work) and compared HO-1 and HO-2 mRNA accumulation in human fibroblasts and keratinocytes [33]. While HO-2 levels are expressed at very low levels in human fibroblasts, this gene is expressed at high levels in keratinocytes. In contrast, keratinocytes show little constitutive or inducible HO-1 activity. The total basal level of HO enzymic activity is three times higher in keratinocytes than in fibroblasts and this correlates with relative levels of ferritin. We propose that HO plays a crucial role in cellular defence against oxidative stress in both types of skin cells, and that the pattern of differential expression of the two HO genes between the different cell types is related to the higher levels of UVB and UVA radiation that penetrate to the basal layer of the epidermis as compared with penetration to the dermal fibroblasts.

In summary, we have shown that glutathione plays a crucial role in protecting cultured skin cells against the oxidative stress generated by both UVA and UVB radiations in cultured skin cells. UVA radiation also leads to an enhancement in ferritin levels which clearly provides increased protection against oxidative damage to membranes. The relevance of this observation to other cellular targets is clearly an important question for the future and one which has direct relevance to understanding degenerative oxidative processes in the skin.

This work is supported by grants from the Swiss National Science Foundation (31–0880–91; 3139–03714893), The League Against Cancer of Central Switzerland and the Association for International Cancer Research (U.K).

References

1. Setlow, R.B., Grist, E., Thompson, K. and Woodhead, A.D. (1993) Proc. Natl. Acad. Sci. U.S.A. **90**, 6666–6670
2. Tyrrell, R.M. (1991) in Oxidative Stress: Oxidants and Antioxidants (Sies, H., ed.), pp. 57–83, Academic Press, London
3. Miguel, A.G. and Tyrrell, R.M. (1983) Carcinogenesis **4**, 375–380
4. Webb, R.B. (1977) Photochem. Photobiol. Rev. **2**, 169–261
5. Tyrrell. R.M. (1976) Photochem. Photobiol. **23**, 13–20
6. Danpure, H.J. and Tyrrell, R.M. (1976) Photochem. Photobiol. **23**, 171–177
7. Tyrrell, R.M. and Pidoux, M. (1986) Photochem. Photobiol. **44**, 561–564
8. Tyrrell, R.M. and Pidoux, M. (1988) Photochem. Photobiol. **47**, 405–412
9. Connor, M.J. and Wheeler, L.A. (1987) Photochem. Photobiol. **46**, 239–245
10. Lautier, D., Lüscher, P. and Tyrrell, R.M. (1992) Carcinogenesis **13**, 227–232
11. Calvin, H.I., Medvedovsky, C. and Worgul, B.V. (1986) Science **233**, 553–555
12. Tyrrell, R.M. and Pidoux, M. (1989) Photochem. Photobiol. **49**, 407–412
13. Kralli, A. and Moss, S.H. (1987) Br. J. Dermatol. **116**, 761–772
14. Sugiyama, M.K., Tzuazuki, K., Matsumoto, K. and Ogura, R. (1992) Photochem. Photobiol. **56**, 31–34
15. Fryer, M.J. (1993) Photochem. Photobiol. **58**, 304–312
16. Trevithick, J.R., Xiong, H., Lee, S., Shun, D.T., Sanford, J.E., Karlik, J.J., Norley, C. and Dilworth, J.R. (1992) Arch. Biochem. Biophys. **296**, 575–582
17. Devary, Y., Gottlieb, R.A., Smeal, T. and Karin, M. (1992) Cell **9**, 565–571
18. Stein, B., Rahmsdorf, H.J., Steffen, A., Litfin, M. and Herrlich, P. (1989) Mol.

Cell. Biol. **9**, 5169–5181

19. Shah, G., Ghosh, R., Amstad, P. and Cerutti, P. (1993) Cancer Res. **53**, 38–45

20. Devary, Y., Gottlieb, R.A., Lau, R. and Karin, M. (1991) Mol. Cell. Biol. **11**, 2804–2811

21. Gillardon, F., Eschenfelder, C., Uhlmann, E., Hartschuh, W. and Zimmermann, H. (1994) Oncogene **9**, 3219–3225

22. Campbell, C., Quinn, A.G., Angus, B., Farr, P.M. and Rees, J.L. (1993) Cancer Res. **53**, 2697–2699

23. Hall, P.A., McKee, P.H., Menage, H.D., Dover, R. and Lane, D.P. (1993) Oncogene **8**, 203–207

24. Liu, M., Dhanwada, K.R., Birt, D.F., Hecht, S. and Pelling, J.C. (1994) Carcinogenesis **15**, 1089–1092

25. Kastan, M.B., Zhan, Q., El-Deing, W.S., Carrier, F., Jacks, T., Walsh, W.V., Plunkert, B.S., Vogelstein, B. and Fornace, A.J. (1992) Cell **71**, 587–597

26. Tyrrell, R.M. and Basu-Modak, S. (1995) Methods Enzymol. **234**, 224–235

27. Keyse, S.M. and Tyrrell, R.M. (1990) Carcinogenesis **11**, 787–791

28. Basu-Modak, S. and Tyrrell, R.M. (1993) Cancer Res. **53**, 4505–4510

29. Stocker, R. and Frei, B. (1991) in Oxidative Stress, Oxidants and Antioxidants (Sies, H., ed.), pp. 213–244, Academic Press, New York

30. Vile, G.F. and Tyrrell, R.M. (1993) J. Biol. Chem. **268**, 14678–14681

31. Vile, G.F., Basu-Modak, S., Waltner, C. and Tyrrell, R.M. (1994) Proc. Natl. Acad. Sci. U.S.A. **91**, 2607–2610

32. Keyse, S.M., Applegate, L.A., Tromvoukis, Y. and Tyrrell, R.M. (1990) Mol. Cell. Biol. **10**, 4967–4969

33. Applegate, L.A., Noel, A., Vile, G.F., Frenk, E. and Tyrrell R.M. (1995) Photochem. Photobiol. **61**, 285–291

Biochem. Soc. Symp. **61**, 55–63
Printed in Great Britain

Thiyl radicals in biological systems: significant or trivial?

B. Kalyanaraman

Biophysics Research Institute, Medical College of Wisconsin, Milwaukee, WI 53226–06059, U.S.A.

Abstract

Thiyl radicals are formed from one-electron oxidation of thiols. Thiyl radicals participate in a number of reactions including electron transfer, hydrogen abstraction and addition reactions with several biological constituents and xenobiotics. Thiyl radicals can be detected by optical spectroscopy or by electron spin resonance (ESR) spectroscopy. Thiyl radicals appear to play a role in the nitrosylation of thiols and protein thiols. The exact mechanism of thiol-induced enhancement of oxidative modification of low-density lipoprotein remains questionable. The proposed role of thiyl radicals in lipid peroxidation needs to be re-examined. It has been proposed that thiyl radicals are detoxified by superoxide dismutase in mammalian cells and by a thiol-specific enzyme in bacterial systems. We propose that thiols or protein thiols act as potent antioxidants in radical-induced damage via formation of thiyl radicals.

Introduction

Thiyl radicals ($RS^\bullet$) are sulphur-centred free radicals that are formed from one-electron oxidation of thiols (RSH). Thiols are well-known radioprotectants, whose major function in radiation-induced biological processes is linked to the ability to 'repair' radical-induced damage to DNA and other vital cellular constituents ($RSH + DNA^\bullet \rightarrow DNA + RS^\bullet$) [1]. Although this repair reaction also produces the reactive thiyl radical, the beneficial effects of restoring the cellular function by repairing the damaged DNA might outweigh the deleterious effects of thiyl radical formation. However, thiyl radicals formed in biochemical oxidation/reduction processes under *in vitro* conditions have been shown to cause enzyme inactivation, lipid peroxidation, etc. Readers are referred to an excellent book based on the Proceedings of a NATO Advanced Study Institute on Sulfur-Centered Reactive Intermediates in Chemistry and Biology, held in Italy [2]. In this chapter, I will discuss some aspects of the following topic, Thiyl radical: significant or trivial?

THIYL WHEEL

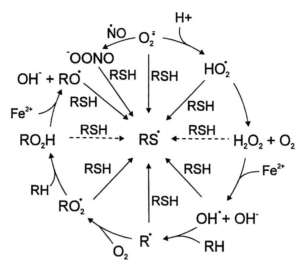

Fig. I. Reactions of thiyl radicals. Dashed arrows $(--- \rightarrow)$ represent indirect oxidants in which H_2O_2 or ROOH are used as a peroxidase substrate (modified from [37]).

Formation and reaction of thiyl radicals

Fig. 1 shows the multiple pathways by which thiyl radicals can be formed in biological oxidations. Reduced oxygen species such as superoxide $(O_2^{\cdot-})$, perhydroxyl radical ($^{\cdot}$OOH), hydroxyl radicals ($^{\cdot}$OH), and peroxyl radicals (ROO$^{\cdot}$) react with RSH to form RS$^{\cdot}$. The rate constants for these reactions, however, vary from $10^3 \, M^{-1} \cdot s^{-1}$ for $O_2^{\cdot-}$ to nearly diffusion-controlled rate for $^{\cdot}$OH.

Peroxidases such as lactoperoxidase or prostaglandin hydroperoxidase as well as myoglobin have been shown to oxidize RSH to RS$^{\cdot}$ using H_2O_2 or ROOH as substrate [3,4]. Although peroxidase-catalysed oxidations of RSH to RS$^{\cdot}$ are 'kinetically sluggish' [2], their rates of formation can be dramatically enhanced by phenols or aminopyrine-like substrate via formation of phenoxyl and cation radicals [5,6]. Such processes are referred to as 'thiol pumping'.

The reaction between nitric oxide ($^{\cdot}$NO)-derived oxidants and thiols is currently of major interest [7]. $^{\cdot}$NO reacts with $O_2^{\cdot-}$ at a diffusion-limited rate to form peroxynitrite ($^{-}$OONO) [8], a powerful oxidant. Peroxynitrite oxidizes both thiols and protein thiols to thiyl radicals, although the extent of the one-electron oxidation mechanism may be a minor pathway [9]. Thiyl radicals are also proposed as intermediates in nitrogen dioxide ($^{\cdot}$NO$_2$)-catalysed oxidation of thiols [10].

Fig. 2 shows the various pathways by which thiyl radicals can initiate oxidation/reduction reactions in biological systems. The rate of production of thiyl radicals in biological systems is usually not high enough to achieve significant

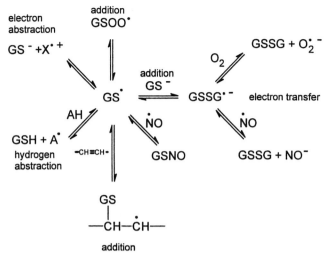

Fig. 2. The oxidation and reduction reactions of glutathionyl radical.
Modified from [37].

steady-state radical concentrations for dimerization reaction to occur. Under normal circumstances, thiyl radicals undergo addition, hydrogen abstraction or electron-transfer reactions as shown for the glutathionyl radical (GS$^\cdot$) (Fig. 2). Evidence for the reaction between GS$^\cdot$ and O_2 to form glutathionyl peroxy radical (GSOO$^\cdot$) has been obtained in chemical and biochemical reactions [11]. The addition reactions of GS$^\cdot$ or GSOO$^\cdot$ with compounds containing an olefinic double bond (i.e. styrene) have been shown to produce epoxides and glutathione–styrene conjugates [12,13,13a]. The addition reaction (Fig. 2) between GS$^\cdot$ and GS$^-$ to form glutathione disulphide radical anion (GSSG$^{\cdot-}$) is significant in that this reaction eventually produces $O_2^{\cdot-}$. Since $O_2^{\cdot-}$ and H_2O_2 can be detoxified by superoxide dismutase, catalase and glutathione peroxidase enzymes, this particular reaction sequela has been hypothesized to be a key detoxification mechanism for most radicals in cells [14]. The addition reaction between GS$^\cdot$ and $^\cdot$NO to form GSNO should be very rapid since it is a radical–radical recombination reaction.

Detection of thiyl radicals

Thiyl radicals generated by pulse radiolysis can be detected by optical spectroscopy or by electron spin resonance (ESR) spectroscopy. However, direct ESR spectroscopy can only be used to detect thiyl radicals in condensed systems at low temperatures, and direct ESR is not suitable for detecting thiyl radicals in solution due to g-anisotropy [15]. Therefore, one has to resort to the spin trapping technique [16]. Spin traps are organic nitrone or nitroso compounds that upon trapping of reactive radicals form more persistent nitroxides. ESR spectra of nitroxide adducts are generally dependent upon the nature of trapped radical. Fig. 3 shows the spin trapping reaction between RS$^\cdot$ and the various spin traps. The reaction between RS$^\cdot$ and 2-methyl-2-nitrosopropane (MNP) yields the corresponding MNP/RS˙ adduct. Although the ESR spectral pattern of MNP/RS˙ adduct is not very characteristic, the g-value of MNP/˙RS adduct should be significantly higher and this particular feature has enabled the identification of thiyl radicals using MNP in photolytic systems. α-Phenyl-*tert*-butyl N-nitrone (PBN) is not a very useful spin trap to detect and characterize small-molecular-mass thiyl radicals. Although the spectral features of PBN/˙RS adducts are not usually very characteristic, PBN has been used to trap high-molecular-mass thiyl radicals, and the resulting PBN–protein thiol adducts exhibit a highly immobilized ESR signal [17], indicating restricted rotation of the nitroxide moiety. The spin trap of choice for detecting thiyl radicals is 5,5-dimethyl-1-pyrolline N-oxide (DMPO). The spectra of DMPO–cysteinyl, DMPO–glutathionyl and DMPO–penicillamine adducts are distinctly different and easily distinguishable. The DMPO–cysteinyl adduct has been isolated and its structure determined by mass spectroscopy [18,19]. The only drawback with DMPO is that the DMPO–hydroxyl and DMPO–glutathionyl adducts, at first glance, exhibit a similar spectral pattern; however, a closer investigation of the spectra will reveal that their intensity patterns are different. DMPO/˙OH exhibits a $1:2:2:1$ pattern, whereas the intensity pattern of DMPO/˙GS is usually $1:1:1:1$ and not $1:2:2:1$.

The novel phosphorylated spin trap (5-diethoxyphosphoryl-5-methyl-1-pyrroline-N-oxide; DEMPMO) developed by Tordo and co-workers has been reported to trap RS˙ to produce ESR spectra from two diastereomers (P. Tordo and B. Kalyanaraman, unpublished work). Although the spectral pattern is more complicated because of the phosphorus hyperfine coupling, the DEPMPO/RS˙ adduct differs from the DEPMPO/˙OH adduct in that the ESR spectrum of the hydroxyl radical is composed of only one stereoisomer. This particular spectral feature can be used to distinguish between the thiyl and hydroxyl radical adducts of DEPMPO.

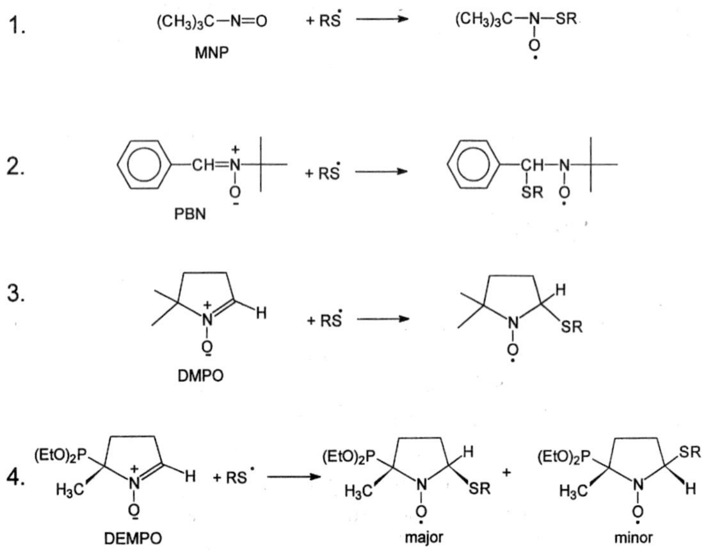

Fig. 3. Reaction between thiyl radicals and spin traps.

DMPO has been used to trap thiyl radicals derived from haemoglobin [21] and serum albumins [22]. Although the ESR spectral pattern is immobilized, it is highly characteristic of protein–thiyl radical trapping. DMPO has been reported to trap low-molecular-mass thiyl radicals at a fairly rapid rate ($k = 10^8\ \mathrm{M^{-1}\cdot s^{-1}}$). Mason and co-workers [14] have shown that thiyl radical-induced O_2 consumption in peroxidase-catalysed reaction is totally inhibited in the presence of DMPO. This implies that DMPO, at concentrations of about 100 mM, should compete very favourably with oxygen for trapping of thiyl radicals. DMPO has also been shown to inhibit other thiyl radical-mediated addition reactions [12].

Thiyl radicals in lipid peroxidation and low-density lipoprotein modification

In a purely homogeneous system, thiyl radicals have been shown to abstract an allylic hydrogen atom from linoleic acid to form a pentadienyl radical using pulse radiolysis [23]. In biological systems, most lipid peroxidation reactions are dependent on the presence of contaminating lipid hydroperoxides and redox-active metal ions. Depending on the reaction conditions (i.e. the concentration of lipid hydroperoxides and metal ions), ascorbic acid can exhibit a pro-oxidant or an antioxidant mechanism. This mechanism is applicable for thiols as well [24]. Thiol-dependent lipid peroxidation is not sensitive to superoxide dismutase [24]. Early on, Gardner and co-workers [25,26] showed that thiols (cysteine or N-acetyl-cysteine) can enhance iron-dependent decomposition of linoleic acid hydro-peroxides (Fig. 4). Although thiyl radicals are formed as intermediates, they only participate in the 'termination' reactions. In the presence of oxygen, RS$^\cdot$ has been shown to form the corresponding thiyl peroxy radical. Under anaerobic conditions, the investigators have isolated and characterized several novel lipid–N-acetylcysteine conjugates by mass spectrometry [25].

More recently, thiols have been shown to augment macrophage-dependent oxidative modification of low-density lipoprotein (LDL) [27,28]. One of the

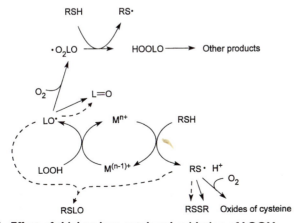

Fig. 4. Effect of thiol on iron-catalysed oxidation of LOOH.

proposed mechanisms involves formation of RS˙, which reacts with O_2 to form RSOO˙ that then abstracts a hydrogen atom of the unsaturated lipid to initiate lipid peroxidation. Invariably, most LDL oxidations are mediated by trace amounts of redox-active metal ions. The extent of oxidative modification of LDL is generally determined by the amount of 'endogenous' lipid hydroperoxides associated with LDL [29]. In general, the initial concentration of lipid hydroperoxides is not measured in most studies. It is known that exceedingly low concentrations of lipid hydroperoxides (that are usually too low to be determined by iodometry) are sufficient to trigger the metal-ion-dependent LDL oxidation. Based on lipid-peroxidation studies in liposomes and microsomes [24], it is conceivable that thiols augment LDL oxidation via mechanisms analogous to those proposed for microsomal lipid peroxidation. As discussed earlier, although DMPO reacts with thiyl radicals fairly rapidly, it does not inhibit the macrophage-dependent oxidation of LDL in the presence of thiols (S. Parthasarathy and B. Kalyanaraman, unpublished work).

Thiyl radicals in S-nitrosylation reactions: reaction between peroxynitrite, thiols and protein thiols

Radi et al. [9] have shown that peroxynitrite ($^-$OONO) oxidizes thiols. Recently, they have shown, by spin trapping with DMPO, that thiyl radicals are formed as intermediates [24]. Although this reaction could be a minor reaction pathway, the production of thiyl radicals may afford a plausible mechanism for formation of nitrosothiols during peroxynitrite-mediated oxidation of thiols [30] as follows:

$$RSH + ONOO^- \xrightarrow{H^+} RS^\bullet + H_2O + {}^\bullet NO_2 \tag{1}$$

$$2RSH + {}^\bullet NO_2 \rightarrow RSNO + RS^\bullet + H_2O \tag{2}$$

$$RS^- + {}^\bullet NO_2 \rightarrow NO_2^- + RS^\bullet \tag{3}$$

$$ONOO^- \rightarrow {}^{-e^-} \rightarrow {}^\bullet NO \ (0.1–1.0\%) \tag{4}$$

$$RS^\bullet + {}^\bullet NO \rightarrow RSNO \tag{5}$$

Alternatively, RS˙ can react with ˙NO_2 to form RSONO, which can undergo a transnitrosylation reaction in the presence of RSH to form RSNO [32a] as follows:

$$RS^\bullet + {}^\bullet NO_2 \rightarrow RSONO \tag{6}$$

$$RSONO + RSH \rightleftharpoons RSOH + RSNO \tag{7}$$

Recently, protein thiols have been shown to form thiyl radicals in the presence of peroxynitrite. Augusto, Radi and co-workers [31,32] had spin-trapped the cysteinyl thiyl radical derived from oxidation of BSA by peroxynitrite. Both DMPO and PBN produced an immobilized spin-adduct characteristic of trapping a thiyl radical from a large-molecular-mass protein [32]. Halliwell, Cross and co-workers [33] have shown that protein thiols present in the plasma undergo rapid oxidation upon treatment with nitrogen dioxide ($^{\bullet}NO_2$). It is conceivable that thiyl radicals are formed as intermediates [10,34].

Wagner et al. [35] have previously suggested that protein thiols could act as the major antioxidant defence against peroxyl radical in human blood plasma. Thiyl radicals are primarily formed as intermediates in human blood plasma during oxidative stress. During oxidative modification of LDL, both lipid and apolipo-protein undergo oxidation. We have discovered that the cysteinyl residues of apolipoprotein B-100 compete with vitamin E for scavenging of peroxyl radical. LDL, in which the hydrophobic cysteinyl residues are blocked, undergoes more rapid oxidation. Spin-trapping data have also shown formation of a protein-derived radical that is tentatively attributed to a thiyl radical formed from oxidation of cysteines.

Detoxification of thiyl radicals

Winterbourn [14] has recently hypothesized that thiyl radicals can be detoxi-fied in cells in the presence of GSH and superoxide dismutase. According to this hypothesis, $O_2^{\bullet-}$ or other radicals ($R^{\bullet}$) oxidize GSH to $GS^{\bullet}$ and the resulting glutathionyl radicals react with GS^- to form the glutathione disulphide radical anion ($GSSG^{\bullet-}$). $GSSG^{\bullet-}$ regenerates $O_2^{\bullet-}$ in the presence of O_2, thus initiating a chain-reaction. Superoxide dismutase eventually dismutates $O_2^{\bullet-}$ to H_2O_2 and oxygen. Thus superoxide dismutase acts as a 'radical sink'.

Studies from Stadtman's laboratory [36] have suggested that thiyl radicals in bacterial systems are detoxified by a thiol-specific antioxidant enzyme. Although the exact function and mechanism of this bacterial enzyme still remain uncertain, it is not clear whether mammalian cells also utilize such an enzymic machinery to detoxify thiyl radicals.

Conclusions and recommendations

Although this review on thiyl radicals is limited in scope and by no means extensive, it is clear that thiyl radicals play an increasing role in biological oxidations/reductions. Based on this limited coverage, the following conclusions and recommendations can be made.

(1) The antioxidant mechanism of protection of protein thiols probably involves formation of thiyl radicals.

(2) Nitrosylation of thiols and protein thiols by $^{\bullet}NO$-derived oxidants is probably mediated by thiyl radicals.

(3) Thiol-induced oxidative modification of LDL is probably not mediated by thiyl radicals.

(4) Spin traps can be used to inhibit thiyl-radical-mediated reactions in biological systems.

(5) Nitrone spin traps may be used to trap protein-associated thiyl radicals.

(6) Although it has been proposed that a thiol-specific detoxification enzyme is needed for detoxification of thiyl radicals in bacterial systems, in mammalian cells thiyl radicals can be detoxified by ascorbate.

(7) More sensitive and specific biological markers for thiyl radicals are needed.

This research was supported by NIH grants RR01008, HL47250, CA49089, and by an Institutional grant sponsored by Gammax Corporation.

References

1. Nucifora, G., Smaller, B., Remko, R. and Avery, E.C. (1972) Radiation Res. **49**, 96–111
2. Chatgiliaboglu, C. and Adams, K.-D. (eds.) (1990) Sulfur-Centered Reactive Intermediates in Chemistry and Biology, NATO-ASI Series A, vol. 197, Plenum, New York
3. Harman, L.S., Carver, D.K., Schrieber, J. and Mason, R.P. (1986) J. Biol. Chem. **261**, 1642–1648
4. Schreiber, J., Foureman, G.L., Hughes, M.F., Mason, R.P. and Eling, T.E. (1989) J. Biol. Chem. **264**, 7936–7943
5. Eling, T.E., Mason, R.P. and Sivarajah, K. (1985) J. Biol. Chem. **260**, 1610–1607
6. Ross, D., Norbeck, K. and Moldeus, P. (1985) J. Biol. Chem. **260**, 15028–15034
7. Gaston, B., Reilly, J., Drazen, J.M. and Frackler, J. (1993) Proc. Natl. Acad. Sci. U.S.A. **90**, 10957–10961
8. Huie, R.E. and Padmaja, S. (1993) Free Radical Res. Commun. **18**, 195–199
9. Radi, R., Beckman, J.S., Bush, R.M. and Freeman, B.A. (1991) J. Biol. Chem. **266**, 4244–4250
10. Pryor, W.A., Church, D.F., Govindan, C.K. and Crank, G. (1982) J. Org. Chem. **47**, 156–159
11. Grierson, L., Hildenbrand, K. and Bothe, E. (1992) Int. J. Radiat. Biol. **62**, 265–277
12. Ortiz de Montello, P.R. and Grab, L.A. (1986) Mol. Pharmacol. **30**, 666–669
13. Stock, B.H., Bend, J.R. and Eling, T.E. (1986) J. Biol. Chem. **261**, 5959–5964
13a. Foureman, G.L. and Eling, T.E. (1989) Arch. Biochem. Biophys. **269**, 55
14. Winterbourn, C.C. (1993) Free Radical Biol. Med. **14**, 85–90
15. Symons, M.C.R. (1974) J. Chem. Soc., Perkin Trans. II, 1618–1622
16. Mason, R.P. (1984) in Spin Labeling in Pharmacology (Holtzman, J.L., ed.), pp. 87–129, Academic Press, New York
17. Graceffa, P. (1983) Arch. Biochem. Biophys. **225**, 802–808
18. Saez, G., Thornalley, P.J., Hill, H.A.O., Hems, R. and Bannister, J.V. (1982) Biochim. Biophys. Acta **719**, 24–31
19. Harman, L.S., Mottley, C. and Mason, R.P. (1984) J. Biol. Chem. **259**, 5606–5611
20. Reference deleted.
21. Kelman, D.J. and Mason, R.B. (1993) Arch. Biochem. Biophys. **306**, 439–442
22. Davies, M.J., Gilbert, B.C. and Haywood, R.M. (1993) Free Radical Res. Commun. **18**, 353–367
23. Schöneich, C., Asmus, K.D., Dillinger, U. and Bruchhausen, F.V. (1989) Biochem. Biophys. Res. Commun. **161**, 113–120
24. Tien, M., Bucher, J.R. and Aust, S.D. (1982) Biochem. Biophys. Res. Commun. **107**, 279–285
25. Gardner, H.W. and Jursinic, P.A. (1981) Biochim. Biophys. Acta **665**, 100–112
26. Gardner, H.W., Plattner, R.D. and Weisleder, D. (1985) Biochim. Biophys. Acta **834**, 65–74
27. Sparrow, C.P. and Olszewski, J. (1993) J. Lipid Res. **34**, 1219–1228

28. Heinecke, J.W., Kawamura, M., Suzuki, L. and Chait, A. (1993) J. Lipid Res. 34, 2051–2061

29. Thomas, C.E. and Jackson, R.L. (1991) J. Pharmacol. Exp. Ther. 256, 1182–1188

30. Moro, M.A., Darley-Usmar, V.M., Goodwin, D.A., Read, N.G., Zamora-Pino, R., Feelisch, M., Radomski, M.W. and Moncada, S. (1994) Proc. Natl. Acad. Sci. U.S.A. 91, 6702–6706

31. Augusto, O., Gatti, R.M. and Radi, R. (1994) Arch. Biochem. Biophys. 310, 118–125

32. Gatti, R.M., Radi, R. and Augusto, O. (1994) FEBS Lett. 348, 287–290

32a. Barnett, D.J., McAninly, J. and Williams, D.L.H. (1994) J. Chem. Soc., Perkin Trans. 2, 1131–1133

33. Halliwell, B., Hu, M.L., Louie, S., Duvall, T.R., Tarkington, B.K., Motchnik, P. and Cross, C.E. (1992) FEBS Lett. 313, 62–66

34. Prütz, W.A., Mönig, H., Butler, J. and Land, E.J. (1985) Arch. Biochem. Biophys. 243, 125–134

35. Wagner, D.D.M., Burton, G.W., Ingold, K.U., Barclay, L.R.C. and Locke, S.J. (1987) Biochim. Biophys. Acta 924, 408–419

36. Yim, M.B., Chae, H.Z., Rhee, S.G., Boon Chock, P. and Stadtman, E.R. (1994) J. Biol. Chem. 269, 1621–1626

37. D'Aquino, M., Bullion, C., Chopra, M., et al. (1994) Methods Enzymol. 233, 34–46

Biochem. Soc. Symp. **61**, 65–72
Printed in Great Britain

The chemistry of lipid alkoxyl radicals and their role in metal-amplified lipid peroxidation

Lawrence J. Marnett and Allan L. Wilcox

Department of Biochemistry, Center in Molecular Toxicology, and The Vanderbilt Cancer Center, Vanderbilt University School of Medicine, Nashville, TN 37232, U.S.A.

Abstract

Reaction of polyunsaturated fatty acid hydroperoxides with metal complexes generates lipid alkoxyl radicals and metal–oxo complexes. Lipid alkoxyl radicals are presumed to be the species responsible for metal-amplified lipid peroxidation because of the chemical analogy of simple organic alkoxyl radicals to the hydroxyl radical. However, polyunsaturated fatty acid alkoxyl radicals exhibit a rich and diverse chemistry that is dominated by intramolecular cyclization to epoxyallylic radicals. Studies described herein demonstrate that the equilibrium between cyclization and ring-opening of epoxyallylic radicals lies overwhelmingly toward cyclization. Thus lipid alkoxyl radicals have a steady-state concentration that is so low that their contribution to metal-amplified lipid peroxidation is insignificant. In fact, the species responsible for metal amplification of lipid peroxidation appears to be the epoxyperoxyl radical formed by coupling the epoxyallylic radical to molecular oxygen.

Introduction

Lipid alkoxyl radicals are the organic analogues of the hydroxyl radical and are anticipated to exhibit similar chemical reactions, i.e. hydrogen atom abstraction (Scheme 1) and addition to double bonds (Scheme 2). However, the products of reaction of lipid alkoxyl radicals generated in simple chemical systems are not consistent with such expectations. In fact, lipid alkoxyl radicals display a rich chemistry that is dominated by unimolecular reactions such as rearrangement and fragmentation rather than the bimolecular reactions depicted in Schemes 1 and 2. This is because the chemistry of these radicals is dictated by the presence of double bonds in the vicinity of the alkoxyl radical centre. Consideration of the

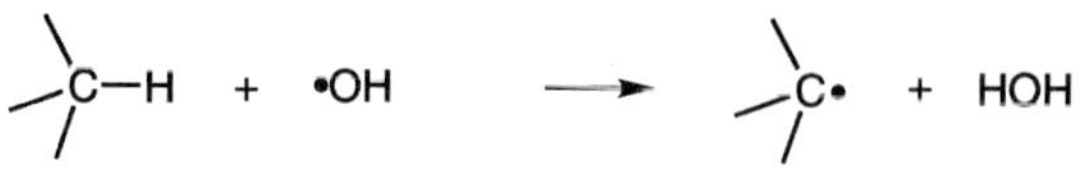

Scheme 1.

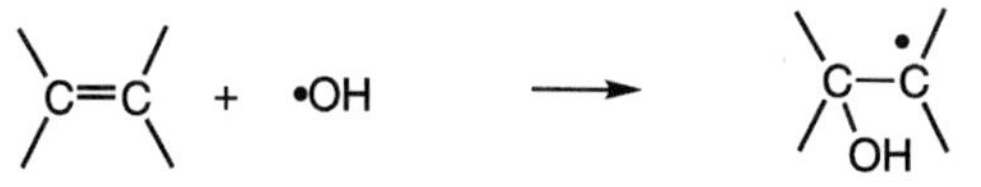

Scheme 2.

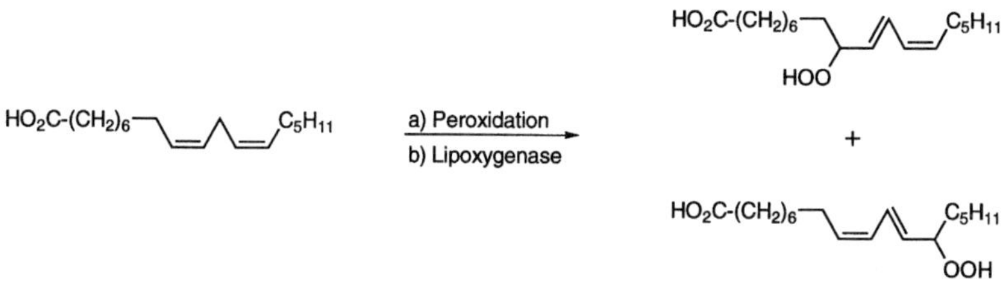

Scheme 3.

chemistry of polyunsaturated fatty acid alkoxyl radicals not only demonstrates the diversity of their reactions but also provides insights into the mechanism of metal-amplified lipid peroxidation, which is believed to be mediated by lipid alkoxyl radicals.

Metal–hydroperoxide reactions

Peroxidation of polyunsaturated fatty acid moieties by autoxidation or enzymic oxidation produces pentadienyl hydroperoxides (Scheme 3). These hydroperoxides are converted into alkoxyl radicals by treatment with metal catalysts; haem complexes are particularly active in this regard. There are two pathways for reduction of organic hydroperoxides by ferric porphyrin complexes [1–6]. Two-electron reduction (heterolytic scission) produces an alcohol and a ferryl–oxo complex in which the iron is formally oxidized by two electrons (Scheme 4). One-electron reduction (homolytic scission) produces an alkoxyl radical and a ferryl–oxo complex in which the iron is oxidized by one electron (Scheme 5). The rate and extent to which a given iron porphyrin or haem protein catalyses heterolytic or homolytic scission are determined by the substituents on the porphyrin, the ligands to the iron, and the polarity and proton-donating ability of the solvent [7–12]. Simple haem complexes (e.g. ferric protoporphyrin IX and ferric tetraphenylporphyrin) produce almost exclusively alkoxyl radical products, whereas haem complexes containing axial imidazole ligands produce various amounts of alcohol and alkoxyl radical products [5,12–16].

Our laboratory has studied the reactions of a series of iron porphyrins with fatty acid hydroperoxides containing different patterns of double-bond substitution in the vicinity of the hydroperoxide. Treatment of these hydroperoxides with

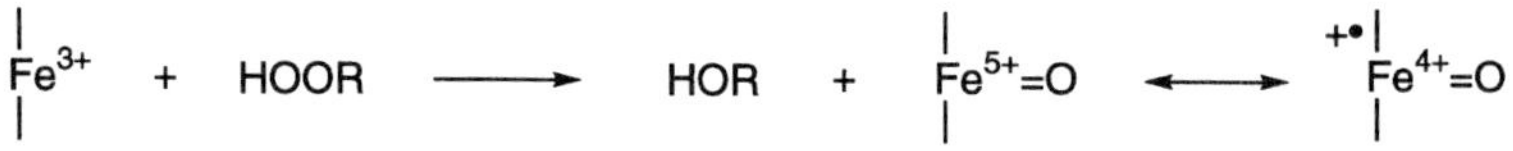

$$Fe^{3+} + HOOR \longrightarrow HOR + Fe^{5+}=O \longleftrightarrow {}^{+\bullet}Fe^{4+}=O$$

Scheme 4.

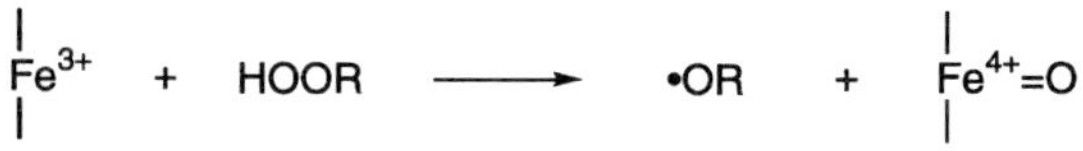

$$Fe^{3+} + HOOR \longrightarrow {}^{\bullet}OR + Fe^{4+}=O$$

Scheme 5.

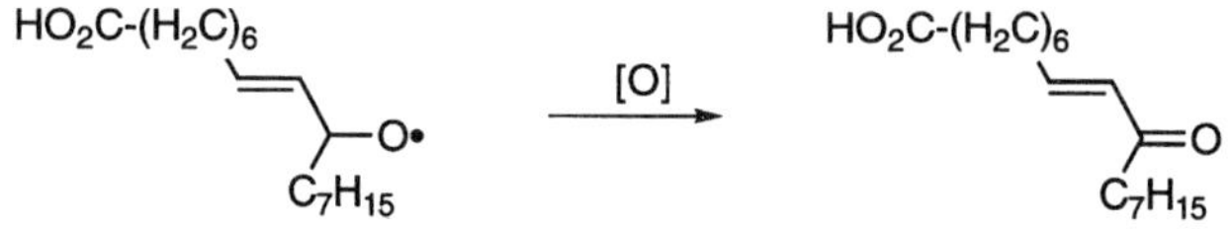

HO$_2$C-(H$_2$C)$_6$ ... -O• $\xrightarrow{\text{[O]}}$ HO$_2$C-(H$_2$C)$_6$ ... =O
C$_7$H$_{15}$ C$_7$H$_{15}$

Scheme 6.

HO$_2$C-(H$_2$C)$_6$ ... -O• $\longrightarrow$ HO$_2$C-(H$_2$C)$_6$ ... =O (H) + •C$_5$H$_{11}$
C$_5$H$_{11}$

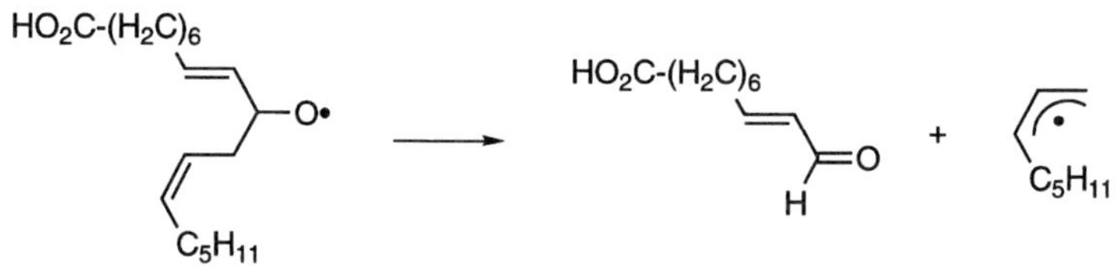

Scheme 7.

ferric protoporphyrin IX in detergent-containing aqueous solutions or with ferric tetraphenylporphyrin in organic solvents reduces the O–O bond by one electron to alkoxyl radicals (Scheme 5). When a double bond is β to the radical, the principal fate is loss of the α-H to form a ketone (Scheme 6) [12]. The oxidizing agent is presumably the ferryl–oxo complex generated by hydroperoxide reduction (Scheme 5). When a double bond is positioned γ to the alkoxyl radical, β-scission to an aldehyde and an allylic radical is the predominant mode of reaction [12,14,17,18] (Scheme 7). The presence of a conjugated diene β to the alkoxyl radical enables cyclization to occur, resulting in the formation of an epoxyallylic radical [16,19–21] (Scheme 8). In the absence of reductants, the major fate of the epoxyallylic radical is coupling to the oxo ligand of the metal–oxo complex to form a series of isomeric epoxyallylic alcohols [19] (Scheme 9). Naturally occurring fatty acid hydroperoxides contain conjugated dienes so the cyclization chemistry depicted in Scheme 8 is important physiologically. In fact, epoxy-alcohols derived from arachidonic acid have been detected in intact human platelets [22].

Certain hydroperoxides derived from arachidonic and eicosapentaenoic acids contain both conjugated dienes and double bonds δ to the hydroperoxides. In these cases, the alkoxyl radical has a choice of intramolecular cyclization or β-scission. Which pathway wins out? To address this question, we reacted 13-hydroperoxyoctadeca-9,11,15-trienoic acid (13-OOH-18:3) with a catalytic amount of ferric tetraphenylporphyrin in dichloromethane [16]. Reaction for

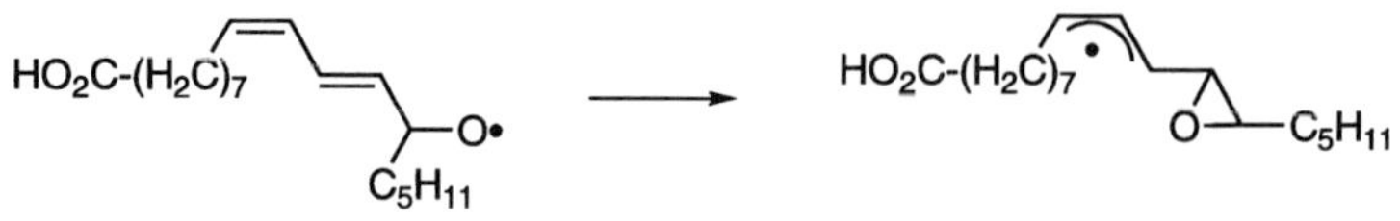

Scheme 8.

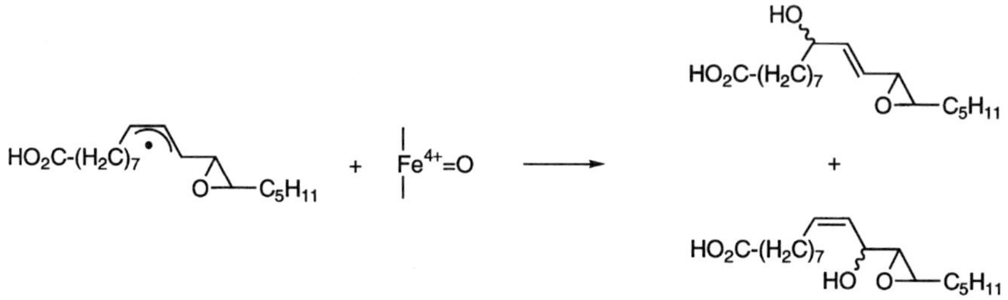

Scheme 9.

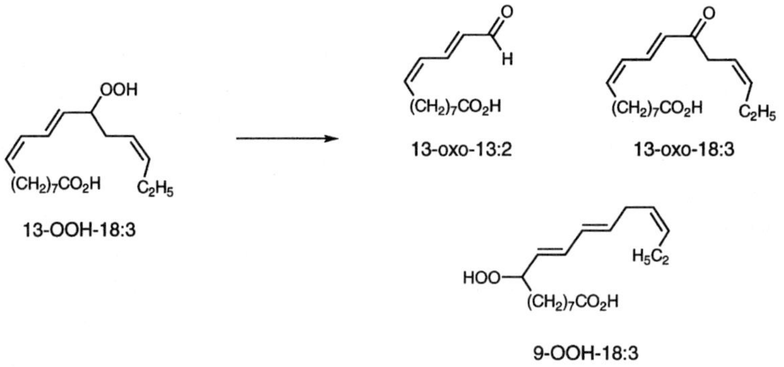

13-OOH-18:3

13-oxo-13:2

13-oxo-18:3

9-OOH-18:3

Scheme 10. Products of reaction of 13-OOH-18:3 with ferric tetraphenylporphyrin in the absence of TBPH.

60 min led to a complex mixture of products containing 4% aldehyde (13-oxo-13:2), 3% ketone (13-oxo-18:3), 22% unreacted starting material, 28% isomerized hydroperoxide (9-OOH-18:3) and 43% unidentified polar products (Scheme 10). The polar material may contain dimeric compounds analogous to previously described epoxyallylic dimers [23,24]. The formation of 9-OOH-18:3 is most probably due to rearrangement of the 13-peroxyl radical formed by H-abstraction from 13-OOH-18:3 by the ferryl–oxo complex [25].

  In another series of reactions, 2,4,6-tri-t-butylphenol (TBPH) was added to support catalytic reduction and to minimize secondary reactions such as hydrogen abstraction from the hydroperoxide by the ferryl–oxo complex [9,26,27]. Inclusion of TBPH (25 mM) caused a dramatic change in the product profile. Straight-phase HPLC analysis indicated that the major product zone (73%) was very non-polar and contained multiple products. 13-Oxo-13:2 and 13-oxo-18:3 were still minor products (4% and 7%, respectively) along with a small amount of rearranged hydroperoxide (3%). The extent of conversion was greater in the presence of TBPH, as only 4% of the starting material was recovered.

Rechromatography of the non-polar product zone revealed the presence of four products with similar spectral properties. Negative ion chemical ionization mass spectra of pentafluorbenzyl esters did not exhibit molecular ions, but contained ions at m/z 489 and m/z 473. The ion at m/z 489 arose from the loss of tri-t-butylphenyl from a putative molecular ion at m/z 734 and the ion at m/z 473 was due to loss of tri-t-butylphenoxyl. ^{1}H-NMR spectra provided evidence for an epoxyaryl ether structure. A correlation spectroscopy (COSY) spectrum revealed weak coupling between two epoxide protons and a vinyl proton. The vinyl proton was in turn coupled to another vinyl proton, which was coupled to a methine proton. These connectivities are consistent with the substitution pattern of an epoxyaryl ether functional group. Similar analysis of the other three non-polar peaks established that each was an epoxyaryl ether (Scheme 11). Double-bond and configurational isomerization account for the different products.

Alkoxyl radical cyclization

The major products of reaction of 13-OOH-18:3 with ferric tetraphenyl-porphyrin in the absence or presence of TBPH are derived by cyclization of the intermediate alkoxyl radical to an epoxyallylic radical. This indicates that cycliza-tion is far more significant than β-scission when alkoxyl radicals have a choice of both pathways. The formation of epoxyaryl ethers in the reaction of 13-OOH-18:3 with ferric tetraphenylporphyrin and TBPH is a dramatic and informative result. The minimum series of reactions necessary to produce epoxyaryl ethers is illustrated in Scheme 12. Homolytic scission of the hydroperoxide by the iron porphyrin produces the alkoxyl radical, which must undergo immediate cyclization to the epoxyallylic radical in order to prevent β-scission to 13-oxo-13:2. The oxidized iron derivative formed by hydroperoxide reduction then oxidizes TBPH

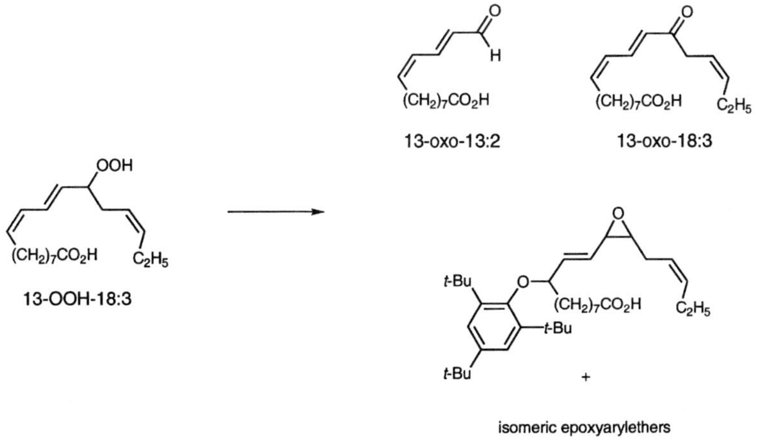

Scheme 11. Products of reaction of 13-OOH-18:3 with ferric tetraphenylporphyrin in the presence of TBPH.

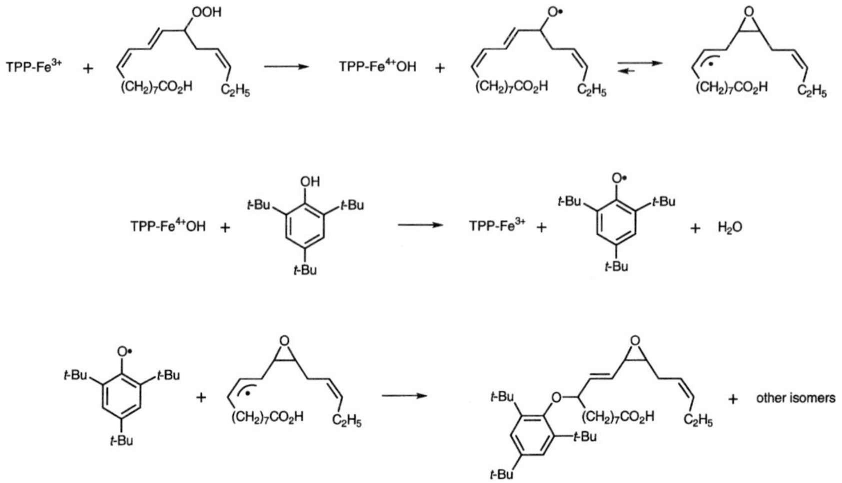

Scheme 12. Mechanism of formation of epoxyaryl ethers in the reaction of 13-OOH-18:3 with ferric tetraphenylporphyrin in the presence of TBPH.

to a phenoxyl radical that couples to the epoxyallylic radical. The ratio of epoxyaryl ethers to aldehyde is nearly 20:1, which emphasizes that the equilibrium between epoxyallylic radical and alkoxyl radical lies substantially towards the epoxyallylic radical. However, these data also require that the rate of equilibration of the two radicals is low, because whenever the epoxyallylic radical opens to the alkoxyl radical it has a significant probability of β-scission to the aldehyde [12,14,17]. The low yield of 13-oxo-13:2 in the presence of TBPH indicates that the epoxyallylic radical opens to the alkoxyl radical slower than the ferryl–oxo complex oxidizes TBPH and the TBPH phenoxyl radical couples to the epoxy-allylic radical. Thus, the pentadienyl alkoxyl radical exists predominantly as the carbon-centred epoxyallylic radical.

Gardner has previously proposed that polyunsaturated fatty acid alkoxyl radicals exist as epoxyallylic radicals because of the predominance of epoxide-containing products relative to alcohol in the reduction of linoleic acid hydroperoxide by ferrous complexes [28]. One limitation of these studies was the absence of a high yield, unimolecular pathway of alkoxyl radical decomposition that could compete with cyclization. The possibility of β-scission in the present case provides such a competitive manifold system. The very low yields of β-scission products in the reaction of 13-OOH-18:3 provide strong evidence for the existence and stability of the epoxyallylic radical.

Metal-amplified lipid peroxidation

These findings provide significant insights into the chemical events respon-sible for lipid peroxidation. Metal-hydroperoxide reactions are known to amplify

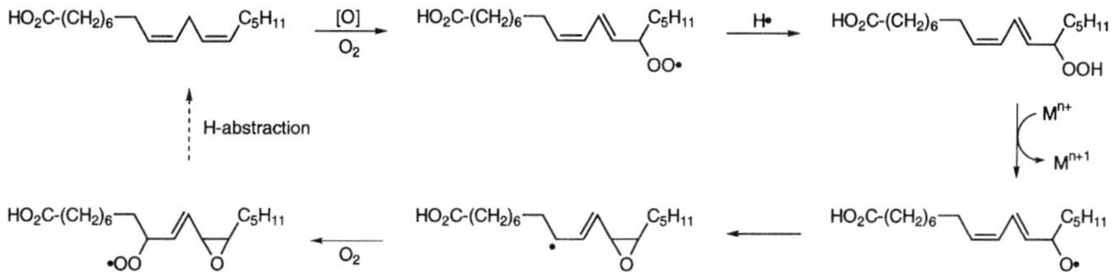

Scheme 13. The role of lipid alkoxyl radicals in metal-amplified lipid peroxidation.

the extent of lipid peroxidation, presumably by formation of alkoxyl free radicals [29]. The alkoxyl free radicals are believed to abstract hydrogen atoms from active methylene groups of the polyunsaturated fatty acid residues of membranes, thereby initiating new radical chains. However, in studies of the metal-catalysed decomposition of polyunsaturated fatty acid hydroperoxides in the presence of microsomal lipids, very low yields of the alcohols that would arise by hydrogen abstraction are obtained [21,28,30]. This paradox can be explained by our finding that the alkoxyl radicals exist primarily as carbon-centred epoxyallylic radicals.

Our findings also help to explain why metal-induced hydroperoxide reduction is an efficient amplifier of lipid peroxidation [31]. Epoxyallylic radicals are more stable than alkoxyl radicals and couple with O_2 to form peroxyl radicals (Scheme 13). Peroxyl radicals are the most stable of the oxygen radicals and are highly selective for abstraction of the active methylene hydrogens of polyunsaturated fatty acids [31–34]. Thus, short-lived alkoxyl radicals that are the initial products of hydroperoxide reduction are converted into long-lived peroxyl radicals that are efficient initiators/propagators of lipid peroxidation.

This work was supported by a research grant and a training grant from the National Institutes of Health (CA47479) (ES07028).

References

1. Bruice, T.C. (1991) Acc. Chem. Res. **24**, 243–249
2. Traylor, T.G., Fann, W.-P. and Bandyopadhyay, D. (1989) J. Am. Chem. Soc. **111**, 8009–8010
3. Arasasingham, R.D., Cornman, C.R. and Balch, A.L. (1989) J. Am. Chem. Soc. **111**, 7800–7805
4. Mansuy, D. (1987) Pure Appl. Chem. **59**, 759–770
5. Labeque, R. and Marnett, L.J. (1989) J. Am. Chem. Soc. **111**, 6621–6627
6. White, R.E. and Coon, M.J. (1980) Annu. Rev. Biochem. **49**, 315–356
7. Traylor, T.G., Tsuchiya, S., Byun, Y.-S. and Kim, C. (1993) J. Am. Chem. Soc. **115**, 2775–2781
8. Traylor, T.G. and Popovitz-Biro, R. (1988) J. Am. Chem. Soc. **110**, 239–243
9. Traylor, T.G. and Xu, F. (1990) J. Am. Chem. Soc. **112**, 178–186
10. Traylor, T.G. and Ciccone, J.P. (1989) J. Am. Chem. Soc. **111**, 8413–8420
11. Reference deleted.
12. Labeque, R. and Marnett, L.J. (1988) Biochemistry **27**, 7060–7070

13. Dix, T.A. and Marnett, L.J. (1985) J. Biol. Chem. 260, 5351–5367
14. Labeque, R. and Marnett, L.J. (1987) J. Am. Chem. Soc. 109, 2828–2829
15. Padbury, G., Sligar, S.G., Labeque, R. and Marnett, L.J. (1988) Biochemistry 27, 7846–7852
16. Wilcox, A.L. and Marnett, L.J. (1993) Chem. Res. Toxicol. 6, 413–416
17. Natrajan, A. and Hecht, S.M. (1991) J. Org. Chem. 56, 5239–5241
18. Chamulitrat, W. and Mason, R.P. (1990) Arch. Biochem. Biophys. 282, 65–69
19. Dix, T.A. and Marnett, L.J. (1983) Science 221, 77–79
20. Dix, T.A. and Marnett, L.J. (1984) Methods Enzymol. 105, 347–352
21. Iwahashi, H., Parker, C.E., Mason, R.P. and Tomer, K.B. (1991) Biochem. J. 276, 447–453
22. Bryant, R.W., Simon, T.C. and Bailey, J.M. (1982) J. Biol. Chem. 257, 14937–14943
23. Kaneko, T. and Matsuo, M. (1985) Chem. Pharm. Bull. 33, 1899–1905
24. Gardner, H.W., Eskins, K., Grams, G. and Inglett, G.E. (1972) Lipids 7, 324–334
25. Mills, K.A., Caldwell, S.E., Dubay, G.R. and Porter, N.A. (1992) J. Am. Chem. Soc. 114, 9689–9691
26. Traylor, T.G., Lee, W.A. and Stynes, D.V. (1984) Tetrahedron 40, 553–568
27. Traylor, T.G. and Xu, F. (1987) J. Am. Chem. Soc. 109, 6201–6202
28. Gardner, H.W. (1991) Biochim. Biophys. Acta (Lipids Lipid Metab.) 1084, 221–239
29. Miller, D.M., Buettner, G.R. and Aust, S.D. (1990) Free Radical Biol. Med. 8, 95–108
30. Schreiber, J., Mason, R.P. and Eling, T.E. (1986) Arch. Biochem. Biophys. 251, 17–24
31. Dix, T.A. and Aikens, J. (1993) Chem. Res. Toxicol. 6, 2–18
32. Ingold, K. (1969) Acc. Chem. Res. 2, 1–9
33. Pryor, W.A. (1986) Annu. Rev. Physiol. 48, 657–667
34. Marnett, L.J. (1987) Carcinogenesis 8, 1365–1373

Biochem. Soc. Symp. **61**, 73–101
Printed in Great Britain

How to characterize an antioxidant: an update

Barry Halliwell

Pharmacology Group, University of London King's College, Manresa Road, London SW3 6LX, U.K.

Abstract

The term antioxidant is widely used but rarely defined. One suggested definition is that an antioxidant is 'a substance that, when present at low concentrations compared with those of an oxidizable substrate, significantly delays or prevents oxidation of that substrate'. Many substances have been suggested to act as antioxidants *in vivo*, but few have been proved to do so. This chapter addresses the criteria necessary to evaluate a proposed antioxidant activity. Simple methods for assessing the possibility of physiologically feasible scavenging of important biological oxygen-derived species (superoxide, hydrogen peroxide, hydroxyl radical, hypochlorous acid, haem-associated ferryl species, radicals derived from activated phagocytes and peroxyl radicals, both lipid-soluble and water-soluble) are presented. Methods that may be used to gain evidence that a compound actually does function as an antioxidant *in vivo* are discussed.

Introduction

The word 'antioxidant' can be defined in various ways. Often, the term is implicitly restricted to chain-breaking antioxidant inhibitors of lipid peroxidation, such as vitamin E. Indeed, food scientists often equate antioxidants to inhibitors of lipid peroxidation. However, free radicals generated *in vivo* damage proteins and DNA as well as lipids, and so the author has introduced a broader definition — an antioxidant is 'any substance that, when present at low concentrations compared with those of an oxidizable substrate, significantly delays or prevents oxidation of that substrate' [1,2]. The term 'oxidizable substrate' includes almost everything found in living cells, including proteins, lipids, carbohydrates and DNA.

When reactive oxygen species (ROS) are generated in living systems, a wide variety of antioxidants comes into play. The term ROS is used in preference to oxygen radicals (since H_2O_2, singlet $O_2{}^1\Delta g$ and HOCl are non-radicals) or oxidants (since superoxide, $O_2^{\cdot-}$, is also a reducing agent). 'Reactive' is a relative term, e.g. $O_2^{\cdot-}$ is more reactive than O_2 but much less so than $^{\cdot}OH$ or HOCl. The relative importance of these antioxidants as protective agents depends upon which ROS is generated, how it is generated, where it is generated and what target of damage is measured. For example, if human blood plasma is tested for its ability to inhibit iron ion-dependent lipid peroxidation, transferrin and caeruloplasmin are found to be the most important protective agents [3,4]. When plasma is exposed to nitrogen dioxide, uric acid seems to exert protection against this oxidizing gas [5]. By contrast, when hypochlorous acid (HOCl) is added to plasma, uric acid plays little role [6]. Similarly, if the oxidative stress is kept the same but a different target of oxidative damage is measured, different answers can result. For example, when plasma is exposed to gas-phase cigarette smoke, lipid peroxidation occurs and ascorbic acid can inhibit [7]. By contrast, ascorbic acid has no effect on oxidative damage to plasma proteins by cigarette smoke, at least as measured by the carbonyl assay [8]. Indeed, some known carcinogens are powerful inhibitors of *in vitro* lipid peroxidation, but can accelerate oxidative DNA damage *in vivo* (discussed in [9]).

The above definition emphasizes the importance of the source of stress and the target ('oxidizable substrate') measured. However, there may be cases which the definition does not include. Thus, plasma albumin may have antioxidant properties, e.g. by binding copper ions and scavenging HOCl [10]. Would it therefore be beneficial to broaden the definition, perhaps to 'an antioxidant is any substance that inhibits oxidative damage to a target under the assay conditions being used?' The risk is that every chemical in the laboratory could then be classified as either an 'antioxidant' and/or 'pro-oxidant', on the basis of assays that have little biological meaning. It is easy to develop some *in vitro* test to support a postulate that compound X is an antioxidant, but very hard to prove that compound X actually works by an antioxidant mechanism *in vivo*.

Antioxidants are of interest to radiation chemists, food scientists, polymer chemists and even to curators of museums [1,11,12], but I shall confine discussion here to the antioxidants known, or proposed, to be important in aerobic organisms. Many reviews have covered the well-established, physiological, antioxidant roles of vitamin E and proteins such as superoxide dismutase (SOD), glutathione peroxidase, catalase and caeruloplasmin, so these will not be discussed here, nor will ascorbic acid.

Many other substances have been proposed to act as antioxidants *in vivo*. They include β-carotene [13], metallothionein [14], carnosine and related compounds [15], mucus [16], phytic acid [17], taurine and its precursors [18–20], bilirubin [21], uric acid [22], oestrogens [23], creatinine [24], ergothioneine (reviewed in [25]), dihydrolipoic acid [26], ovothiols [27], ubiquinol [28], polyamines [29], retinol [30], flavonoids and other phenolic compounds of plant origin [31], and melatonin [32]. Some drugs administered to humans, such as non-steroidal anti-inflammatory drugs (reviewed in [33]), desferrioxamine [34] and N-acetylcysteine [35] could have antioxidant properties *in vivo* (also see other chapters in this volume).

In evaluating the likelihood of a proposal that a given compound can act directly as an antioxidant *in vivo*, it is important to ask the right questions, as

Table 1. Questions to ask when evaluating the proposed role of an 'antioxidant' *in vivo*.

1. What biomolecule is the compound supposed to protect? Is the compound present *in vivo* at or near that biomolecule at sufficient concentration?
2. How does it protect — by scavenging ROS, by preventing their formation or by repairing damage?
3. Is antioxidant protection the primary biological role of the molecule or a secondary role? For example, SOD has probably evolved as an antioxidant enzyme [36]. By contrast, transferrin has probably evolved as an iron transport protein, although the binding of iron ions to transferrins stops them accelerating radical reactions [37], giving these proteins an important secondary role in extracellular antioxidant defence.
4. If the antioxidant acts by scavenging a ROS, can the antioxidant-derived radicals themselves do biological damage?
5. Can the antioxidant cause damage in biological systems different from those in which it exerts protection?

summarized in Table 1. Some quite simple experiments can be performed *in vitro* to answer certain of these questions, and the results can allow one to rule out the proposed antioxidant ability in several cases. The purpose of the present review is to outline a battery of fairly simple experiments that may be used to approach this problem.

Biologically important reactive oxygen species

In testing putative antioxidant activity it is important to use biologically relevant ROS and sources generating such species. One relevant species is superoxide, $O_2^{\cdot-}$, which is known to be formed *in vivo* [1,36,38].

Superoxide formed *in vivo* is largely, if not completely, converted, by SOD-catalysed or non-enzymic dismutation, into H_2O_2. Some enzymes, such as glycolate oxidase, also produce H_2O_2 directly [1,39]. Unlike $O_2^{\cdot-}$, H_2O_2 is able to cross biological membranes [1]. Both $O_2^{\cdot-}$ and H_2O_2 can find some targets within cells at which they can do direct damage [36,39,40], but on the whole their reactivity is limited [41]. Thus only a few compounds, other than specific enzymes such as SOD and catalase, are able to remove $O_2^{\cdot-}$ and H_2O_2 at rapid rates. For example, many thiols react with H_2O_2 and with $O_2^{\cdot-}$, but the rate constants for these reactions are low, usually $< 10^3\ M^{-1} \cdot s^{-1}$ [35,41]. Thus very high thiol concentrations (often $> 1\ mM$) would be required to achieve significant scavenging. It is therefore unlikely that most thiol compounds administered to humans as drugs (such as *N*-acetylcysteine or penicillamine) could act *in vivo* by scavenging $O_2^{\cdot-}$ or H_2O_2, simply because such high drug concentrations are not achieved in body fluids. GSH is present at intracellular concentrations in the high millimolar range, but the reaction of GSH with $O_2^{\cdot-}$ or H_2O_2 has been claimed to be capable of producing reactive sulphur-containing radicals that might be capable of doing more damage than the $O_2^{\cdot-}$ and H_2O_2 would by themselves [42,43]. It is perhaps therefore fortunate that reactions of $O_2^{\cdot-}$ and H_2O_2 with thiols are slow.

Hydroxyl radical

Much of the damage done by $O_2^{\cdot-}$ and H_2O_2 *in vivo* is thought to be due to their conversion into much more reactive species (reviewed in [1,44]). After a long debate, it seems to be established firmly that one of these highly reactive species is hydroxyl radical, $\cdot OH$ [1,44,45].

Formation of $\cdot OH$ from $O_2^{\cdot-}$ can be achieved by at least four different mechanisms. One requires traces of catalytic transition metal ions, of which iron seems likely to be the most important *in vivo*, although copper ions also play a role (reviewed in [44]). In systems containing $O_2^{\cdot-}$, H_2O_2 and iron ions, reactive species additional to $\cdot OH$, including perferryl and ferryl, might also be formed, although direct chemical evidence for their existence in aqueous Fenton systems is lacking. With copper ion/H_2O_2 systems the chemistry is even less clear — debate continues as to whether $\cdot OH$ is formed at all, or if it is formed in addition to a reactive copper(III) species [e.g. $Cu(OH)_2^+$] [44–47]. A second mechanism is that background exposure to ionizing radiation causes a steady low rate of $\cdot OH$ formation within cells, by splitting of water [48]. Another means of forming $\cdot OH$ (or a species that resembles it closely) is the reaction of $O_2^{\cdot-}$ with the free radical nitric oxide ($NO^\cdot$), a reaction which proceeds at a rate comparable with that of $O_2^{\cdot-}$ with SOD [49]. Indeed, $NO^\cdot$ is one of the few molecules that $O_2^{\cdot-}$ reacts with quickly [49]

$$O_2^{\cdot-} + NO^\cdot \rightarrow ONOO^- \qquad (1)$$

The product, peroxynitrite, may cause direct biological damage (e.g. by oxidizing -SH groups [50]) and, at physiological pH, it can protonate and decompose to a range of noxious products, which are identical with (or closely resemble) nitronium ion (NO_2^+), the free radical gas nitrogen dioxide ($NO_2^\cdot$) and $\cdot OH$ [50,51].

A fourth mechanism for making $\cdot OH$ involves HOCl. Reaction of HOCl with $O_2^{\cdot-}$ makes $\cdot OH$; the rate constant is close to $10^7\,M^{-1}\cdot s^{-1}$ [52]

$$HOCl + O_2^{\cdot-} \rightarrow \cdot OH + O_2 + Cl^- \qquad (2)$$

Reactions of hydroxyl radicals

Hydroxyl radical is fearsomely reactive: it combines with almost all molecules found in living cells, with rate constants of 10^9–$10^{10}\,M^{-1}\cdot s^{-1}$ [53]. Thus almost everything in a cell is an $\cdot OH$ scavenger: no specific molecule has evolved for this role. Hence a suggestion that, for example, plasma metallothionein [14] acts to scavenge $\cdot OH$ *in vivo* seems chemically unlikely. The rate constant for scavenging (at $<10^{10}\,M^{-1}\cdot s^{-1}$) may be high, but the molar concentration of metallothionein in plasma is far less than that of substances that are also capable of rapidly scavenging $\cdot OH$, such as albumin (rate constant also $>10^{10}\,M^{-1}\cdot s^{-1}$ [54]). Glucose is not quite as good as an $\cdot OH$ scavenger (rate constant [53] about $10^9\,M^{-1}\cdot s^{-1}$) but its presence at 4.5 mM would allow it to compete favourably with metallothionein in plasma. In the same way, suggestions that several anti-inflammatory drugs act *in vivo* by scavenging $\cdot OH$ formed at sites of inflammation are unlikely to be true: in almost all cases the drug does not accumulate to a high enough concentration *in vivo* [33,55]. A possible exception is salicylate [56].

Antioxidants affecting hydroxyl radical formation

It seems much more likely that an antioxidant acting to interfere with damage caused by ·OH *in vivo* will act not by direct ·OH scavenging, but by scavenging H_2O_2, blocking formation of $O_2^{·-}$ and/or H_2O_2, or by binding the transition metal ions needed for ·OH formation from $O_2^{·-}$ and H_2O_2. The latter may be achieved by two mechanisms. First, binding of the metal ions may so alter their redox potential and/or accessibility that they cannot participate in ·OH formation: this appears to be true of iron ions bound to transferrin or lactoferrin [37] and of copper ions bound to caeruloplasmin [57], although recent studies on caeruloplasmin suggest that some re-evaluation of the biological functions of this protein is needed [58]. Metallothionein could also help to sequester copper and other transition metal ions in 'safe' forms. In the same way, the iron chelator desferrioxamine, at the concentrations actually achieved *in vivo* during therapeutic administration, is far more likely to protect against damage mediated by ·OH by binding iron ions and preventing ·OH formation than by scavenging this radical directly [34].

A second possibility is that binding of a 'catalytic' transition metal ion to an 'antioxidant' does not prevent the redox reactions, but that these reactions are directed on to the antioxidant, so sparing a more important target [59]. Because ·OH is highly reactive, it will combine with the biological molecules that are present at or very close to its site of formation, and so the location of 'catalytic' transition metal ions *in vivo* is an important determinant of the actual cellular damage that is caused by oxidative stress [1,44,60–65]. Hence the presence of copper or iron ions bound to DNA *in vivo* can lead to DNA damage by site-specific Fenton chemistry [44,47,62,63], whereas binding of metal ions to membranes will facilitate lipid peroxidation [61,64]. When copper ions bind to plasma albumin, Fenton-type reactions can still occur on the binding sites and the protein is damaged [59,65]. However, albumin is much less significant as a target of damage than are the membranes of erythrocytes [64], other blood cells or vascular endothelial cells, so that the binding of copper ions to albumin may represent a protective mechanism, since the damaged albumin can be replaced quickly [10]. Binding of copper ions to the amino acid histidine in plasma might also be a protective mechanism: formation of ·OH radicals detectable in free solution is suppressed [66], but the histidine is destroyed [67]. Both albumin and histidine might thus represent safe temporary transport forms for copper ions in plasma, until they can be cleared from the circulation by the liver. Histidine-containing dipeptides, found in many mammalian tissues, might also act as copper ion chelators [68].

Peroxyl radicals

Attack of ·OH upon biological molecules can proceed by addition, hydrogen atom abstraction or electron-transfer reactions (reviewed in [1,48,53]). In all cases, a radical is formed from the biomolecule attacked. Detailed studies have been carried out on the radicals that can result from attack of ·OH upon lipids [1,69],

DNA (for reviews see [48,70,71]) and proteins [48,72–75]. In many cases, carbon-centred radicals are produced, that can then react with O_2 to give peroxyl radicals, e.g.

$$R-H \xrightarrow{\cdot OH} H_2O + R^{\cdot} \xrightarrow{O_2} RO_2^{\cdot} \tag{3}$$

Formation of peroxyl radicals is the major chain-propagating step in lipid peroxidation [1,69], but they can also be formed in non-lipid systems, such as proteins [74–76].

Reaction of $\cdot OH$ with thiols can produce thiyl radicals ($RS^{\cdot}$), which can then combine with oxygen to give reactive oxysulphur radicals such as $RSO^{\cdot}$ and $RSO_2^{\cdot}$ (thiyl peroxyl): the exact chemistry of these reactions is still uncertain [48,77,78]. Oxysulphur radicals resulting from attack of $\cdot OH$ upon penicillamine appear to be capable of inactivating α_1-antiproteinase [79], and probably of damaging other proteins [48,77,78]. But could $\cdot OH$ radicals ever react with penicillamine in $vivo$ in patients taking this drug? At first sight, no: the concentration of penicillamine present in their body fluids is far less than 1 mM, and so it could never compete effectively with endogenous molecules for any $\cdot OH$ generated [55]. However, penicillamine readily binds iron and copper ions and so it might bind available catalytic metal ions in rheumatoid synovial fluid, directing $\cdot OH$ formation on to itself and generating sulphur radicals.

Peroxyl radical scavenging

Scavengers able to remove peroxyl radicals might be effective in the aqueous phase (e.g. dealing with radicals from DNA, thiols, proteins, etc.) or in the hydrophobic (membrane and lipoprotein interior) phase. Glutathione (GSH) reacts rapidly (rate constants $\sim 10^7$–10^{-8} $M^{-1} \cdot s^{-1}$) with radicals resulting from attack of $\cdot OH$ upon DNA [48,80]. Indeed, 'repair' of DNA-derived radicals in irradiated cells is thought to be the major mechanism accounting for the radio-protective action of GSH [48,80], although damage potentially resulting from the $GS^{\cdot}$ radical and its derivatives must not be ignored [42,77,78].

The scavengers of peroxyl radicals that operate in the hydrophobic interior of biological membranes, are, of course, the chain-breaking antioxidant inhibitors of lipid peroxidation. The most important of these in $vivo$ is α-tocopherol [81,82]. The main biological function of α-tocopherol in humans seems to be that of acting as an antioxidant, although the possibility of additional functions must not be neglected [81]. Some other compounds present in membranes may be able to act as chain-breaking antioxidants, but it is uncertain if this is their major physiological function: perhaps they are oxidized simply because they happen to be there. Thus peroxidation of mitochondrial membranes results in loss of ubiquinol, and this loss appears to protect the lipid and delay the loss of vitamin E [83]. Hence ubiquinol has been suggested to be an important antioxidant in mitochondria [28,83,84]. Of course, the fact that excessive loss of ubiquinol will inhibit mitochondrial electron transport and ATP synthesis, and that this could conceivably be more damaging than lipid peroxidation, must be considered. Ubiquinol has been suggested to be an important antioxidant in human low-density lipoproteins (LDLs) [85] but the fact that there is less than one molecule per human LDL particle (Table 2) suggests that it cannot be essential in $vivo$.

Retinol [30] and lycopene [87,88] in membranes might also be attacked by free radicals during membrane lipid peroxidation simply because of their location, as might β-carotene within membranes. β-Carotene inhibits peroxidation of lipids only at low O_2 concentrations [13,89], but this is not without biological relevance since many human tissues have low intracellular O_2 concentrations *in vivo*. When LDLs isolated from plasma undergo peroxidation, oxidation of lipids does not reach its maximum rate until tocopherols, lycopene, retinol and β-carotene have been oxidized [90]. Does this mean that retinol, β-carotene and lycopene are selectively accumulated in LDL in order to act as antioxidants? Probably not, since there is less than one molecule of β-carotene per LDL particle *in vivo* (Table 2). By contrast, about seven α-tocopherol molecules are present per LDL particle (Table 2), consistent with its important physiological role as a chain-breaking antioxidant [81,82,87].

Pro-oxidant effects of lipid antioxidants

Many lipid-soluble chain-breaking antioxidants can have pro-oxidant properties under certain circumstances *in vitro*, often because they can bind Fe(III) or Cu(II) ions and reduce them to Fe^{2+} or Cu^+. Even α-tocopherol can be made to exert pro-oxidant effects *in vitro* [91,92] and this has also been observed in food

Table 2. Composition of native human low-density lipoproteins (LDL). Data abstracted from Esterbauer *et al.* [87]. Obviously, the LDL composition of a given individual will depend to a considerable extent on their diet. For example, consumption of large amounts of PUFA will increase their content in LDL.

Constituent	Mean amount (molecules/LDL particle)
Total lipids	
Phospholipids	700
Phosphatidylcholine	450
Triacylglycerols	170
Free cholesterol	600
Cholesterol ester	1600
Antioxidants	
α-Tocopherol	7–8 (range 3–15)*
γ-Tocopherol	0.5
Ubiquinol 10	0.10–0.50†
Putative antioxidants	
β-Carotene	0.3
α-Carotene	0.12
Lycopene	0.16
Lutein and zeaxanthin	0.02
Phytofluene	0.05

*Range in subjects not consuming vitamin E supplements.
†Ref. [86] reports ubiquinol levels higher than those in [87].

systems [93]. The α-tocopherol radical is capable of abstracting H atoms from polyunsaturated fatty acids (PUFAs) [94] although it does so at a rate orders of magnitude slower than for peroxyl radicals. Propyl gallate, an antioxidant sometimes used in the food industry, has limited solubility in water, but this is enough to allow it to accelerate both ˙OH formation from H_2O_2 by Fenton chemistry and DNA damage by the antibiotic bleomycin, in both cases by its ability to reduce Fe(III) to Fe^{2+} [95,96]. Many plant phenolics (especially flavonoids) have been styled as 'antioxidants' because they inhibit lipid peroxidation — hence the appearance of 'bioflavonoids' (plus or minus vitamin C) on the shelves of health-food stores. However, several plant phenolics can accelerate oxidative damage to non-lipid biomolecules such as DNA *in vitro* [97–99]. They can do this by reducing metal ions and/or by oxidizing to produce $O_2^{˙-}$ and H_2O_2 [97–99]. Thus an antioxidant in one system is not an antioxidant in all systems, and this must be borne in mind when evaluating 'natural' antioxidants: 'natural' does not equate to 'safe'.

Phagocyte-derived ROS

Activated neutrophils, macrophages, eosinophils and monocytes produce $O_2^{˙-}$ and H_2O_2. Most, if not all, of the H_2O_2 arises by dismutation of $O_2^{˙-}$, the first product of the NADPH oxidase enzyme complex [38,100].

If neutrophil-derived $O_2^{˙-}$ and H_2O_2 are involved in producing oxidative damage to tissues, antioxidant protection could be achieved not only by scavenging these species, but also by agents that block the respiratory burst and stop their formation. Thus several anti-inflammatory drugs have been suggested to interfere with phagocyte functioning (reviewed in [33]). However, very few of these claims meet the criterion that the drug at the concentrations actually achieved *in vivo* during normal therapeutic regimes must slow the respiratory burst that is triggered by using physiologically relevant stimuli, such as opsonized bacteria. Agents for which interference with the respiratory burst may be a feasible contributor to their action *in vivo* include piroxicam [101,102], certain antimalarials [103] and some diphenylene iodonium derivatives [104].

Hypochlorous acid

Activated neutrophils contain and secrete the enzyme myeloperoxidase, which uses H_2O_2 to oxidize chloride ions into the powerful oxidant HOCl [105]. Human eosinophils contain a similar enzyme, which prefers bromide (Br^-) ions as a substrate and presumably produces HOBr [106]. Hypohalous acids contribute to the mechanisms by which neutrophils and eosinophils attack ingested bacteria or parasites respectively, but the extent of the contribution is uncertain [38,100,107]. HOCl produced outside the phagocyte might also contribute to tissue damage. For example, it is a powerful oxidant of -SH groups on cell surfaces and so can interfere with membrane transport systems [108,109]. HOCl can also oxidize an essential methionine residue in $α_1$-antiproteinase (formerly called $α_1$-antitrypsin). $α_1$-Antiproteinase is an important inhibitor of serine proteases, such as elastase, in human body fluids. Oxidation of the methionine causes this protein to lose its protease inhibitory capacity, so facilitating proteolytic injury in the surrounding area, e.g. damage to elastic fibres in lung by elastase [105,110]. The rate of inactivation of α_1-antiproteinase by HOCl is extremely fast, being complete within minutes [110]. As discussed previously, HOCl can react with $O_2^{\cdot-}$ to make $^\cdot OH$ [52]. In addition, HOCl appears to interact with H_2O_2 to facilitate oxidative damage to lipids [111].

However, because HOCl is highly reactive, it can also combine with many of the other molecules in its immediate vicinity. Thus when HOCl is added to human plasma, α_1-antiproteinase is not inactivated because the HOCl preferentially reacts with other plasma components present at greater concentrations than those of α_1-antiproteinase [112]. These components include albumin and ascorbic acid [112,113]. Indeed, ascorbic acid at physiological concentrations is a powerful scavenger of HOCl, being able to protect α_1-antiproteinase against inactivation [113]. Scavenging of HOCl by albumin may well be due to rapid reaction with -SH groups on this protein [6]. The bilirubin bound to circulating albumin does not contribute significantly to the HOCl-scavenging ability [114], although bilirubin may help to prevent unsaturated fatty acids, transported in an albumin-bound form in the blood, from becoming peroxidized [21]. Oxidized albumin may be rapidly cleared from the circulation and degraded [10,115].

Hypochlorous acid scavengers

Several papers have examined the ability of anti-inflammatory drugs to scavenge HOCl [116–119]. It was concluded that almost all of the drugs examined could react with HOCl *in vivo*, but only a few drugs would, at the concentrations present *in vivo*, be capable of reacting fast enough to protect important biological targets from attack by HOCl. Thus HOCl scavenging *in vivo* in patients treated with the drugs examined would only be feasible in the case of thiol compounds (penicillamine, *N*-acetylcysteine), phenylbutazone and amino-salicylates [117]. Again, even if these drugs are oxidized *in vivo* by HOCl, the possibility of forming toxic products as a result of oxidation must not be ignored [119–122].

An antioxidant protecting against damage by HOCl might do so not only by scavenging HOCl but also by inhibiting myeloperoxidase. Thus several thiols are not only good scavengers of HOCl, but also act as competing substrates for myeloperoxidase and therefore slow down HOCl formation [118,119,122]. Aminosalicylates and dapsone may also inhibit myeloperoxidase [123]. Ascorbic acid probably also acts as an alternative substrate for myeloperoxidase, but its effects on HOCl production are complex [124]. The plant phenol 4-hydroxy-3-methoxyacetophenone (apocynin) inhibits neutrophil $O_2^{\cdot-}$ release *in vitro*, apparently because it is oxidized by myeloperoxidase to generate the 'real' inhibitory agent [125].

Haem proteins

Ferryl is a powerfully oxidizing oxo-iron species in which the iron has an oxidation number of 4. It might be formed in Fenton systems (possibly as an intermediate in $^\cdot OH$ formation). Haem-associated ferryl species are well-known to be generated by reaction of certain haem proteins (horseradish peroxidase, myoglobin and probably haemoglobin) with H_2O_2 [126–130]. Mixtures of myoglobin or haemoglobin with H_2O_2 are capable of accelerating lipid peroxidation [130–132], a property that may involve initiation of peroxidation by the ferryl species and/or by various amino acid radicals on the protein [133,134]. In addition, incubation of myoglobin and haemoglobin with an excess of H_2O_2 causes haem breakdown to release iron ions [135–137]. Both ferryl formation, and the release of iron ions able to accelerate free radical reactions, from haemoglobin might account for the observation that bleeding into a site of inflammation exacerbates tissue injury [138]. Formation of ferrylmyoglobin as a result of production of H_2O_2 upon reoxygenation of ischaemic heart tissues may contribute to myocardial reoxygenation injury [139,140]. Cytochrome c can also accelerate lipid peroxidation in the presence of peroxides, presumably by similar mechanisms [141,142].

Hence agents that scavenge ferryl species might prevent lipid peroxidation stimulated by ferryl haem proteins. They might also prevent decomposition of the proteins to release catalytic iron ions. Ascorbic acid seems especially effective in this respect, presumably by being preferentially oxidized and so reducing the iron in the haem ring back to a ferric (or even a ferrous) state [143,144]. Thus ascorbic acid inhibits lipid peroxidation stimulated by mixtures of haem proteins and H_2O_2, and also slows or prevents haem degradation [142–145].

Other species capable of reacting with ferryl haem include thiols and uric acid (reviewed in [146]), although the potential pro-oxidant effects of radicals resulting from one-electron oxidation of not only thiols but also of uric acid must be considered. For example, radicals resulting from the attack of ˙OH upon uric acid can inactivate yeast alcohol dehydrogenase [147] or human α_1-antiproteinase [148]. Hence, tests of the ability of a substance to scavenge haem-associated ferryl species are relevant in the evaluation of antioxidant activity, particularly if antioxidants are being developed for use against myocardial reoxygenation injury.

Singlet oxygen

Oxygen has two singlet states, but the $^1\Delta g$ state is probably the most important in biological systems (reviewed in [1]). Singlet O_2 $^1\Delta g$ has no unpaired electrons and is therefore not classified as a radical, but it is known to be a powerful oxidizing agent, able to combine directly with many molecules that are unreactive with ground-state O_2, such as PUFAs [1]. The term 'singlet O_2' is used in the rest of this review to refer to both $^1\Delta g$ and $^1\Sigma g^+$ states collectively.

Singlet oxygen can be produced on or in the skin as a result of photosensitization reactions triggered by certain drugs [149–152], cosmetics [151], plant toxins [153] or by the porphyrins that accumulate in some forms of porphyria [154]. It is also formed when O_3 reacts with constituents of human body fluids [155]. Singlet O_2 is important in the 'phototherapy' of certain diseases, e.g. the use of psoralens to treat psoriasis [149] and of haematoporphyrin derivatives in lung cancer [156]. Singlet O_2 may also be generated in the lens of the eye and may contribute to the development of cataract [157].

However, whether singlet O_2 is produced as a major tissue-damaging species in the deeper tissues of the body is uncertain. Suggestions that singlet O_2 is produced by non-enzymic dismutation of $O_2^{˙-}$ or during the respiratory burst of phagocytic cells have not received much experimental support [158–160]. During peroxidation of membrane lipids, singlet O_2 (or at least a species closely resembling it) is produced, probably largely by the self-reaction of lipid peroxyl radicals (reviewed in [161]).

$$\text{\diagdown}\!CHO_2^{\bullet} + \text{\diagdown}\!CHO_2^{\bullet} \rightarrow {}^1O_2 + \text{\diagdown}\!C{=}O + \text{\diagup}\!C{-}OH \tag{4}$$

This singlet O_2 could conceivably react with further PUFA side-chains and contribute to the overall peroxidation process [160]. However, singlet O_2 seems only to make a minor contribution in most peroxidation systems, possibly because lipid peroxyl radicals do not accumulate to high concentrations in membranes and so their self-reaction is kinetically disfavoured.

Methodology: how to test for antioxidant activity

A substance might exert antioxidant activity *in vivo* by direct free-radical scavenging, by inhibiting formation of ROS and/or by altering levels of endogenous antioxidant defences. Over the years, the author's laboratory, like many others, has evolved a strategy for examining the biological feasibility of the first two mechanisms. This 'screening' approach can be used to rule out direct antioxidant activity *in vivo*: a compound that is poorly effective *in vitro* will not be any better *in vivo*. It is essential to examine the action of a compound over a physiologically relevant concentration range. For example, if compound X is present *in vivo* at concentrations <1 mM, its ability to inhibit lipid peroxidation only at concentrations >20 mM is irrelevant unless there is good reason to suspect that it concentrates at a particular site *in vivo*. One must also bear in mind that, if acting as a scavenger, an 'antioxidant' may itself give rise to damaging radical species.

Scavenging of superoxide

Superoxide is easily produced by radiolysis of water in the presence of O_2 and formate ions. Pulse radiolysis allows examination of the spectrum of any products formed when $O_2^{\bullet-}$ reacts with a putative antioxidant [162]. However, pulse radiolysis is unsuitable for measuring most reactions of $O_2^{\bullet-}$ in aqueous solution, since the reaction rates are usually lower than the overall rate of non-enzymic dismutation of $O_2^{\bullet-}$. This limits measurements of rate constants to those of $10^5 \, M^{-1} \cdot s^{-1}$ or greater. Unfortunately, the rate constants for the reaction of $O_2^{\bullet-}$ with most biological molecules, except ascorbate [163], $NO^{\bullet}$ [49] and SOD, are less than this. Stopped-flow methods can be used to study these slower reactions (e.g. [164]). However, provided that suitable control experiments are done, good approximations to rate constants may be achieved using simple test-tube systems. Thus a mixture of hypoxanthine and xanthine oxidase at pH 7.4 generates $O_2^{\bullet-}$ [165] which reacts with cytochrome *c* and Nitro-Blue tetrazolium (NBT) with defined rate constants, namely 2.6×10^5 and $6 \times 10^4 \, M^{-1} \cdot s^{-1}$ respectively. Any added molecule capable of reacting with $O_2^{\bullet-}$ will decrease the rates of cytochrome *c* or NBT reduction, and analysis of the inhibition produced allows calculation of an approximate rate constant [166]. This simple method has been used in attempts to establish rate constants for the reactions of desferrioxamine [166], taurine [167], carnosine [168], lipoic acid [169] and *N*-acetylcysteine [35] with $O_2^{\cdot-}$. It should be noted that the method cannot distinguish between a reaction of the added compound with $O_2^{\cdot-}$ or a much faster reaction with the small amount of $HO_2^{\cdot}$ in equilibrium with $O_2^{\cdot-}$ at pH 7.4 [35]. The potassium salt of superoxide ($K^+O_2^{\cdot-}$) is available commercially and may be used as an alternative source of $O_2^{\cdot-}$ [164,170].

Some controls are essential in using these simple 'test-tube' methods to investigate scavenging of $O_2^{\cdot-}$, particularly in systems using xanthine oxidase.

(i) It must be checked that the substance under test does not inhibit $O_2^{\cdot-}$ generation, e.g. by inhibiting xanthine oxidase. This can be checked by measuring uric acid formation (using HPLC, or spectrophotometrically).

(ii) It must be checked that the substance does not itself reduce cytochrome *c* or NBT. This is a particular problem with cytochrome *c*, which is easily reduced (e.g. by ascorbic acid and by thiols at high concentrations), especially at alkaline pH. My experience is that it is less of a problem with NBT, provided that pH values of 7.4 or less are used.

(iii) One must consider the possibility that a radical formed by attack of $O_2^{\cdot-}$ on a substance could itself reduce cytochrome *c* or NBT. This will be revealed as deviations from linear competition kinetics at high scavenger concentrations. Thus the nitroxide radical formed when $O_2^{\cdot-}$ reacts with desferrioxamine [171] can probably reduce cytochrome *c*.

Hydrogen peroxide

H_2O_2 is easily and sensitively measured by using peroxidase-based assay systems. The most common employs horseradish peroxidase, which uses H_2O_2 to oxidize scopoletin into a non-fluorescent product [172,173]. Thus if a putative scavenger is incubated with H_2O_2 and the reaction mixture sampled for analysis of H_2O_2 at various times, rates of loss of H_2O_2 can be measured to allow calculation of rate constants. The essential control is to check that the substance being tested is not itself a substrate for peroxidase, which could compete with scopoletin and cause an artefactual inhibition. Thus ascorbic acid and thiol compounds can be oxidized by horseradish peroxidase; hence they can often interfere seriously with peroxidase-based assay systems. In order to check if a substance might be oxidized by peroxidase, one should look for changes in the absorption spectrum when the compound is added to a peroxidase–H_2O_2 mixture: radicals derived by peroxidase-dependent oxidations often have spectra very different from those of the parent compounds, and there will be spectral changes in the peroxidase itself if it is oxidizing the compound under test. Superoxide radical can inactivate peroxidase (forming compound III) and may compromise measurement of H_2O_2 in systems generating $O_2^{\cdot-}$. This can be avoided by addition of SOD [174].

If the compound does interfere with peroxidase-based systems, other assays for H_2O_2 can be used. Thus H_2O_2 can be estimated by simple titration with acidified potassium permanganate or by measuring the O_2 release (1 mol of O_2 per 2 mol of H_2O_2) when a sample of the reaction mixture is injected into an O_2 electrode containing buffer and a large amount of catalase [1]. Varma [175] has described a sensitive radiochemical assay for H_2O_2, based on its ability to decarboxylate ^{14}C-labelled 2-oxoglutarate to $^{14}CO_2$ (measured by scintillation counting). However, this assay produces unexpectedly large H_2O_2 concentrations in urine and other human body fluids and so many scientists are sceptical of it. Electrodes that detect H_2O_2 have been described (e.g. [176]), although they are subject to interference.

Hydroxyl radical: the deoxyribose assay

The definitive technique for measuring the rate constant for reaction of a substance with ·OH, and for studying the products of that reaction, is pulse radiolysis [162]. Most compounds react with ·OH with rate constants of 10^9–10^{10} $M^{-1} \cdot s^{-1}$.

If pulse radiolysis facilities are not available, approximate rate constants can often be calculated using the 'deoxyribose method'. Hydroxyl radicals are generated by a mixture of ascorbic acid, H_2O_2 and Fe^{3+}-EDTA. Those radicals not scavenged by other components of the reaction mixture attack the sugar deoxyribose, degrading it into a series of fragments, some or all of which react on heating with thiobarbituric acid (TBA) at low pH to give a pink chromogen [177] which is an adduct of TBA with malondialdehyde [178]. If a scavenger of ·OH is added to the reaction mixture, it will compete with deoxyribose for the ·OH radicals and inhibit deoxyribose degradation, to an extent depending on the scavenger's concentration and on its rate constant for reaction with ·OH. Competition plots allow this rate constant to be calculated, assuming that deoxyribose reacts with ·OH with a rate constant of 3.1×10^9 $M^{-1} \cdot s^{-1}$ [179].

The deoxyribose assay works well with most substances. Essential controls include checking that (i) the substance does not react rapidly with H_2O_2, which could block ·OH formation. This has rarely been a problem because H_2O_2 is poorly reactive. (ii) The substance is not a powerful iron chelator, capable of removing iron ions from EDTA. Again, this is rarely a problem. (iii) Attack of ·OH upon the substance does not produce TBA-reactive material. A control should be performed in which deoxyribose is omitted from the reaction mixture. (iv) The substance does not interfere with measurement of deoxyribose degradation products. This can be checked by showing that it does not inhibit when added to the reaction mixture at the end of the incubation, with the TBA and acid.

Inhibition of metal ion-dependent hydroxyl radical formation

As argued previously, direct scavenging of ·OH is a generally unlikely mode of antioxidant action *in vivo*, simply because very high concentrations of scavenger are required to compete with biological molecules for any ·OH generated. It is therefore of interest to examine the ability of a putative antioxidant to chelate metal ions in such a way that it interferes with metal ion-dependent generation of ·OH, particularly that involving iron ions bound to a target ('site-specific' Fenton chemistry). The deoxyribose method affords a way of doing this also. When iron ions are added to the reaction mixture as $FeCl_3$ (not chelated to EDTA), some of them bind to deoxyribose [180,181]. The bound iron ions still participate in Fenton chemistry, but any ·OH radicals formed immediately attack the sugar and are not released into free solution [182]. Hydroxyl radical scavengers, at moderate concentrations, do not inhibit this deoxyribose degradation because they cannot compete with the deoxyribose for ·OH generated by bound iron ions [182]. The only substances that do inhibit in this assay are those that bind iron ions strongly enough to remove them from the deoxyribose [55,182]. Hence this assay [subject to controls (i), (iii) and (iv) above] indicates the potential ability of a compound to interfere with 'site-specific' generation of ˙OH radicals catalysed by bound iron ions. Indeed, the assay has been used to evaluate the abilities of anti-inflammatory drugs [55], taurine and its precursors [167] and carnosine, homocarnosine or anserine [168] to act in this way.

It must be emphasized that this version of the deoxyribose assay measures a combination of two factors: the ability to remove iron ions from deoxyribose and to render those iron ions inactive or poorly active in generating ˙OH. Thus EDTA removes iron ions from deoxyribose, but iron-EDTA chelates are very effective in generating ˙OH (for reasons discussed in [183]) so that the deoxyribose is still degraded — this time by ˙OH in 'free solution', rather than by ˙OH formed upon the deoxyribose molecule.

If a compound inhibits site-specific radical damage to deoxyribose by chelating iron ions and rendering them less active in producing ˙OH, two possibilities can account for the latter property. First, the inhibitor–metal ion complex may be incapable of reacting with $O_2^{˙-}$ or H_2O_2, so blocking ˙OH formation. Secondly, it may be that the inhibitor–metal ion complex still undergoes redox reactions, but that the ˙OH is largely intercepted by the inhibitor and is not allowed to escape into free solution, i.e. damage is directed on to the inhibitor and away from the deoxyribose. To distinguish between these mechanisms, one can examine the fate of the inhibitor in the reaction mixture. For example, HPLC analysis should show whether or not the inhibitor is undergoing degradation as the reaction proceeds. An example may be found in ref. [184].

To summarize, the deoxyribose method performed in the absence of EDTA represents an approximate, but simple, test of the ability of a compound to interfere with iron ion-dependent site-specific Fenton chemistry.

Water-soluble peroxyl radicals

To what extent water-soluble peroxyl radicals contribute to oxidative damage *in vivo* is uncertain, since they react quickly with ascorbic acid [185]. Indeed, a recent study of the reactivity of peroxyl radicals produced as a result of attack of ˙OH on several anti-inflammatory drugs in the presence of O_2 suggested that such radicals are, in general, of limited reactivity [79]. However, damage to biological targets by several such radicals has been demonstrated [79,185,186] and a complete 'screen' of antioxidant ability should therefore include an assessment of the capacity of a putative antioxidant to scavenge peroxyl radicals. How can this be done? Peroxyl radicals derived from anti-inflammatory drugs can easily be generated by pulse radiolysis under appropriate conditions, and their scavenging by antioxidants studied [185,186]. The ability of antioxidants to scavenge electron spin resonance (ESR)-detectable peroxyl radicals is an additional approach [187].

Another method of examining peroxyl radical scavenging is the TRAP assay, introduced by Ingold and colleagues [188,189] and much used (in this or adapted versions) in studies of antioxidants in body fluids (e.g. refs. [188–192]). Peroxyl radicals are generated at a controlled rate by the thermal decomposition of a water-soluble 'azo initiator', such as 2,2′-azo*bis*(2-amidinopropane)-dihydrochloride (AAPH). They are allowed to react with a lipid, whereupon they cause peroxidation. Thus by analysing the effect of a water-soluble antioxidant on the rate of peroxidation, a relative rate for its reaction with peroxyl radicals can be measured [193]. A suspension of linoleic acid, or an ester of it, is frequently used as lipid substrate. Studies of the ability to protect linoleic acid or other lipids against peroxidation by AAPH-derived radicals have been used to show, for example, that ascorbic acid is an excellent scavenger of water-soluble peroxyl radicals [188–191] whereas desferrioxamine is a much poorer scavenger [193].

Lipid-soluble peroxyl radicals

It has often proved difficult to generate 'clean' lipid-soluble peroxyl radicals *in vitro*. One exception is trichloromethylperoxyl [194,195], formed by exposing a mixture of carbon tetrachloride (CCl_4), propan-2-ol and buffer to ionizing radiation, so producing hydrated electrons ($e_{aq.}^-$) and $^{\cdot}OH$

$$e_{aq.}^- + CCl_4 \rightarrow {^{\cdot}CCl_3} + Cl^- \tag{5}$$

$$^{\cdot}OH + CH_3CHOHCH_3 \rightarrow H_2O + CH_3\dot{C}OHCH_3 \tag{6}$$

$$CH_3\dot{C}OHCH_3 + CCl_4 \rightarrow CH_3COCH_3 + \dot{C}Cl_3 + H^+ \tag{7}$$

$$^{\cdot}CCl_3 + O_2 \rightarrow CCl_3O_2^{\cdot} \tag{8}$$

Rate constants for the reaction of several known and putative antioxidants with $CCl_3O_2^{\cdot}$ have been published [196] (Table 3 gives some examples). However

Table 3. Second-order rate constants for reaction of various compounds with trichloromethylperoxyl radicals. Results are means of three or more determinations that varied by $\leq 5\%$.

Compound	Rate constant ($M^{-1} \cdot s^{-1}$)
Ascorbic acid	1.2×10^8
Carnosol	$(1–3) \times 10^6$
Haloperidol	No reaction detected
Quercetin	3.9×10^7
Myricetin	4.0×10^7
Morin	3.0×10^8
Fisetin	4.1×10^8
Butylated hydroxyanisole	3.0×10^7
α-Tocopherol	4.9×10^8
Prochlorperazine	4.0×10^8
Promethazine	3.0×10^8
Chlorpromazine	3.0×10^8
Methotrimeprazine	4.0×10^8
Propyl gallate	1.7×10^7
Trolox C	2.2×10^8

Data from ref. [196].

CCl_3O_2· may be somewhat more reactive than non-halogenated peroxyl radicals [194,195], and so the results should not be taken as indicative of reactions for other peroxyl radicals that can be generated *in vivo*.

Studies of lipid peroxidation

Peroxyl radicals are the major chain-propagating species in the process of lipid peroxidation in membranes [1]. Thus a direct test of antioxidant ability is to examine the ability of a substance to inhibit peroxidation of membranes such as erythrocytes, tissue homogenates [197], liposomes [198] or microsomes [199]. Although such studies are widely performed, several points must be considered in interpreting them. First, the lipid systems are usually maintained under ambient partial pressure of O_2, although some putative antioxidants (e.g. β-carotene) work better at lower O_2 concentrations [13]. Variable results may arise because rapid peroxidation often depletes O_2 in the reaction mixture.

Secondly, how should peroxidation be measured? O_2 uptake is one possibility (reviewed in [1]). The TBA test is widely used and works well in liposomal and microsomal systems [198,199]. However, it is essential to ensure that the apparent antioxidant effect of an added compound is not due to interference with the TBA test itself. Table 4 shows why this control is necessary: much of the apparent antioxidant effect of carnosine and anserine in inhibiting microsomal lipid peroxidation is still seen when these compounds are added with the TBA and acid, i.e. they are interfering with the assay [168]. Detailed reviews of methods for measuring lipid peroxidation in biological material have been published [1,200–202] so I will not dwell on these points here.

The third major point to consider is how peroxidation of the lipid substrate can be started. If a water-soluble azo initiator such as AAPH is used, it will be difficult to distinguish whether an antioxidant acts by direct scavenging of the AAPH-derived peroxyl radicals, or by scavenging of the lipid peroxyl radicals within the lipid substrate. This problem is not overcome by treating the membrane with a lipid-soluble azo initiator such as 2,2'-azo*bis*(2,4-dimethylvaleronitrile) (AMVN). Although the hydrophobic AMVN decomposes within the membrane interior to form peroxyl radicals, it is still difficult to distinguish whether an antioxidant that has entered the membrane is acting by scavenging the AMVN-derived radicals, or the (more biologically important) peroxyl radicals arising from the fatty acid side-chains within the membrane.

Peroxidation can also be accelerated by adding iron salts to membranes [199,203], e.g. as Fe^{2+}, $FeCl_3$ plus ascorbate or $FeCl_3$-ADP plus NADPH (in the case of microsomes). In metal ion-dependent systems, an added antioxidant might act not only by scavenging peroxyl radicals but also by binding iron ions and stopping them from accelerating peroxidation. However, these two possibilities can be distinguished. If the antioxidant is acting by metal binding, it will not be consumed during the reaction, as can be shown by direct analysis (e.g. by HPLC). A chain-breaking antioxidant is consumed as it reacts with peroxyl radicals in the membrane. Chain-breaking antioxidants at low concentrations often introduce a lag period into the peroxidation process, corresponding to the time taken for the antioxidant to be consumed, whereas metal-binding antioxidants would be expected to give a constant inhibition through the reaction.

Table 4. Action of the putative antioxidants anserine and carnosine on lipid peroxidation: interference with the TBA assay. Peroxidation of rat-liver microsomes was studied, using a standard TBA test as described in [168]. Desferrioxamine exerted its inhibitory effect during the incubation: when added with the TBA reagents it had little effect. By contrast, much of the apparent inhibition of lipid peroxidation by carnosine and anserine is due to interference with the TBA test. Results abstracted from [168].

Peroxidation stimulated by adding	Extent of peroxidation (A_{532})	12 mM Carnosine		12 mM Anserine		0.2 mM Desferrioxamine	
		Added at start of expt.	Added during TBA assay only	Added at start of expt.	Added during TBA assay only	Added at start start of expt.	Added during TBA assay only
Fe^{3+}/ascorbate	1.18 (100%)	75	61	80	53	84	7
Fe^{3+}-ADP/NADPH	1.22 (100%)	79	54	81	40	80	0
Fe^{3+}	1.05 (100%)	66	58	54	50	75	5
Fe^{3+}-ADP	1.13 (100%)	69	56	62	48	75	13

Inhibition by antioxidant added (%)

Much lipid peroxidation *in vivo* is probably metal ion-dependent, often involving iron and sometimes, as in the case of lipoproteins, copper. I therefore feel that the most biologically relevant evaluation of ability to inhibit lipid peroxidation is achieved by testing a putative antioxidant against metal ion-stimulated lipid peroxidation in liposomes, lipoproteins, microsomes or other biological membranes, paying particular attention to possible artefacts in the assay methods used and to checking what is actually happening to the antioxidant in the reaction mixture.

Microsomal peroxidation assays

Microsomal fractions will already contain variable amounts of endogenous antioxidants, such as α-tocopherol [199] and some added antioxidants might not act directly, but by 'recycling' endogeneous antioxidants (e.g. ref. [204]). For example, dihydrolipoate had no inhibitory effect on iron/ascorbate-dependent peroxidation in liposomes (in fact, it accelerated peroxidation somewhat [169]), but it could recycle vitamin E radical in microsomes [205]. If microsomal lipid peroxidation is started by adding NADPH plus Fe^{3+}-ADP to the microsomes [203], a control should also be performed to check that an added compound does not inhibit enzymic reduction of the iron complex. This is usually done by measuring consumption of NADPH. Addition of NADPH to microsomes also activates the cytochrome *P*-450 system, which is capable of metabolizing certain antioxidants. For example, the observed inhibitory effect of chlorpromazine on NADPH-dependent peroxidation of microsomes was claimed to be due to its conversion into antioxidant hydroxylated derivatives by microsomal mixed-function oxidases [206].

Peroxidation may also be started by adding Fe^{3+}/ascorbate mixtures to microsomes or liposomes. For microsomes, this avoids problems with the mixed function oxidase system, but it should be noted that ascorbate may well be capable of chemically reducing lipid-soluble radicals (derived by reaction of the antioxidant with peroxyl radicals), back to the antioxidant molecule, so facilitating antioxidant action. Such a reaction will only occur, of course, if the antioxidant-derived radicals become accessible for reduction at the membrane surface, as has been shown to be the case for α-tocopheryl radicals in membranes, and in LDLs isolated from human plasma [87,204,205,207]. Thus it is possible that the antioxidant activity of some lipid-soluble chain-breaking antioxidants might appear to be greater in systems containing ascorbic acid, as has been observed with some plant phenolics [99]. Hence it is wise to compare antioxidant ability using peroxidation started by several different mechanisms. This is particularly important when using isolated lipoproteins. The importance of checking that an antioxidant in lipid systems does not exert pro-oxidant effects in non-lipid systems has already been stressed.

Phagocyte-derived ROS

Methods for isolating phagocytic cells and measuring their production of $O_2^{\cdot-}$ and H_2O_2 are well described in the literature (e.g. refs. [100,107]). Standard methods [38,107] can be used to check the ability of compounds to interfere with phagocyte ROS production after triggering the respiratory burst. It is essential to ensure that compounds do not interfere with the methods used to measure ROS production, e.g. by directly reducing cytochrome c or by interfering with peroxidase-based measurement of H_2O_2 (see previous sections). The concentrations of compounds tested must also be comparable with those present *in vivo*.

Hypochlorous acid scavenging assays

Compounds can also be tested for their potential to interfere with tissue damage by HOCl, which could be achieved by scavenging HOCl and/or by inhibiting its production by myeloperoxidase. Myeloperoxidase can be assayed in several ways including standard tests of peroxidase activity [1] (e.g. its ability to oxidize guaiacol to a chromogen in the presence of H_2O_2 [208]) or by specific measurements of HOCl production using monochlorodimedon (discussed in [209]). Often the former type of assay is easier to use in looking for inhibition, since the latter type of assay is prone to interference if compounds that can also act as HOCl scavengers are tested. If an apparent inhibition of myeloperoxidase is found, it should be checked whether the compound is really inhibiting myeloperoxidase or is simply acting as a competing substrate (perhaps being oxidized to damaging products).

If it has been established that a compound does not inhibit myeloperoxidase directly, then scavenging of HOCl can be examined using myeloperoxidase/H_2O_2/Cl^- as a source of this substance. More simply, HOCl can be made as required by acidifying commercial sodium hypochlorite (Na^+OCl^-) to pH 6.2 and using its molar absorption coefficient at 235 nm to calculate its concentration [210]. Thus a concentration of the putative antioxidant that is achievable *in vivo* can be mixed with α_1-antiproteinase, a protein that is highly susceptible to attack by HOCl. A good scavenger of HOCl should protect α_1-antiproteinase against inactivation when HOCl is added subsequently. Such a method has been used to show that 5-aminosalicylate [117], *N*-acetylcysteine [35], ascorbic acid [113], lipoic and dihydrolipoic acids [169,211], some anti-inflammatory drugs [117], bile pigments [114], hypotaurine [167], mercaptopropionylglycine [212] and tetracycline [213] could conceivably act as scavengers of HOCl *in vivo*. This is not, of course, proof that they actually do scavenge HOCl *in vivo*. A series of controls is necessary, to show that the substance under test does not: (i) itself inactivate elastase; (ii) interfere with the ability of α_1-antiproteinase to inactivate elastase; or (iii) re-activate α_1-antiproteinase that has been inactivated by HOCl.

If a substance fails to protect α_1-antiproteinase against inactivation by HOCl in this assay system, there are two possible explanations. First, its reaction with HOCl may be too slow, or non-existent. Secondly, its reaction with HOCl may form a 'long-lived' oxidant that is also capable of inactivating α_1-antiproteinase [214]. Taurine has been shown to do this and the possibility must always be considered for other compounds [214,215]. The spectra of various chloramines have been published [214] and it is also of interest to see if putative antioxidants can scavenge such products.

Singlet oxygen

Singlet O_2 can be easily generated by photosensitization reactions, but it is important to ensure that any damage caused to a biological molecule in such systems is due to singlet O_2 rather than by direct interaction with the excited state of the sensitizer or by reactions involving other oxidants, such as $O_2^{\cdot-}$ and $^{\cdot}OH$, that can sometimes be generated in illuminated pigment-containing systems [1]. A technique has been described [216] in which singlet O_2 is generated by an immobilized sensitizer and allowed to diffuse a short distance to react with the target molecule. This system has proved to be useful for studying biological damage produced by singlet O_2 [217] and it should be easily applicable to studies of quenching and scavenging activity. Singlet O_2 can also be generated by the thermal decomposition of endoperoxides, such as 3,3'-(1,4-naphthylidene)dipropanoate [88] and such sources have been used to examine the reactions of singlet O_2 with human plasma [218].

Haem proteins/peroxides

Mixtures of H_2O_2 and haemoglobin or myoglobin stimulate peroxidation of fatty acids and of microsomes, apparently by the action of both amino acid radicals and haem-associated ferryl species. The ability of a substance to react with activated haem proteins can be examined spectrophotometrically, by looking for loss of the ferryl myoglobin (or haemoglobin) spectrum as the compound reduces it to the ferrous or ferric state [141–146,219]. A good 'quencher' of ferryl, such as ascorbate, will inhibit ferryl-dependent peroxidation of fatty acids or membrane lipids [141–146,219]. In using this assay it is essential to check that the compound does not act as a chain-breaking antioxidant as well.

Exposure of haem proteins to a large molar excess of H_2O_2 causes haem breakdown and iron ion release [135–137]. Some antioxidants, such as ascorbic acid, prevent this process by reducing the ferryl species. The ability to inhibit release of iron ions provides an additional assay method for testing the effect of putative antioxidants on haem protein–H_2O_2 systems.

Peroxynitrite

Peroxynitrite (eqn. 1) can be simply prepared (reviewed in [50]) and its reaction with biological molecules investigated. Careful control of pH is essential and the effects produced depend on the bicarbonate content of the system [50,220]. The effects of addition of peroxynitrite to human plasma have recently been described [220].

Proving that a putative antioxidant is important *in vivo*

The battery of tests outlined above enables one to examine the possibility that a given compound could act as a direct antioxidant in one or more ways *in vivo*. The tests may clearly show that an antioxidant role is unlikely. Alternatively, they could show that an antioxidant action is feasible, in that the compound shows protective action at concentrations within the range present *in vivo*. In the latter case, how then can one prove that the compound actually does act as an antioxidant *in vivo*?

In some cases involving naturally occurring antioxidants, it has been possible to remove the compound and look for increased oxidative damage. Thus mutants of *Escherichia coli*, genetically engineered to lack both MnSOD and FeSOD, show severe damage when grown aerobically [221,222], and damage can be minimized by introducing a gene coding for SOD, even mammalian CuZnSOD [223]. These and other experiments clearly illustrate the physiological antioxidant role of SOD. For antioxidants of dietary origin, the effect of removing them from the diet can sometimes be studied. Thus examination of patients with disorders of intestinal fat absorption has shown that severe deficiency of vitamin E in humans produces neurological symptoms that are consistent with, although certainly not yet proved to be caused by, increased oxidative damage *in vivo* [224].

For most putative antioxidants, such as uric acid, this approach has not been feasible. Evidence consistent with an antioxidant role *in vivo* can then be provided by at least two types of method. First, is the compound depleted under conditions of oxidative stress? Thus ascorbic acid is rapidly oxidized at sites of oxidative stress, e.g. in synovial fluid from the knee-joints of patients with rheumatoid arthritis [225,226]. Presumably ascorbate is acting to scavenge ROS derived from the many activated phagocytes present [226]. Ascorbate is also rapidly oxidized in the plasma of patients with adult respiratory distress syndrome, in which there is often massive infiltration of neutrophils into the lung, where they become activated [227]. However, antioxidant action *in vivo* need not necessarily result in depletion of the antioxidant. Thus the α-tocopheryl radical can be 'repaired' by ascorbic acid as discussed previously.

Secondly, if a compound acts as a radical scavenger, it might be degraded to form specific products whose concentrations increase during oxidant stress and can be measured. Thus oxidation of uric acid by ˙OH, HOCl or ferryl species produces a range of products, including allantoin, cyanuric acid and parabanic acid [228]. Increased allantoin concentrations have been detected in the plasma of patients with rheumatoid arthritis [229], a disease in which formation of ROS *in vivo* is known to be increased [1]. This perhaps suggests that uric acid is exerting at least some scavenging activity *in vivo*.

As far as the ability of administered 'foreign' compounds (such as drugs) to act as antioxidants *in vivo* is concerned, specific assays are now becoming available to measure rates of damage to protein, DNA and lipid due to oxidative attack *in vivo* (see above). The steady-state and total body oxidative damage can now be approximated, which gives the nutritionist a tool to examine the effects of putative antioxidants, both synthetic and derived from the diet, on oxidative damage in the human body.

References

1. Halliwell, B. and Gutteridge, J.M.C. (1989) Free Radicals in Biology and Medicine, 2nd edn., Clarendon Press, Oxford, U.K.
2. Halliwell, B. (1990) Free Radical Res. Commun. 9, 1–32
3. Halliwell, B. and Gutteridge, J.M.C. (1990) Arch. Biochem. Biophys. 280, 1–8
4. Gutteridge, J.M.C. and Quinlan, G.J. (1992) Biochim. Biophys. Acta 1159, 248–254
5. Halliwell, B., Hu, M.L., Louie, S., Duvall, T.R., Tarkington, B.R., Motchnik, P. and Cross, C.E. (1992) FEBS Lett. 313, 62–66

6. Hu, M.L., Louie, S., Cross, C.E., Motchnik, P. and Halliwell, B. (1992) J. Lab. Clin. Med. **121**, 257–262

7. Frei, B., Forte, T.M., Ames, B.N. and Cross, C.E. (1991) Biochem. J. **277**, 133–138

8. Reznick, A.Z., Cross, C.E., Hu, M., Suzuki, Y.J., Khwaja, S., Safadi, A., Motchnik, P.A., Packer, L. and Halliwell, B. (1992) Biochem. J. **286**, 607–611

9. Wiseman, H. and Halliwell, B. (1993) FEBS Lett. **322**, 159–163

10. Halliwell, B. (1988) Biochem. Pharmacol. **37**, 569–571

11. Scott, G. (1988) Free Radical Res. Commun. **5**, 141–147

12. Daniels, V. (1988) Free Radical Res. Commun. **5**, 213–220

13. Burton, G.W. and Ingold, K.U. (1984) Science **224**, 569–573

14. Thornalley, P.J. and Vasak, M. (1985) Biochim. Biophys. Acta, **827**, 36–44

15. Boldyrev, A.A., Dupin, A.M., Bunin, A.Y., Babizhaev, M.A. and Severin, S.E. (1987) Biochem. Int. **15**, 1105–1113

16. Cross, C.E., Halliwell, B. and Allen, A. (1984) Lancet **i**, 1328–1330

17. Graf, E. (1983) J. Am. Oil Chem. Soc. **60**, 1861–1867

18. Banks, M.A., Martin, W.G., Pailes, W.H. and Castranova, V. (1989) J. Appl. Physiol. **66**, 1079–1086

19. Wright, C.E., Tallan, H.H., Lin, Y.Y. and Gaull, G.E. (1989) Annu. Rev. Biochem. **55**, 427–453

20. Schurr, A. and Rigor, B.M. (1987) FEBS Lett. **224**, 4–8

21. Stocker, R., Glazer, A.N. and Ames, B.N. (1987) Proc. Natl. Acad. Sci. U.S.A. **84**, 5918–5922

22. Ames, B.N., Cathcart, R., Schwiers, E. and Hochstein, P. (1981) Proc. Natl. Acad. Sci. U.S.A. **78**, 6858–6862

23. Sugioka, K., Shimosegawa, Y. and Nakano, M. (1987) FEBS Lett. **210**, 37–39

24. Glazer, A.N. (1988) FASEB J. **2**, 2487–2491

25. Hartman, P.E. (1990) Methods Enzymol. **186**, 310–318

26. Suzuki, Y.J., Tsuchiya, Y. and Packer, L. (1991) Free Radical Res. Commun. **15**, 255–263

27. Holler, T.P. and Hopkins, P.B. (1988) J. Am. Chem. Soc. **110**, 4837–4838

28. Landi, L., Cabrini, L., Sechi, A.M. and Pasquali, P. (1984) Biochem. J. **222**, 463–466

29. Tadolini, B. (1988) Biochem. J. **249**, 33–36

30. D'Aquino, M., Dunster, C. and Willson, R.L. (1989) Biochem. Biophys. Res. Commun. **161**, 1199–1203

31. Ratty, A.K. and Das, N.P. (1988) Biochem. Med. Metab. Biol. **39**, 69–79

32. Tan, D.X., Chen, L.D., Poeggeler, B., Manchester, L.C. and Reiter, R.J. (1993) Endocr. J. **1**, 57–60

33. Halliwell, B., Hoult, J.R.S. and Blake, D.R. (1988) FASEB J. **2**, 2867–2873

34. Halliwell, B. (1989) Free Radical Biol. Med. **7**, 645–651

35. Aruoma, O.I., Halliwell, B., Hoey, B.M. and Butler, J. (1989) Free Radical Biol. Med. **6**, 593–597

36. Fridovich, I. (1983) Annu. Rev. Pharmacol. Toxicol. **23**, 239–257

37. Aruoma, O.I. and Halliwell, B. (1987) Biochem. J. **241**, 273–278

38. Curnutte, J.T. and Babior, B.M. (1987) Adv. Human Genet. **6**, 229–297

39. Chance, B., Sies, H. and Boveris, A. (1979) Physiol. Rev. **59**, 527–605

40. Flint, D.H., Tuminello, J.F. and Emptage, M.H. (1993) J. Biol. Chem. **268**, 22369–22376
41. Bielski, B.H.J. (1985) J. Phys. Chem. Ref. Data **14**, 1041–1100
42. Wefers, H. and Sies, H. (1983) Eur. J. Biochem. **137**, 29–36
43. Schoneich, C., Asmus, K.D., Dillinger, U. and Bruchhausen, Fv. (1989) Biochem. Biophys. Res. Commun. **161**, 113–120
44. Halliwell, B. and Gutteridge, J.M.C. (1990) Methods Enzymol. **186**, 1–85
45. Sutton, H.C. and Winterbourn, C.C. (1989) Free Radical Biol. Med. **6**, 53–60
46. Masarwa, M., Cohen, H., Meyerstein, D., Hickman, D.L., Bakac, A. and Espenson, J.H. (1988) J. Am. Chem. Soc. **110**, 4293–4297
47. Aruoma, O.I., Halliwell, B., Gajewski, E. and Dizdaroglu, M. (1991) Biochem. J. **273**, 601–604
48. von Sonntag, C. (1987) The Chemical Basis of Radiation Biology, Taylor and Francis, London
49. Huie, R.E. and Padmaja, S. (1993) Free Radical Res. Commun. **18**, 195–199
50. Beckman, J.S., Chen, J., Ischiropoulos, H. and Crow, J.P. (1994) Methods Enzymol. **233**, 229–240
51. van der Vliet, A., O'Neill, C.A., Halliwell, B., Cross, C.E. and Kaur, H. (1994) FEBS Lett. **339**, 89–92
52. Candeias, L.P., Patel, K.B., Stratford, M.R.L. and Wardman, P. (1993) FEBS Lett. **333**, 151–153
53. Anbar, M. and Neta, P. (1967) Int. J. Appl. Rad. Isotopes **18**, 495–523
54. Smith, C.A., Halliwell, B. and Aruoma, O.I. (1993) Food Chem. Toxicol. **30**, 483–489
55. Aruoma, O.I. and Halliwell, B. (1988) Xenobiotica **18**, 459–470
56. Grootveld, M. and Halliwell, B. (1988) Biochem. J. **237**, 499–504
57. Gutteridge, J.M.C. and Stocks, J. (1981) CRC Crit. Rev. Clin. Lab. Sci. **14**, 257–329
58. Ehrenwald, E., Chisholm, G.M. and Fox, P.L. (1994) J. Clin. Invest. **93**, 1493–1501
59. Marx, G. and Chevion, M. (1986) Biochem. J. **236**, 397–400
60. Larramendy, M., Mello-Filho, A.C., Leme Martins, E.A. and Meneghini, R. (1987) Mutat. Res. **178**, 57–63
61. Hebbel, R.P. (1988) Clin. Haematol. **14**, 129–140
62. Imlay, J.A. and Linn, S. (1988) Science **240**, 1302–1309
63. Dizdaroglu, M., Nackerdien, Z., Chao, B.C., Gajewski, E. and Rao, G. (1991) Arch. Biochem. Biophys. **285**, 388–390
64. Hochstein, P., Sree Kumar, K. and Forman, S.J. (1980) Ann. N.Y. Acad. Sci. **355**, 240–248
65. Gutteridge, J.M.C. and Wilkins, S. (1983) Biochim. Biophys. Acta **759**, 38–41
66. Rowley, D.A. and Halliwell, B. (1983) Arch. Biochem. Biophys. **225**, 279–284
67. Uchida, K. and Kawakishi, S. (1986) Biochem. Biophys. Res. Commun. **138**, 659–665
68. Kohn, R., Yamamoto, Y., Cundy, K.C. and Ames, B.N. (1988) Proc. Natl. Acad. Sci. U.S.A. **85**, 3175–3179
69. Gardner, H.W. (1989) Free Radical Biol. Med. **7**, 65–86
70. Halliwell, B. and Aruoma, O.I. (eds.) (1993) DNA and Free Radicals, Ellis-

Horwood, Chichester
71. Steenken, S. (1989) Chem. Rev. **89**, 503–520
72. Whitburn, K.D., Shieh, J.J., Sellers, R.M., Hoffman, M.Z. and Taub, I.A. (1982) J. Biol. Chem. **257**, 1860–1869
73. Nagy, I.Z. and Floyd, R.A. (1984) Biochim. Biophys. Acta **790**, 238–250
74. Davies, M.J., Gilbert, B.C. and Haywood, R.M. (1993) Free Radical Res. Commun. **18**, 353–367
75. Dean, R.T., Gieseg, S. and Davies, M.J. (1993) Trends Biochem. Sci. **18**, 437–441
76. Ambe, K.S. and Tappel, A.L. (1961) J. Food Sci. **26**, 448–451
77. Asmus, K.D. (1987) in Radioprotectors and Anticarcinogens (Slater, T.F., ed.), pp. 23–42, Academic Press, London
78. Sevilla, M.D., Yan, M., Becker, D. and Gillich, S. (1989) Free Radical Res. Commun. **6**, 21–24
79. Aruoma, O.I., Halliwell, B., Butler, J. and Hoey, B.M. (1989) Biochem. Pharmacol. **38**, 4353–4357
80. Fahey, R.C. (1988) Pharmacol. Ther. **39**, 101–108
81. Diplock, A.T. (1985) in Fat-Soluble Vitamins (Diplock, A.T., ed.), pp. 154–224, Heinemann, London
82. Burton, G.W. and Ingold, K.U. (1986) Acc. Chem. Res. **19**, 194–201
83. Noack, H., Kube, U. and Augustin, W. (1994) Free Radical Res. **20**, 375–386
84. Kagan, V., Serbinova, E. and Packer, L. (1990) Biochem. Biophys. Res. Commun. **169**, 351–357
85. Stocker, R., Bowry, V.W. and Frei, B. (1991) Proc. Natl. Acad. Sci. U.S.A. **88**, 1646–1650
86. Frei, B. and Gaziano, J.M. (1993) J. Lipid Res. **34**, 2135–2145
87. Esterbauer, H., Gebicki, J., Puhl, H. and Jürgens, G. (1992) Free Radical Biol. Med. **13**, 341–390
88. Di Maschio, P., Kaiser, S. and Sies, H. (1989) Arch. Biochem. Biophys. **274**, 532–538
89. Vile, G. and Winterbourn, C.C. (1988) FEBS Lett. **238**, 356–357
90. Esterbauer, H., Striegl, G., Puhl, H. and Rotheneder, M. (1989) Free Radical Res. Commun. **6**, 67–75
91. Yamamoto, K. and Niki, E. (1988) Biochim. Biophys. Acta **958**, 19–23
92. Maiorino, M., Zamburtini, A., Roveri, A. and Ursini, F. (1993) FEBS Lett. **330**, 174–176
93. Cillard, J., Cillard, P. and Cormier, J. (1980) J. Am. Oil. Chem. Soc. **57**, 255–261
94. Mukai, K., Morimoto, H., Okauchi, Y. and Nagaoka, S. (1993) Lipids **28**, 753–756
95. Gutteridge, J.M.C. and Xaio-Chang, F. (1981) FEBS Lett. **123**, 71–74
96. Aruoma, O.I., Evans, P.J., Kaur, H., Sutcliffe, L. and Halliwell, B. (1990) Free Radical Res. Commun. **10**, 143–157
97. Ochiai, M., Nagao, M., Wakabayashi, K. and Sugimura, T. (1984) Mutat. Res. **129**, 19–24
98. Srivastava, A.K. and Padmanaban, G. (1987) Biochem. Biophys. Res. Commun. **118**, 1515–1522

99. Laughton, M.J., Halliwell, B., Evans, P.J. and Hoult, J.R.S. (1989) Biochem. Pharmacol. **38**, 2859–2865

100. Hurst, J.K. and Barrette, W.C., Jr. (1989) CRC Crit. Rev. Biochem. Mol. Biol. **24**, 271–328

101. Biemond, P., Swaak, A.J.G., Penders, J.M.A., Beindorff, C.M. and Koster, J.F. (1986) Ann. Rheum. Dis. **45**, 249–255

102. Kaplan, H.B., Edelson, H.S., Korchak, H.M., Given, W.P., Abramson, S. and Weissman, G. (1984) Biochem. Pharmacol. **33**, 371–378

103. Hurst, N.P., French, J.K., Bell, A.L., Nuki, G., O'Donnell, M.L., Betts, W.H. and Cleland, L.G. (1986) Biochem. Pharmacol. **35**, 3083–3089

104. Cross, A.R. (1990) Free Radical Biol. Med. **8**, 71–93

105. Weiss, S.J. (1989) N. Engl. J. Med. **320**, 365–376

106. Mayeno, A.N., Curran, A.J., Roberts, R.L. and Foote, C.S. (1989) J. Biol. Chem. **264**, 5660–5668

107. Sbarra, A.J. and Strauss, R.R. (eds.) (1989) in The Respiratory Burst and its Physiological Significance, Plenum Press, New York

108. Fliss, H. (1988) Mol. Cell. Biochem. **84**, 177–188

109. Albrich, J.M., Gilbaugh III, J.H., Callahan, K.B. and Hurst, J.K. (1989) J. Clin. Invest. **78**, 177–184

110. Clark, R.A., Stone, P.J., El Hag, A., Calore, J.D. and Franzblau, C. (1981) J. Biol. Chem. **256**, 3348–3353

111. van der Vliet, A., Hu, M.L., O'Neill, C.A., Cross, C.E. and Halliwell, B. (1994) J. Lab. Clin. Med. **124**, 701–707

112. Wasil, M., Halliwell, B., Hutchison, D.C.S. and Baum, H. (1987) Biochem. J. **243**, 219–223

113. Halliwell, B., Wasil, M. and Grootveld, M. (1987) FEBS Lett. **213**, 15–18

114. Stocker, R. and Peterhans, E. (1989) Free Radical Res. Commun. **6**, 57–66

115. Olszowska, E., Olszowski, S., Zgliczynski, J.M. and Stelmaszynska, T. (1989) Int. J. Biochem. **21**, 799–805

116. Aruoma, O.I., Wasil, M., Halliwell, B., Hoey, B.M. and Butler, J. (1987) Biochem. Pharmacol. **36**, 3739–3742

117. Wasil, M., Halliwell, B., Moorhouse, C.P., Hutchison, D.C.S. and Baum, H. (1987) Biochem. Pharmacol. **36**, 3847–3850

118. Cuperus, R.A., Muijsers, A.O. and Wever, R. (1985) Arthritis Rheum. **28**, 1228–1233

119. Matheson, N.R. (1982) Biochem. Biophys. Res. Commun. **108**, 259–265

120. Kalyanaraman, B. and Sohnle, P.G. (1985) J. Clin. Invest. **75**, 1618–1622

121. Uetrecht, J.P. (1989) Pharmacol. Rev. **6**, 265–273

122. Svensson, B.E. and Lindvall, S. (1988) Biochem. J. **249**, 521–530

123. Von Ritter, C., Grisham, M.B. and Granger, D.N. (1989) Gastroenterology **96**, 811–816

124. Marquez, L.A. and Dunford, H.B. (1990) J. Biol. Chem. **265**, 6074–6078

125. Hart, B.A.T., Simons, J.M., Knaan-Shanzer, S., Bakker, N.P.M. and Labadie, R.P. (1990) Free Radical Biol. Med. **9**, 127–131

126. Ortiz de Montellano, P.R. (1987) Acc. Chem. Res. **20**, 289–294

127. Whitburn, K.D. (1988) Arch. Biochem. Biophys. **267**, 614–622

128. Aviram, I., Wittenberg, B.A. and Wittenberg, J.B. (1978) J. Biol. Chem. **253**, 5685–5689

129. Petersen, R.L., Symons, M.C.R. and Taiwo, F.A. (1989) J. Chem. Soc. Faraday Trans. I, **85**, 2435–2443

130. Kanner, J., German, J.B. and Kinsella, J.E. (1987) CRC Crit. Rev. Food Sci. Nutr. **25**, 317–364

131. Grisham, M.B. (1985) J. Free Radical Biol. Med. **1**, 227–232

132. Gutteridge, J.M.C. (1987) Biochim. Biophys. Acta **917**, 219–223

133. Rao, S.I., Wilks, A., Hamberg, M. and Ortiz de Montellano, P. (1994) J. Biol. Chem. **269**, 7210–7216

134. Kelman, D.J., De Gray, J.A. and Mason, R.P. (1994) J. Biol. Chem. **269**, 7458–7463

135. Gutteridge, J.M.C. (1986) FEBS Lett. **201**, 291–295

136. Puppo, A. and Halliwell, B. (1988) Biochem. J. **249**, 185–190

137. Puppo, A. and Halliwell, B. (1988) Free Radical Res. Commun. **4**, 415–422

138. Yoshino, S., Blake, D.R., Hewitt, S., Morris, C. and Bacon, P.A. (1985) Ann. Rheum. Dis. **44**, 485–490

139. Mitsos, S.E., Kim, D., Lucchesi, B.R. and Fantone, J.C. (1988) Lab. Invest. **59**, 824–830

140. Galaris, D., Cadenas, E. and Hochstein, P. (1989) Free Radical Biol. Med. **6**, 473–478

141. Radi, R., Turrens, J.F. and Freeman, B.A. (1991) Arch. Biochem. Biophys. **288**, 118–125

142. Evans, P.J., Akanmu, D. and Halliwell, B. (1994) Biochem. Pharmacol. **48**, 2173–2179

143. Kanner, J. and Harel, S. (1985) Arch. Biochem. Biophys. **237**, 314–321

144. Rice-Evans, C., Okunade, G. and Khan, R. (1989) Free Radical Res. Commun. **7**, 45–54

145. Evans, P.J., Cecchini, R. and Halliwell, B. (1992) Biochem. Pharmacol. **44**, 981–984

146. Giulivi, C. and Cadenas, E. (1994) Methods Enzymol. **233**, 189–202

147. Kittridge, K.J. and Willson, R.L. (1984) FEBS Lett. **170**, 162–164

148. Aruoma, O.I. and Halliwell, B. (1989) FEBS Lett. **244**, 76–80

149. Pathak, M.A. (1982) J. Natl. Cancer Inst. **69**, 163–170

150. Epstein, J.H. (1982) J. Natl. Cancer Inst. **69**, 265–268

151. Hall, R.D., Buettner, G.R., Motten, A.G. and Chignell, C.F. (1987) Photochem. Photobiol. **46**, 295–300

152. Hasan, T. and Khan, A.U. (1986) Proc. Natl. Acad. Sci. U.S.A. **85**, 4604–4606

153. Dodge, A.D. and Knox, J.P. (1986) Pest. Sci. **17**, 579–586

154. Mathews-Roth, M.M. (1987) Fed. Proc. Fed. Am. Soc. Exp. Biol. **46**, 1890–1893

155. Kanofsky, J.R. and Sima, P.D. (1993) Photochem. Photobiol. **58**, 335–340

156. Cortese, D.A. and Kinsey, J.H. (1984) Chest **86**, 8–13

157. Goosey, J.D., Zigler, J.S., Jr., Matheson, I.B.C. and Kinoshita, J.H. (1981) Invest. Ophthal. Vis. Sci. **20**, 679–683

158. Arudi, R.L., Bielski, B.H.J. and Allen, A.O. (1984) Photochem. Photobiol. **39**, 703–706

159. Nagano, T. and Fridovich, I. (1985) Photochem. Photobiol. **41**, 33–37

160. Kanofsky, J.R., Wright, J., Miles-Richardson, G.E. and Tauber, A.I. (1984) J. Clin. Invest. **74**, 1489–1495

161. Wefers, H. (1987) Bioelectrochem. Bioenerg. **18**, 91–104

162. Butler, J., Hoey, B.M. and Lea, J.S. (1988) in Free Radicals, Methodology and Concepts (Rice-Evans, C. and Halliwell, B., eds.), pp. 457–479, Richelieu Press, London

163. Nishikimi, M. (1975) Biochem. Biophys. Res. Commun. **63**, 463–468

164. Bull, C., McClune, G.J. and Fee, J.A. (1983) J. Am. Chem. Soc. **105**, 5290–5300

165. McCord, J.M. and Fridovich, I. (1969) J. Biol. Chem. **244**, 6049–6055

166. Halliwell, B. (1985) Biochem. Pharmacol. **34**, 229–233

167. Aruoma, O.I., Halliwell, B., Hoey, B.M. and Butler, J. (1988) Biochem. J. **256**, 251–255

168. Aruoma, O.I., Laughton, M.J. and Halliwell, B. (1989) Biochem. J. **264**, 863–869

169. Scott, B.C., Aruoma, O.I., Evans, P.J., O'Neill, C., van der Vliet, A., Cross, C.E., Tritschler, H. and Halliwell, B. (1994) Free Radical Res. **20**, 119–133

170. Henry, L.E.A., Halliwell, B. and Hall, D.O. (1976) FEBS Lett. **66**, 303–306

171. Davies, M.J., Donkor, R., Dunster, C.A., Gee, C.A., Jonas, S. and Willson, R.L. (1987) Biochem. J. **246**, 725–729

172. Boveris, A., Martino, E. and Stoppani, A.O.M. (1977) Anal. Biochem. **80**, 145–158

173. Corbett, J.T. (1989) J. Biochem. Biophys. Methods **18**, 297–308

174. Kettle, A.J., Carr, A.C. and Winterbourn, C.C. (1994) Free Radical Biol. Med. **17**, 161–164

175. Varma, S.D. (1989) Free Radical Res. Commun. **5**, 359–368

176. Tatsuma, T., Okawa, Y. and Watanabe, T. (1989) Anal. Chem. **61**, 2352–2355

177. Halliwell, B. and Gutteridge, J.M.C. (1981) FEBS Lett. **128**, 347–352

178. Cheeseman, K.H., Beavis, A. and Esterbauer, H. (1988) Biochem. J. **252**, 649–653

179. Halliwell, B., Gutteridge, J.M.C. and Aruoma, O.I. (1987) Anal. Biochem. **165**, 215–219

180. Aruoma, O.I., Grootveld, M. and Halliwell, B. (1987) J. Inorg. Biochem. **29**, 289–299

181. Aruoma, O.I., Chaudhary, S.S., Grootveld, M. and Halliwell, B. (1989) J. Inorg. Biochem. **35**, 149–155

182. Gutteridge, J.M.C. (1984) Biochem. J. **224**, 761–767

183. Grootveld, M. and Halliwell, B. (1986) Free Radical Res. Commun. **1**, 243–250

184. Gutteridge, J.M.C., Zs-Nagy, I., Maidt, L. and Floyd, R.A. (1990) Arch. Biochem. Biophys. **277**, 422–428

185. Willson, R.L. (1985) in Oxidative Stress (Sies, H., ed.), pp. 41–72, Academic Press, London

186. Hiller, K.O., Hodd, P.L. and Willson, R.L. (1983) Chemico-Biol. Int. **47**, 293–305

187. Greenley, T.L. and Davies, M.J. (1992) Biochim. Biophys. Acta **1116**, 192–203

188. Wayner, D.D.M., Burton, C.W. and Ingold, K.U. (1986) Biochim. Biophys. Acta **884**, 119–123

189. Wayner, D.D.M., Burton, G.W., Ingold, K.U., Barclay, L.R.C. and Locke, S.J. (1987) Biochim. Biophys. Acta **924**, 408–419

190. Thurnham, D.I., Situnayake, R.D., Koottathep, S., McConkey, B. and Davis, M. (1987) in Free Radicals, Oxidant Stress and Drug Action (Rice-Evans, C., ed.), pp. 169–192, Richelieu Press, London

191. Frei, B., Stocker, R. and Ames, B.N. (1988) Proc. Natl. Acad. Sci. U.S.A. **85**, 9748–9752

192. Lindeman, J.N.H., Zoeeren-Grobben, D.V., Schriver, J., Speek, A.J., Poorthuis, B.H.J. and Berger, H.M. (1989) Pediat. Res. **26**, 20–24

193. Darley-Usmar, V.M., Hersey, A. and Garland, L.G. (1989) Biochem. Pharmacol. **38**, 1465–1469

194. Lal, M., Schoneich, C., Monig, J. and Asmus, K.D. (1988) Int. J. Radiat. Biol. **54**, 773–779

195. Alfassi, Z.B., Huie, R.E. and Neta, P. (1993) J. Phys. Chem. **97**, 6835–6838

196. Aruoma, O.I., Spencer, J.P.E., Butler, J. and Halliwell, B. (1994) Free Radical Res. **22**, 187–190

197. Stocks, J., Gutteridge, J.M.C., Sharp, R.J. and Dormandy, T.L. (1974) Clin. Sci. Mol. Med. **47**, 215–222

198. Gutteridge, J.M.C. (1977) Anal. Biochem. **82**, 76–82

199. Wills, E.D. (1969) Biochem. J. **113**, 325–332

200. Gutteridge, J.M.C. (1986) Free Radical Res. Commun. **1**, 173–184

201. Halliwell, B. and Chirico, S. (1993) Am. J. Clin. Nutr. **57** (Suppl.), 715S–725S

202. Packer, L. (ed.) (1994) Methods Enzymol. **233**, pages 163, 174, 182, 273, 289, 303, 310, 314, 319, 324, 332, 338, 425

203. Minotti, G. and Aust, S.D. (1987) Chem. Phys. Lipids **44**, 191–208

204. Wefers, H. and Sies, H. (1988) Eur. J. Biochem. **174**, 353–357

205. Scholich, H., Murphy, M.E. and Sies, H. (1989) Biochim. Biophys. Acta **1001**, 256–261

206. Eluashvili, I.A., Pashinova, T.P., Bogdanova, E.D., Kagan, V.E. and Prilipko, L.L. (1977) Byull. Eksp. Biol. Med. **84**, 323–326

207. Liebler, D.C., Kling, D.S. and Reed, D.J. (1986) J. Biol. Chem. **261**, 12114–12119

208. Iwamoto, H., Kobayashi, T., Hasegawa, E. and Morita, Y. (1987) J. Biochem. (Tokyo) **101**, 1407–1412

209. Kettle, A.J. and Winterbourn, C.C. (1988) Biochim. Biophys. Acta **957**, 185–191

210. Green, T.R., Fellman, J.H. and Eicher, A.L. (1985) FEBS Lett. **192**, 33–36

211. Haenen, G.R.M.M. and Bast, A. (1991) Biochem. Pharmacol. **42**, 2246–2249

212. Puppo, A., Cecchini, R., Aruoma, O.I., Bolli, R. and Halliwell, B. (1990) Free Radical Res. Commun. **10**, 371–381

213. Wasil, M., Halliwell, B. and Moorhouse, C.P. (1988) Biochem. Pharmacol. **37**, 775–778

214. Weiss, S.J., Lampert, M.B. and Test, S.T. (1983) Science **222** 625–628

215. Thomas, E.L., Grisham, M.B., Melton, D.F. and Jefferson, M.M. (1985) J. Biol. Chem. **260**, 3321–3329

216. Midden, W.R. and Wang, S.Y. (1983) J. Am. Chem. Soc. **105**, 4129–4135

217. Dahl, T.A., Midden, W.R. and Hartman, P.E. (1988) Mut. Res. **201**, 127–136

218. Wagner, J.R., Motchnik, P.A., Stocker, R., Sies, H. and Ames, B.N. (1993) J. Biol. Chem. **268**, 18502–18506

219. Kanner, J. and Harel, S. (1987) Free Radical Res. Commun. **3**, 309–317

220. van der Vliet, A., Smith, D., O'Neill, C.A., Kaur, H., Darley-Usmar, V., Cross, C.E. and Halliwell, B. (1994) Biochem. J. **303**, 295–301

221. Touati, D. (1989) Free Radical Res. Commun. **8**, 1–9

222. Schellhorn, H. and Hassan, H.M. (1988) Can. J. Microbiol. **34**, 1171–1176

223. Natvig, D.O., Imlay, K., Touati, D. and Hallewell, R.A. (1989) J. Biol. Chem. **262**, 14697–14701

224. Harding, A.E., Matthews, S., Jones, S., Ellis, C.J.K., Booth, I.W. and Muller, D.P.R. (1985) N. Engl. J. Med. **313**, 32–35

225. Lunec, J. and Blake, D.R. (1985) Free Radical Res. Commun. **1**, 31–39

226. Blake, D.R., Hall, N.D., Treby, D.A., Halliwell, B. and Gutteridge, J.M.C. (1981) Clin. Sci. **61**, 483–486

227. Cross, C.E., Forte, T., Stocker, R., Louie, S., Yamamoto, Y., Ames, B.N. and Frei, B. (1990) J. Lab. Clin. Med. **115**, 396–404

228. Kaur, H. and Halliwell, B. (1990) Chem-Biol. Interact. **73**, 235–247

229. Grootveld, M. and Halliwell, B. (1987) Biochem. J. **243**, 803–808

Biochem. Soc. Symp. **61**, 103–116
Printed in Great Britain

Plant polyphenols: free radical scavengers or chain-breaking antioxidants?

Catherine Rice-Evans

Free Radical Research Group, Division of Biochemistry and Molecular Biology, UMDS–Guy's Hospital, St. Thomas Street, London SE1 9RT, U.K.

Abstract

There is increasing interest in the biological effects of tea- and wine-derived polyphenols and many studies *in vitro* and *in vivo* are demonstrating their antioxidant properties. Tea is a major source of dietary polyphenols and an even richer source of the flavanols, the catechins and catechin/gallate esters. Although there are limited studies on the bioavailability of the polyphenols, the absorption of flavanols in humans has been shown. The studies described in this chapter discuss the relative antioxidant potentials of the polyphenolic flavonoids *in vitro* against radicals generated in the aqueous phase in comparison with their relative effectiveness as antioxidants against propagating lipid peroxyl radicals, and how their activity influences that of α-tocopherol in low-density lipoproteins exposed to oxidative stress.

Introduction

There is considerable evidence from chemical, biological, human and epidemiological studies for a role for antioxidant nutrients (vitamins E and C and β-carotene) in the maintenance of health and in contributing to protection from cancer, cataract and cardiovascular disease. One epidemiological study of particular interest is the WHO cross-cultural European epidemiological study showing a highly significant inverse correlation between mortality from ischaemic heart disease and vitamin E levels in the blood (lipid-normalized) with $r^2 = 0.62$ [1,2]. The study also reveals a slope across Europe, with relatively higher blood vitamin E levels and enhanced protection from heart diseases in the population of the countries of Southern Europe and vice versa for Northern Europe. In addition, intake of vitamin E supplements has been correlated with a reduced risk of cardiovascular disease [3,4].

There is a considerable amount of epidemiological evidence (reviewed in [5]) revealing an association between those with diets rich in fresh fruit and vegetables and a decreased risk of cardiovascular disease and certain forms of cancer. Until relatively recently it was generally assumed that the active dietary constituents contributing to these protective effects are the antioxidant nutrients. But more recent work is highlighting the additional role of the polyphenolic components of the higher plants [6,7] which may act as antioxidants or agents of other mechanisms contributing to anti-carcinogenic or cardioprotective actions.

Flavonoids constitute a large class of compounds, ubiquitous in plants, containing a number of phenolic hydroxyl groups attached to ring structures, conferring the antioxidant activity [6]. Plant polyphenols are multifunctional and can act as reducing agents, hydrogen-donating antioxidants, metal chelators and singlet oxygen quenchers. Estimates of our daily intake range from about 20 mg to 1 g [7]. Table 1 shows some of the dietary sources of flavonoids. The flavanols, particularly the catechin family, and the flavonols quercetin, kaempferol and their glycosides are major constituents of the beverages green and black tea and red wine. Quercetin is also a predominant component of onions and apples, and myricetin and quercetin of berries. The flavanones are mainly found in citrus fruits. Little is known about the bioavailability and absorption and metabolism in man and it is likely that different groups of flavonoids have different pharmacokinetic properties. In this article we shall focus on the catechins and the flavonol quercetin.

Table 1. Some dietary sources of polyphenolic flavonoids.

Flavonoid	Source
Flavanols	
Catechin	Green and black tea, red wine.
Epicatechin	
Epigallocatechin	
Epicatechin gallate	
Epigallocatechin gallate	
Flavanones	
Naringenin	Eucalyptus
Taxifolin	Citrus fruits
Flavones	
Chrysin	Fruit skins
Apigenin	Parsley, celery
Flavonols	
Kaempferol	Endive, leak, broccoli, radish, teas, grapefruit
Myricetin	Cranberry, grapes (white and black), red wine
Quercetin	Onion, lettuce, broccoli, tomato, cranberry, berries, apple skin, grapes, olive oil, teas
	Red wine* (Chianti > Pinot Noir > Rioja = Bordeaux) [7]

*1990 vintage.

Table 2. French Paradox. From ref. [8].

Region	Plasma cholesterol (mg/dl)	Mortality from coronary heart disease (per 10^4)
France (General)	216	102
Toulouse region	224	78
U.S.A. (Stanford)	209	182
U.K.	240	380

The French paradox

The constituents of red wine are factors of particular interest due to the intrigue created by the French paradox. The Southern French have a very low incidence of coronary heart disease despite their high-fat diet and smoking tendencies [8] (Table 2). One of the features that has been highlighted relates to the high consumption of red wine by the French and the question as to whether the polyphenolic antioxidants from this dietary source contribute to the protection from coronary heart disease along with the antioxidants in olive oil and high intake of antioxidant nutrients from the fresh fruit- and vegetable-rich Mediterranean diet. Indeed, red wine has been shown to inhibit the oxidation of low-density lipoproteins (LDLs) in *in vitro* studies [9]. Of course, sight should not be lost of the fact that the high intake of monounsaturated fatty acids also decreases plasma cholesterol and has been reported to reduce the oxidizability of LDL (*ex vivo*).

Zutphen study

In support of flavonoids exerting a protective effect *in vivo* are the findings of a Dutch epidemiological study showing that coronary heart disease in elderly males is inversely correlated with their intake of flavonoids [7]. Most of their dietary flavonoids derived from tea (48% of the flavonoid intake), onions (29%), apples (7%) and red wine (1%). The risk of death from coronary heart disease in the lower tertile of flavonoid intake was about 2.4 times that of the upper tertile. It still remains to be established to what extents the antioxidant and anti-thrombotic properties of the polyphenols contribute to this protection.

Determinants of radical scavenging potential

The chemical properties of polyphenols in terms of the availability of the phenolic hydrogens as hydrogen-donating radical scavengers defines their antioxidant activity. The two basic conditions that must be satisfied for a polyphenolic substance to be defined as an antioxidant are: (i) when present in low concentrations relative to the substrate to be oxidized they can delay, retard or prevent the autoxidation or free radical-mediated oxidation [10]; and (ii) the resulting radical formed after scavenging must be stable; polyphenols can be stabilized through intramolecular hydrogen bonding or by further oxidation [11].

Three criteria for effective radical scavenging by the polyphenols [12,13] are: (i) the *o*-dihydroxy structure in the B ring which confers higher stability to the

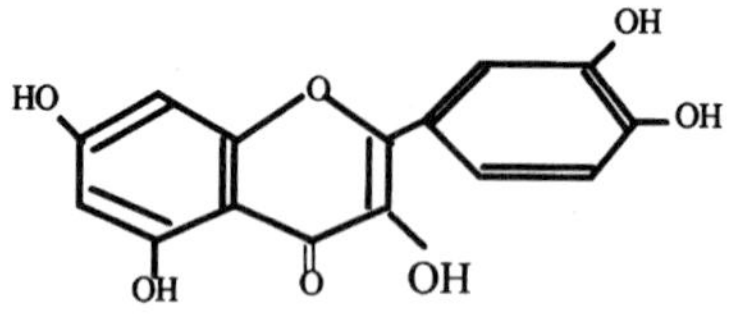

flavonol
(quercetin)

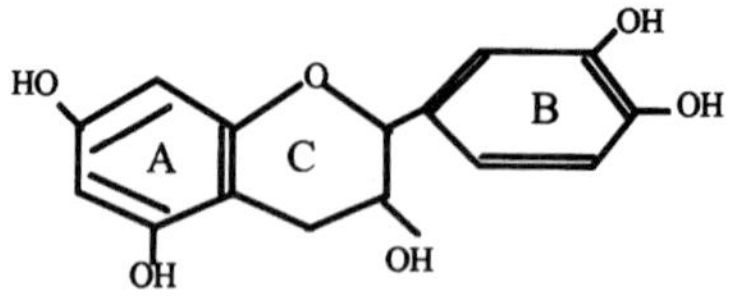

flavanol
(catechin)

Fig. 1. Comparative structures of representative flavonoids, quercetin a typical flavonol and catechin a typical flavanol.

radical form and participates in electron delocalization; (ii) the 2,3 double bond in conjugation with 4-oxo function in the C ring responsible for electron delocalization from the B ring; and (iii) the 3- and 5-OH groups with 4-oxo function in A and C rings for maximum radical scavenging potential.

Thus, as indicated in Fig. 1, it is reasonably expected that the flavonols (e.g. quercetin) are more effective antioxidants than the flavanols (e.g. catechin) since quercetin satisfies all the above determinants whereas catechin lacks aspects of the structural advantages of quercetin and other flavonols and only satisfies determinant (i).

The phenoxyl radical formed by reaction of a phenolic antioxidant with a lipid radical is stabilized by delocalization of unpaired electrons around the aromatic ring. The o-dihydroxy substitution in the B ring is important for stabilizing the resulting free radical form (as well as for metal chelating activity). The possibility exists for stabilization of radical forms though the 3-OH, 5-OH and 4-oxo groups and conjugation from the A ring to the B ring through the additional 2,3 unsaturation in the C ring. This type of reaction is mainly seen with peroxyl (aliphatic) radicals reacting with phenolic antioxidants, as pointed out by Bors et al. [12]. Polyphenols, depending on their precise structure and the proximity or adjacence of hydroxyl groups, also have the possibility of chelating metal ions and preventing metal-catalysed formation of initiating radical species. The two points of attachment of metal ions, such as copper, to the flavonoid molecule are the o-diphenol in the 3′,4′-dihydroxy position in ring B and the ketol structure, 4-oxo, 3-OH, in the C ring of the flavonols [14].

Thus, the specific mode of inhibition of oxidation by the individual polyphenols is not clear but they may act by (i) chelating metal ions via the o-dihydroxy phenolic structure; (ii) scavenging lipid alkoxyl and peroxyl radicals by acting as chain-breaking antioxidants, e.g. as hydrogen donors

$$ROO^{\cdot} + AH \rightarrow ROOH + A^{\cdot}$$

$$RO^{\cdot} + AH \rightarrow ROH + A^{\cdot}$$

or (iii) by regenerating α-tocopherol through reduction of the α-tocopheroxyl radical.

Biological properties of bioflavonoids

Flavonoids and other plant phenolics are reported to have multiple biological activities [15,16] including anticarcinogenic, anti-inflammatory, antibacterial, immune-stimulating, anti-allergic, antiviral, and oestrogenic effects, and as inhibitors of cyclo-oxygenase, lipoxygenase and phospholipase A_2 [17–20]. The chemistry of the flavonoids is predictive of their free radical-scavenging activity since the reduction potentials of flavonoid radicals are lower than those of alkyl peroxyl radicals and the superoxide radical, which means that flavonoids may inactivate these oxyl species and prevent the deleterious consequences of their reactions [20,21]. Their antioxidant activity is also reported: as scavengers of superoxide radical [22–25] although there is conflicting evidence [12,26]; as peroxyl radical scavengers [27,28]; inhibitory effects on lipid peroxidation [29–31]; and inhibition of LDL oxidation induced by copper ions and macrophages [32,33] with half-maximal inhibition induced by compounds ranging in concentration from 1–10 μM. In studies on model systems (erythrocyte membranes and rat liver microsomes), the catechins from tea have revealed high activity, with greatest protection from lipid oxidation by epigallocatechin gallate and epicatechin gallate, the latter being ten times more effective than vitamin E [34]. Others have evaluated the antioxidant activity of flavonoids by investigating their effects in cells in culture. In their studies, pretreatment of cells followed by exposure to reactive oxygen species resulted in the proposed concentrations required for protection being quercetin < kaempferol < catechin. Higher concentrations of quercetin and kaempferol induced toxicity in cells.

Catechin, epicatechin and quercetin have been shown to have powerful antioxidative capacities to approximately the same extents in phospholipid bilayers exposed to aqueous oxygen radicals [31], although the electron-donating ability of catechin is lower than that of quercetin. On the other hand, quercetin is more effective than catechin as an antioxidant in protecting LDLs from oxidation in copper-mediated peroxidation systems (B. Scott, G. Paganga, B. Halliwell and C. Rice-Evans, unpublished work). Furthermore, these flavonoids have been shown to conserve endogenous α-tocopherol in LDL and quercetin is the most effective of the compounds studied [33]. It has been proposed that flavonoids located near the surface of phospholipid structures are ideally located for scavenging oxygen radicals generated in the aqueous phase.

Another property of polyphenols is their metal-chelating potential which may also play a role in the protection against iron- and copper-induced free radical reactions and preventing metal-catalysed formation of initiating radical species [35,36]. There are reports of the pro-oxidant activity of some polyphenols in which high concentrations (25–100 μM) accelerate hydroxyl radical production and DNA damage in vitro, mediated by iron-EDTA but not by iron-ADP or iron itself [35,37]. Others have shown that high concentrations (100 μM) of the flavonols gossypetin and myricetin can modify LDL through non-oxidative processes probably involving covalent modification of the apolipoprotein B_{100} [38]. These are very high relative concentrations of flavonoid:LDL and it is very unlikely that these compounds achieve such high concentrations in vivo.

There is increasing interest in the biological effects of other wine- and tea-derived polyphenols and many in vitro and in vivo studies are demonstrating their antioxidant properties [39,40]. Tea is a rich source of dietary polyphenols and a main dietary source of flavonol glycosides. Tea is an even richer source of the flavanols, the catechins, and it has been shown that green tea constituents [(+)-catechin], are absorbed though the human gut [41,42]. The studies described in this chapter discuss the relative antioxidant potentials of the polyphenolic flavonoids against radicals generated in the aqueous phase in relation to their relative effectiveness as antioxidants against propagating lipid peroxyl radicals, and how their activity influences that of α-tocopherol.

Antioxidant potentials of polyphenols

Antioxidant activity against radicals in the aqueous phase

The total antioxidant activity (TAA) or the Trolox equivalent antioxidant activity (TEAC) is defined as the concentration of Trolox solution with equivalent antioxidant potential to a 1 mM concentration of the compound under investigation [43,44]. The chemical basis of the assay is the generation of a long-lived specific radical cation chromophore based on the peroxidative activity of metmyoglobin and the interaction with the phenothiazine compound, 2,2′-azinobis-(3-ethyl benzthiazoline-6-sulphonic acid) (ABTS) in the presence of hydrogen peroxide to form the ABTS$^{·+}$ radical cation with an absorption maximum at 734 nm. The TEAC reflects the ability of the putative antioxidant to scavenge the ABTS$^{·+}$ radical cation compared with that of Trolox, the water-soluble vitamin E analogue.

The structures of the catechins and gallate/catechin compounds are shown in Fig. 2. These are the main catechins found in fresh leaf and green tea, mostly in the epi-configuration. Catechins with three hydroxyl groups on the B ring are referred to as gallocatechins. Catechin gallates contain gallic acid and are esterified at the OH group on the pyran (C) ring. The antioxidant potentials of the catechin/gallate family of polyphenols are given in the form of their TEAC values in Table 3. The results show that for this series of structures the compounds with

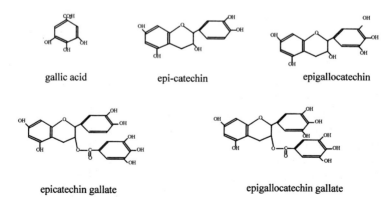

gallic acid   epi-catechin   epigallocatechin

epicatechin gallate   epigallocatechin gallate

Fig. 2. Chemical structures of the catechins and catechin-gallate esters.

Table 3. Relative antioxidant potentials of the catechins and catechin/gallate esters in comparison with vitamins E and C.

	TEAC (mM)	Number of OH groups
Catechin	2.40±0.05 (9)	3,5,7,3',4'
Epicatechin	2.50±0.02 (6)	3,5,7,3',4'
Gallic acid	3.01±0.05 (7)	3,4,5
Epigallocatechin	3.82±0.06 (6)	3,5,7,3',4',5'
Epigallocatechin gallate	4.75±0.06 (9)	5,7,3',4',3",4",5"
Epicatechin gallate	4.93±0.02 (9)	5,7,3',4',3",4",5"
Vitamin C	0.99±0.04 (5)	
Vitamin E	0.97±0.01 (5)	

the most hydroxyl groups exert the greatest antioxidant activity, with the catechin isomers at 2.4 mM and 2.5 mM, more than twice as effective as vitamins E and C (TEAC = 1 mM) [45]. The values for the catechin-gallate esters reflect the additional contribution from the tri-hydroxy phenolic component of gallic acid. Quercetin (Scheme 1a) has an identical number of hydroxyl groups in the same positions as catechin, but also contains the 2,3-double bond in the C ring and the 4-oxo group. This structural advantage confers an enhancement of the TEAC value to 4.7 ± 0.10 mM ($n = 6$). Thus the catechin structure with a TEAC value of 2.4 ± 0.05 mM ($n = 9$), still more than twice as effective as α-tocopherol or ascorbate, can be modified to enhance its antioxidant potential to 4.7 by two different types of structural modification: as in quercetin by incorporation of the 2,3-double bond and the 4-oxo function both in the C ring, allowing electron delocalization and stabilization of the radical form; and as in epigallocatechin gallate (4.75 ± 0.06 mM, $n = 9$) by ester linkage via the 3-OH group to gallic acid carboxylate group enhancing the number of available hydrogens and incorporation of an additional 5'-OH group in the B ring (Fig. 2). On the other hand, kaempferol (TEAC 1.34 ± 0.08 mM, $n = 6$) lacks the o-dihydroxy structure in the B ring (Scheme 1b), decreasing the hydrogen-donating potential; in this case the presence of the 2,3-double bond in the C ring is less relevant since the monophenolic B ring is not such an effective hydrogen donor. Blocking the 3-hydroxyl group in the C ring as a glycoside, as in rutin (quercetin rutinoside) decreases the antioxidant activity to a value of 2.4 ± 0.06 mM ($n = 7$) (Scheme 1b). Taxifolin, lacking the 2,3-double bond, responds almost as catechin with a TEAC of 1.9 ± 0.03 mM ($n = 6$) as predicted.

Antioxidant activity against radicals generated in the lipophilic phase

The oxidation of LDLs is used as a model for investigating the efficacy of the polyphenols as chain-breaking antioxidants. Free radical-mediated peroxidation of polyunsaturated fatty acids leads to the formation of lipid hydroperoxides through a chain reaction of peroxidation (Scheme 2). Oxidative and reductive decomposition of peroxides mediated by haem-proteins or transition metal ions can amplify the peroxidation process (Scheme 3). The presence of chain-breaking antioxidants

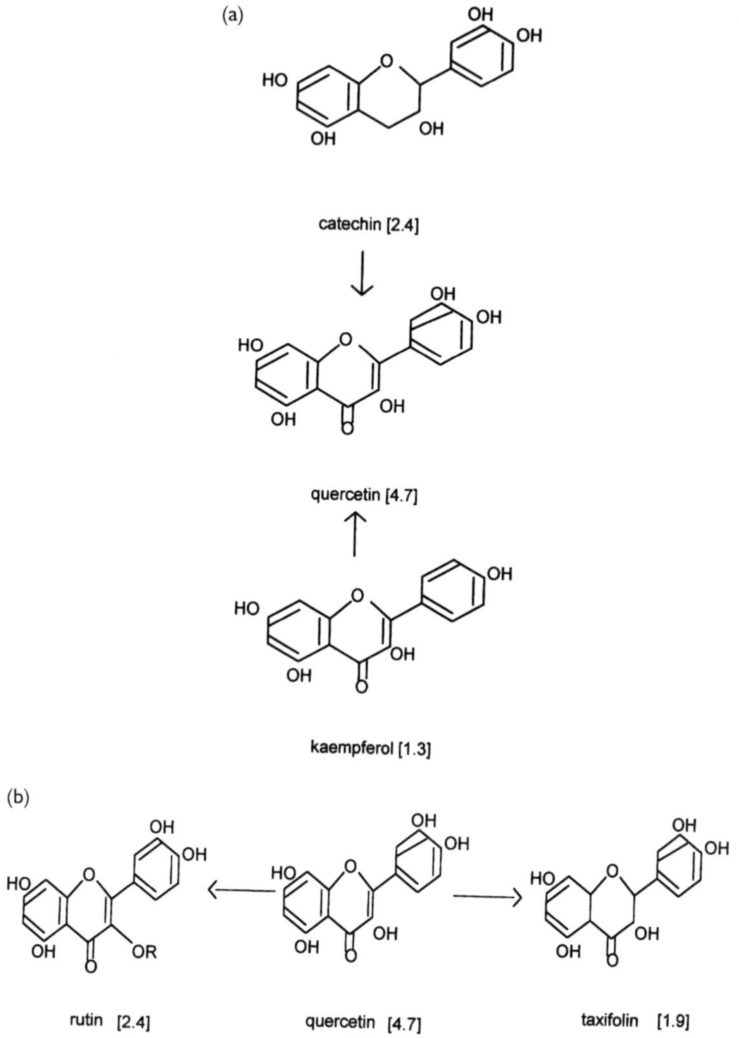

(a)

catechin [2.4]

↓

quercetin [4.7]

↑

kaempferol [1.3]

(b)

rutin [2.4]   quercetin [4.7]   taxifolin [1.9]

Scheme 1. Structure relationships and total antioxidant potentials of quercetin in comparison with catechin and kaempferol (a) and with rutin and taxifolin (b).

can intercept this peroxidation process by reducing the alkoxyl or peroxyl radicals to alkoxides or hydroperoxides, the hydroperoxides re-entering the cycle until the antioxidants are consumed. It has been proposed that alkoxyl radicals rearrange through their own reactivity to epoxides [46]. The oxidative interaction of LDL with haem proteins is hydroperoxide-dependent [47], and, without the addition of initiating species, these agents will slowly cycle the endogenous peroxides within the LDL and amplify the peroxidation process (Scheme 4). In order to study the antioxidant activity of polyphenols as scavengers of propagating lipid peroxyl radicals, no initiating species were added, but metmyoglobin was applied to

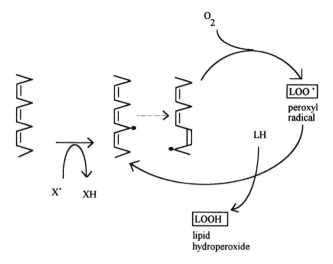

Scheme 2. The initiation of the peroxidation of a polyunsaturated fatty acid.

$$\text{LOOH} + \text{HX - Fe}^{\text{III}} \rightarrow \text{LO}^\bullet + \text{HX } [\text{Fe}^{\text{IV}} = \text{O}]^{2+} + \text{H}^+$$

$$\rightarrow \text{LOO}^\bullet + \text{HX Fe}^{\text{II}} + \text{H}^+$$

$$\text{LOOH} + \text{HX - Fe}^{\text{II}} \rightarrow \text{LO}^\bullet + \text{HX- Fe}^{\text{III}} + \text{OH}^-$$

$$\text{LOOH} + \text{Cu}^{\text{II}} \quad \rightarrow \quad \text{LOO}^\bullet + \text{Cu}^{\text{I}} + \text{H}^+$$

$$\text{LOOH} + \text{Cu}^{\text{I}} \quad \rightarrow \quad \text{LO}^\bullet + \text{Cu}^{\text{II}} + \text{OH}^-$$

Scheme 3. The oxidative and reductive decomposition of lipid hydroperoxides mediated by haem proteins or transition metal ions.

propagate the decomposition of the minimal levels of endogenous pre-formed lipid hydroperoxides. Copper ions were avoided in order to eliminate the confounding effects of the polyphenols as metal-chelators.

In LDL, on oxidation, the aldehydic decomposition products of peroxidation can be assessed as markers of the oxidation of the polyunsaturated fatty acids. They can bind to the apolipoprotein B_{100} on the surface of the LDL, specifically the amino groups, altering the charge and recognition properties, and these modifications can be monitored as changes in electrophoretic mobility as a further indication of the oxidative modification of the LDL. Thus the extent of inhibition of LDL oxidation by the polyphenols can be assessed. The relative effectiveness of the catechin/gallate polyphenols in inhibiting LDL oxidation is shown in Table 4. The data show that gallic acid is the least effective, requiring about 1.2 μM for

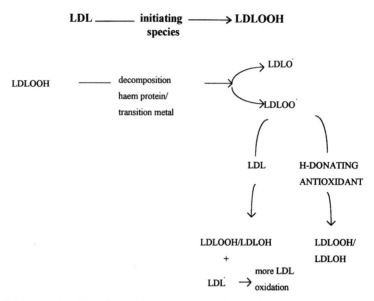

Scheme 4. A schematic representation of the fate of LDL hydroperoxides.

Table 4. The abilities of the catechin/gallate polyphenols as chain-breaking antioxidants against propagating lipid peroxides. [LDL] = 125 μg/ml; metmyoglobin 5 μM; incubation time 5 h.

	Concentration for 50% inhibition of peroxidation (μM)
Epicatechin gallate	0.25
Epicatechin	0.30
Catechin	0.30
Epigallocatechin gallate	0.38
Epigallocatechin	0.75
Gallic acid	1.2

50% inhibition of maximal oxidation, epigallocatechin 0.75 μM, whereas catechin, epicatechin, epicatechin gallate (ECG) and epigallocatechin gallate (EGCG) were all very similar with values ranging from 0.25 to 0.38 μM. A similar sequence is seen in the inhibition of altered relative electrophoretic mobility, as expected.

The catechin/gallate family of compounds was also studied for their ability to spare vitamin E and protect it from oxidation. LDL contains a number of endogenous antioxidants including α- and γ-tocopherols, β-carotene, lycopene, etc. The reduction potentials of flavonoid radicals are higher than that of Trolox which means that their reaction with vitamin E is thermodynamically feasible [48]. Monitoring the consumption of vitamin E in LDL when challenged with a pro-oxidant in the form of metmyoglobin in the presence of the polyphenols (2 μM)

Table 5. Effects of catechin and catechin-gallate esters (2 μM) on the time to consumption of α-tocopherol in LDL on pro-oxidant challenge with 5 μM metmyoglobin. [LDL] = 125 μg/ml.

Additions	Time (h)
Control (no catechin)	1
Gallic acid	1.5
Epigallocatechin	1.5
Epicatechin	2
Epicatechin gallate	4
Epigallocatechin gallate	4

demonstrates (Table 5) that gallic acid and epigallocatechin are indeed the least effective in sparing the vitamin E, reflecting their lesser contribution to increasing the resistance of LDL to oxidation, whereas the delay in consumption of the LDL-vitamin E was prolonged by EGCG and ECG. Flavonoid aglycones are rather lipophilic antioxidants although generally more hydrophilic than α-tocopherol. It has been hypothesized that catechins might be localized near the membrane surface scavenging aqueous radicals and preventing the consumption of tocopherol, whereas α-tocopherol mainly acts as a chain-breaking lipid peroxyl radical scavenger within the LDL [31].

The study of the catechins is particularly important for the understanding of the antioxidant properties of tea, since the total polyphenolic content of green and black teas is 44–45%, of which the catechins constitute 26.7% of the tea solid content of freeze-dried green tea, i.e. approx. 60% of the total polyphenolic composition of green tea [49].

Conclusions

These studies along with those from other laboratories help to identify the active ingredients in beverages, vegetables and fruit that may protect against radical damage and LDL oxidation, implicated in the pathogenesis of coronary heart disease, platelet aggregation and endothelium-dependent vasodilatation of the arteries. This might be useful information not only from the point of view of identifying appropriate foods that are rich in these protective components for the consumer but also presents opportunities for the development of safe food products and additives with appropriate antioxidant properties. Evidence exists that catechin is absorbed by the human gut [42] and that quercetin might reach levels of up to 1 μM in human plasma [50] although the findings are conflicting. Others studies have reported that quercetin after oral administration in humans is not detected in plasma or urine but $\sim$50% is recovered in the faeces suggestive of extensive degradation [51]. Dietary studies in rats have shown a reduction in mammary tumours [52] and suggested only 20% is absorbed from the gastro-intestinal tract [53]. Others report that the major portion of ingested flavonoids (44%) is present in the gastrointestinal tract before excretion in the bile. However, there is a paucity of information on the absorption, metabolism and excretion of these compounds in man and much work needs to be done in this area.

The findings described here are based in part on the following work: Salah, N., Miller, N.J., Paganga, G., Tijburg, L., Bolwell G.P. and Rice-Evans, C. (1995) Arch. Biochem. Biophys. **322**. The author gratefully acknowledges the collaboration of Peter Bramley and John Pridham, Royal Holloway, University of London. The Ministry of Agriculture Fisheries and Food, the Biotechnology and Biological Sciences Research Council and Unilever are acknowledged for funding the research in the author's laboratory.

References

1.   Gey, K.F., Puska, P., Jordan, P. and Moser, K. (1991) Am. J. Clin. Nutr. **53**, 326S–334S
2.   Gey, K.F. (1994) in Free Radicals in the Environment, Medicine and Toxicology (Nohl, H., Esterbauer, H. and Rice-Evans, C., eds.), Richelieu Press, London
3.   Rimm, E.B., Stampfer, M.J., Asherio, A., Giovannucci, E., Colditz, G.A. and Willett, W. (1993) N. Engl. J. Med. **328**, 450–456
4.   Stampfer, M.J., Hennekens, C.H., Manson, J.A., Colditz, G.A., Rosner, B. and Willett, W.C. (1993) N. Engl. J. Med. **328**, 444–449
5.   Block, G. (1992) Nutr. Rev. **50**, 207–213
6.   Harborne, J.B. (1986) in Plant Flavonoids in Biology and Medicine (Cody, B., Middleton, E. and Harborne, J.B., eds.), pp. 15–24, Alan Liss, New York
7.   Hertog, M.G.L., Fesrens, E.J.M., Hollman, P.C.H., Katan, M.B. and Kromhout, D. (1993) Lancet **342**, 1007–1011
8.   Renaud, S. and De Lorgeril, M. (1992) Lancet **339**, 1523–1526
9.   Frankel, E.N., Kanner, J., German, J.B., Parks, E. and Kinsella, J.E. (1993) Lancet **341**, 454–457
10. Halliwell, B. (1990) Free Radical Res. Commun. **9**, 1–32
11. Shahidi, F. and Wanasundara, P.K.J. (1992) Crit. Rev. Food Sci. Nutr. **32**, 67–103
12. Bors, W., Heller, W., Michel, C. and Saran, M. (1990) Methods Enzymol. **186**, 343–355
13. Sichel, G., Corsaro, C., Scalia, M., Di Bilio, A.J. and Bonomo, R.P. (1991) Free Radical Biol. Med. **11**, 1–8
14. Kuhnau, J. (1976) World Rev. Nutr. Diet **24**, 117–191
15. Ho, C.-T., Chen, Q., Shi, H., Zhang, K.-Q. and Rosen, R.T. (1992) Prev. Med. **21**, 520–525
16. Kinsella, J.E., Frankel, E., German, B. and Kanner, J. (1993) Food Technol. **47**, 85–89
17. Brown, J.P. (1980) Mutat. Res. **75**, 243–277
18. Middleton, E. and Kardaswani, C. (1992) Biochem. Pharmacol. **43**, 1167–1179
19. Mabry, T.J., Markham, K.R. and Chari, V.M. (1982) in The Flavanoids, Advances in Research (Harborne, J.R. and Mabry, T.J., eds.), pp. 52–134, Chapman and Hall, London

20. Jovanovic, S.V., Jankovic, I. and Josimovic, L. (1992) J. Am. Chem. Soc. **114**, 9018–9021
21. Wardman, P. (1989) J. Phys. Chem. Ref. Data **18**, 1637
22. Hanasaki, Y., Ogawa, S. and Fukui, S. (1994) Free Radical Biol. Med. **16**, 845–850
23. Cotelle, N., Bernier, J.L., Henichart, J.P., Catteau, J.P., Gaydou, E. and Wallet, J.C. (1992) Free Radical Biol. Med. **13**, 211–219
24. Yuting, C., Rongliang, Z., Zhongjian, J. and Yong, J. (1990) Free Radical Biol. Med. **9**, 19–21
25. Zhou, Y.C. and Zheng, R.L. (1991) Biochem. Pharmacol. **42**, 1177–1179
26. Tsujimoto, Y., Hashizume, H. and Yamazaki, M. (1993) Int. J. Biochem. **25**, 491–494
27. Erben-Russ, M., Michel, C., Bors, W. and Saran, M. (1987) J. Phys. Chem. **91**, 2362–2365
28. Jovanovic, S.V., Steenken, S., Tosic, M., Marjanovic, B. and Simic, M.G. (1994) J. Am. Chem. Soc. **116**, 4846–4851
29. Fraga, C.G., Martino, V.S., Ferraro, G.E., Coussio, J.D. and Boveris, A. (1987) Biochem. Pharmacol. **36**, 717–720
30. Negre-Salvayre, A., Alomar, Y., Troly, M. and Salvayre, R. (1991) Biochim. Biophys. Acta **1096**, 291–300
31. Terao, J., Piskuli, M. and Yao, Q. (1994) Arch. Biochem. Biophys. **308**, 278–284
32. Mangiapane, H., Thomson, J., Salter, A., Brown, S., Bell, G.P. and White, D.A. (1992) Biochem. Pharmacol. **43**, 445–450
33. De Whalley, C., Rankin, S.M., Hoult, J.R., Jessup, W. and Leake, D. (1990) Biochem. Pharmacol. **39**, 1743–1750
34. Namiki, M. and Osawa, T. (1986) Basic Life Sci. **39**, 131–142
35. Laughton, M.J., Evans, P.J., Moroney, M.A., Hoult, J.R.S. and Halliwell, B. (1991) Biochem. Pharmacol. **42**, 1673–1681
36. Morel, I., Lescoat, G., Cognel, P., Sergent, O., Pasdelop, N., Brissot, P., Cillard, P. and Cillard, J. (1993) Biochem. Pharmacol. **45**, 13–19
37. Aruoma, O.I., Murcia, A., Butler, J. and Halliwell, B. (1993) J. Agric. Food Chem. **41**, 1880–1885
38. Rankin, S.M., De Whalley, C.V., Hoult, J.R.S., Jessup, W., Wilkins, G., Collard, J. and Leake, D.S. (1993) Biochem. Pharmacol. **45**, 67–75
39. Ruch, R.J., Cher, S.J. and Klaunig, J.E. (1989) Carcinogenesis **10**, 1003–1008
40. Namiki, M. (1990) Crit. Rev. Food Sci. Nutr. **29**, 273–300
41. He, Y.H. and Kies, C. (1994) Plant Food Human Nutr. **46**, 221–229
42. Das, N.P. (1971) Biochem. Pharmacol. **20**, 3435–3445
43. Miller, N.J., Rice-Evans, C., Davies, M.J., Gopinathan, V. and Milner, A. (1993) Clin. Sci. **84**, 407–412
44. Rice-Evans, C. and Miller, N.J. (1994) Methods Enzymol. **234**, 279–283
45. Rice-Evans, C., Miller, N.J., Bolwell, G.P., Bramley, P.M. and Pridham, J.B. (1995) Free Radical Res. **22**, 375–383
46. Wilcox, A.L. and Marnett, L.J. (1993) Chem. Res. Toxicol. **6**, 413–416
47. Hogg, N., Rice-Evans, C., Darley-Usmar, V., Wilson, M.T., Paganga, G. and Bourne, L. (1994) Arch. Biochem. Biophys. **314**, 39–44
48. Steenken, S. and Neta, P. (1982) J. Phys. Chem. **86**, 3661–3667
49. Wang, Z.Y., Huang, M.-T., Lou, Y.-R., Xie, J.-G., Reuhl, K., Newmark, H., Ho,

C.-T., Yang, C.S. and Conney, A.H. (1995) Cancer Res. in the press

50. Hollman, P.C.H., Dijkshoorn, H., Venema, D.P. and Katan, M.B. (1993) Proc. ILSI Int. Symp. Antioxidants Dis. Prevention, Sweden, 30.6–30.7

51. Gugler, R., Leschik, M. and Dengler, H.T. (1975) Eur. J. Clin. Pharmacol. 9, 229–234

52. Verma, A.K., Johnson, J.A., Gould, M.N. and Tanner, M.A. (1988) Cancer Res. 48, 5754–5788

53. Ueno, I., Kohno, M., Haraikawa, K. and Hirono, I. (1984) J. Pharmacobio-Dyn. 7, 798–803

Biochem. Soc. Symp. **61**, 117–126
Printed in Great Britain

Plant carotenoids and related molecules: important dietary antioxidants

Norman I. Krinsky

Department of Biochemistry, School of Medicine, and the Human Nutrition Research Center on Aging, Tufts University, Boston, MA 02111–1837, U.S.A.

Abstract

The antioxidant effects of dietary carotenoids such as β-carotene have been well documented in various systems *in vitro*, using either organic solvents or membrane systems. However, the biologically relevant studies of the effects of β-carotene on low-density lipoprotein (LDL) oxidation are still controversial, as are those studies using LDL from individuals supplemented with large amounts of β-carotene. These findings do not agree with the epidemiological evidence which suggests that individuals who consume fruits and vegetables rich in carotenoids, or who have relatively high serum carotenoid levels, are at a lower risk of developing coronary heart disease. What is apparent is that studies that have looked at antioxidant protection in the whole organism have demonstrated a decrease in markers of lipid peroxidation after β-carotene supplementation. Maybe those studies trying to pin-point the antioxidant site of carotenoids *in vivo* have been looking at the wrong tissue.

Introduction

The antioxidant properties of carotenoids were reviewed extensively in 1989 [1], and as the interest in this area of carotenoid action continues to grow, have been subject to several recent reviews [2–5]. In addition to trying to learn about the chemistry involved during the process of antioxidation, many investigators try to deduce the possible role of carotenoids as biological antioxidants. Despite the frequency with which the antioxidant action of carotenoids is invoked to explain the epidemiological observations of carotenoid protection of both cancer [6–9] and cardiovascular diseases [10–12], the evidence linking an antioxidant property of carotenoids and disease protection is still tenuous [13]. The following sections will review some of the more recent information that studies the effects of carotenoids, primarily β-carotene, under conditions where an antioxidant action might be expected.

Antioxidant effects *in vitro*

There have been many systems used to investigate the antioxidant effectiveness of carotenoids. Among these are experiments carried out in free solution (homogeneous or heterogeneous) or in artificial (liposome) or natural (microsomes, mitochondria, or red blood cell) membranes. Oxidation has been initiated by generating free radicals, using either pulse-radiolysis or chemical radical initiators, or through enzyme-generated lipid peroxidation, or autoxidation of lipids.

Using methyl linoleate dissolved in a hexane:isopropanol (1:1, v/v) solution, Terao was able to demonstrate that the addition of the carotenoids, astaxanthin, canthaxanthin, zeaxanthin and β-carotene (Fig. 1), effectively inhibited 2,2′-azo*bis*(2,4-dimethylvaleronitrile) (AMVN)-initiated lipid peroxidation [14]. The oxo-carotenoids, astaxanthin and canthaxanthin, were more effective antioxidants than β-carotene or zeaxanthin, and in AMVN-initiated autoxidation reactions, the oxo-carotenoids were oxidized more slowly than β-carotene or zeaxanthin.

These observations have been supported by Jørgensen and Skibsted [15] working in both CHCl₃ and in a lipid/water phase, who demonstrated that the order of antioxidant effectiveness in CHCl₃ is astaxanthin > canthaxanthin > β-carotene > zeaxanthin, which also supports the idea that the carbonyl carotenoids are more effective *in vitro* antioxidants. They suggested that the basis for the increased effectiveness of astaxanthin was due to increased resonance stabilization of the presumed carbon-centred radical through the formation of an intra-

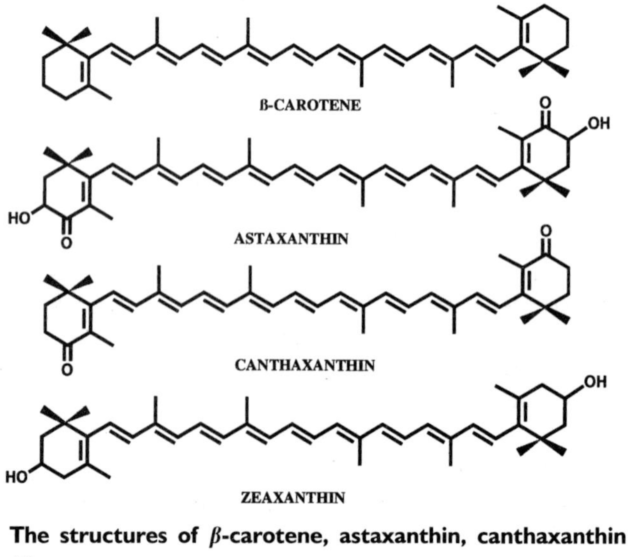

Fig. 1. The structures of β-carotene, astaxanthin, canthaxanthin and zeaxanthin.

molecular hydrogen bond between the C-3 hydroxyl group and the C-4 carbonyl. However, that would not explain increased effectiveness of canthaxanthin. They also studied metmyoglobin-induced lipid peroxidation in a lipid/water system, and did not observe any difference in antioxidant efficiency with these carotenoids. Finally, they studied the effect of oxygen tension in the lipid/water system, and found an inverse relationship between oxygen tension and antioxidant activity, similar to that reported by Burton [16].

Additionally, carotenoids exist as geometric isomers, since they can assume either a *trans* or *cis* configuration about many of the in-chain double bonds. Very little is known about any possible differences in antioxidant activity between such isomers, although Levin and Mokady have suggested that the 9-*cis* isomer of β-carotene may be a more effective *in vitro* antioxidant than the all-*trans* isomer [17].

There have been many other reports of carotenoids displaying antioxidant activity *in vitro*, and those reported up to 1992 have been reviewed previously [3,5]. More recent reports are discussed below.

Micelles have been used to study the effectiveness of carotenoids as antioxidants. Pryor and his associates have used SDS micelles, and they find virtually no activity for β-carotene (0.3% of α-tocopherol), which they attribute to the inaccessible physical location of the β-carotene in these micelles [18]. Canfield and Valenzuela have also used micelles, and find that β-carotene, added in tetrahydrofuran (THF), inhibits lipoxygenase-initiated linoleic acid oxidation, as determined by conjugated diene formation [19].

Liposomes have also been used for many years [20], and several new studies have appeared recently. A very interesting approach was used by Tsuchiya *et al.* who used the loss of fluorescence of either phycoerythrin or *cis*-parinaric acid to evaluate both water- and lipid-soluble antioxidants [21,22]. Using this system, they reported that several carotenoids are very effective antioxidants, although it is still difficult to understand how each carotenoid molecule can quench 30 peroxyl radicals [23].

Low-density lipoprotein (LDL) oxidation

Since the report appeared that the vast majority of the β-carotene present in human plasma is associated with LDL [24], there have been many suggestions regarding a possible role for β-carotene in this lipoprotein. Since β-carotene can quench radical species [20,25], many investigations have focused on the possible antioxidant effect of β-carotene in LDL. These studies have been carried out under *in vitro* conditions, with β-carotene added directly to LDL or to plasma, or in *in vivo* experiments, following supplementation of volunteers or patients with various doses of β-carotene.

In vitro effects on LDL oxidation

The *in vitro* studies, involving the direct addition of β-carotene to LDL, remain controversial (Table 1). The ability of β-carotene to inhibit free radicals led Morel *et al.* to investigate a possible antioxidant function in LDL [26]. These

Table 1. In vitro effects of β-carotene (β-C) on LDL oxidation. Abbreviations: THF, tetrahydrofuran; TBARS, thiobarbituric acid-reactive substances; AAPH, 2,2'-azobis(2-amidinopropane) dihydrochloride; DMSO, dimethyl sulphoxide.

Solvent	Concentration (μM)	Time (h)	Oxidant	Marker	Effect	Reference
(A) No effect						
β-C in ethanol	18	—	Dialysis	TBARS	None	[26]
				Cytotoxicity	None	[26]
β-C and LDL	10–50	—	Co-cultures: smooth muscle and endothelial cells	Monocyte migration	None	[27]
β-C and co-cultures	5	16	Co-cultures: smooth muscle and endothelial cells	Monocyte migration	Decreased	[27]
β-C in THF in plasma	0.54	3	Cu	Lag phase	None	[28]
β-C in THF in plasma	0.54	3	AAPH	Lag phase	None	[28]
β-C in THF or hexane	0.54	3	Cu	Lag phase	None	[28]
(B) Antioxidant effect						
β-C in ethanol	0.5–2.0	0	Cu	TBARS	Decreased	[29]
			Macrophages	LDL degradation	Decreased	[29]
β-C in DMSO/ethanol	40	5	Cu	TBARS	Decreased	[30]
	40	5	Cu, followed by macrophages	LDL degradation	Decreased	[30]
β-C in liposomes	19	3	Cu	TBARS	Decreased	[31]

workers observed that dialysis of LDL induced lipid peroxidation and subsequent cytotoxicity when fibroblasts were exposed to the oxidized LDL. Antioxidants such as α-tocopherol or butylated hydroxytoluene were able to prevent the lipid peroxidation, but β-carotene was ineffective. Several other groups have added β-carotene, in various solvents or carriers, incubated with LDL for various periods of time and exposed these mixtures to different oxidants, and still failed to demonstrate any protection by the added β-carotene [27,28].

In contrast, three laboratories have reported an antioxidant effect of added β-carotene. Jialal et al. [29] added β-carotene directly to LDL and initiated lipid oxidation by treatment with Cu^{2+}. Under these conditions, they report that the β-carotene was 20-fold more effective than an equivalent amount of added α-tocopherol in preventing lipid peroxidation, as measured by thiobarbituric acid-reactive substance (TBARS) formation. They also reported that these β-carotene-treated LDL particles showed decreased degradation by macrophages, when compared with placebo-treated LDL. Naruszewicz et al. [30] reported that Cu^{2+} treatment resulted in less TBARS formation, and less LDL degradation by macrophages, in those LDL samples treated with β-carotene. In addition, Lavy et al. [31] exposed LDL to liposomes containing β-carotene and reported that this treatment led to a decrease in the TBARS formed when this LDL was treated with Cu^{2+}.

How can such differences be explained? It is possible that different amounts of β-carotene actually entered the LDL particle, although none of these studies determined how well the β-carotene was incorporated under these in vitro conditions. Another possibility is that LDL simply serves to carry β-carotene, and other carotenoids, to sites where it might more readily demonstrate an antioxidant action. One such example is described below.

Navab et al., who were unable to demonstrate an effect on LDL-induced monocyte transmigration when β-carotene was added directly to LDL [27], were able to demonstrate clearly that the addition of β-carotene to these co-cultures inhibited LDL-initiated monocyte transmigration [27]. These findings suggest that the normal LDL oxidation brought about by the aortic cells is inhibited when the cells contain the antioxidants, in contrast to the LDL containing the antioxidants.

In vivo effects on LDL oxidation

The results of studies involving LDL isolated from individuals supplemented with β-carotene and then exposed to oxidizing conditions are shown in Table 2. The vast majority of these studies indicate that such in vivo loading of LDL with β-carotene does not lead to protection against oxidation. The earliest studies reported either no change [32], or a slight increase in the lag period of Cu-induced LDL oxidation [33]. Abbey et al. [34] had observed an increase in the lag time, but they had supplemented their subjects with vitamin E and vitamin C, in addition to β-carotene, and thus it is not possible to tell which component of the mixture was active. Reaven et al. [35] pursued their investigations by looking at the effect of supplementation on the ability of LDL to enhance monocyte adherence to co-cultures of endothelial and smooth-muscle cells, but found no effect. Of great interest was their attempt to demonstrate a protective effect of β-carotene against singlet oxygen attack on LDL. β-Carotene is one of the best

Table 2. *In vitro* effects of β-carotene on LDL oxidation.

Subjects	Supplementation (mg/day)	Period (days)	Oxidant	Marker	Effect	Reference
(a) No effect						
Smokers	40	14				
	then 20					
Volunteers	60	84	Cu	Lag time	None	[32]
		90	Cu	Lag time	None	[33]
			Macrophage	LDL degradation	None	
Volunteers	15	28	Cu	Conjugated dienes	None	[35]
	then 30	14	$^1O_2$ or macrophage co-cultures	TBARS	None	
				Adherent monocytes	None	
Volunteers*	0.5/kg body weight	28	Cu	Conjugated dienes	None	[47]
Volunteers	100	6				
	then 50–100 q.e.d.	21	AAPH	Lag phase	Decreased	[28]
			Cu	Lag phase	None	
(b) Antioxidant effect						
Women (depleted)	0.06	68	Cu	Hydrocarbons	Increased	[39]
Women (repleted)	15	28	Cu	Hydrocarbons	Increased	
Cystic fibrosis patients	0.5/kg body weight	90	Cu	Lag phase	Increased	
				Maximum rate	Increased	
				Maximum conjugated diene	None	

*Ingested 0.5 ml of ethanol/kg body weight.

singlet oxygen quenchers found in nature [36], and has been demonstrated to function as such *in vivo* [37,38]. To initiate singlet oxygen reactions, Reaven *et al.* added Rose Bengal to LDL, and illuminated these samples. Under these conditions, there was no difference in the appearance of TBARS in LDL from control or supplemented subjects. This is actually a surprising result, but may be explained either by the low concentration of β-carotene in LDL, even in the case of supplemented individuals, or by a localization phenomenon, with the singlet oxygen generated by the photosensitized reaction acting at a site other than that occupied by the β-carotene. In one instance, supplementation with β-carotene led to a decrease in the lag phase of Cu-treated LDL, although this effect was not seen during 2,2'-azo*bis*(2-amidinopropane) dihydrochloride-induced oxidation [28].

On the other hand, two groups have reported a protective action of supplementary β-carotene on LDL oxidation. In both cases, extremely β-carotene-depleted LDL was used to demonstrate an antioxidant effect. Dixon *et al.* [39] placed a group of women on a carotene-depleted diet for 68 days, during which time their plasma TBARS increased dramatically. These women were then repleted with >15 mg/day β-carotene, and an additional dosage (amount not specified) of mixed carotenoids was administered during the last 12 days of the repletion period. Repletion led to a significant decrease in the production of hexanal, pentanal, and pentane, as measured by gas chromatography, following Cu-treatment of isolated LDL.

A very similar effect was reported by Winklhofer-Roob *et al.* [40] using LDL isolated from cystic fibrosis patients supplemented with β-carotene at 0.5 mg/kg body weight for 90 days. Under these circumstances, the lag phase of Cu-initiated LDL oxidation was increased, although no change was observed in the maximum rate or maximum formation of conjugated dienes.

In both of the above cases, the investigators started out with LDL particles that were quite deficient in carotenoids, and this may explain why they were able to find an antioxidant effect of supplementary β-carotene, as opposed to the other studies reported in Table 2 that reported no effect.

Antioxidant effects *in vivo*

In addition to the two cases reported above for *in vivo* antioxidant effects of β-carotene in LDL following supplementation, there are only a few more studies that have addressed this issue. In two cases, breath pentane output (BPO) was measured as a means of evaluating whole body antioxidant status following β-carotene supplementation. BPO arises during peroxidative reactions of ω-6 polyunsaturated fatty acids. Gottlieb *et al.* placed two groups of healthy volunteers on a carotenoid-free liquid diet for a 2 week period, during which time their serum β-carotene levels decreased by 54–67%. These two groups were then repleted with synthetic β-carotene at either 15 or 120 mg/day for 4 weeks. In both groups, the repletion period resulted in a drop in the BPO output, although it only achieved significance with the 120 mg/day dose [41]. This was surprising, in view of the fact that this group had demonstrated earlier that both doses of β-carotene led to a significant decrease in the total body lipid peroxides, as determined by measuring TBARS in serum [42].

Another approach was utilized by Allard *et al.* [43], who investigated BPO in smokers, where evidence has clearly indicated that they have lower plasma levels of a variety of antioxidants, including β-carotene [44]. In this double-blind study, both smokers and non-smokers were supplemented with 20 mg/day β-carotene or a placebo, for a 28 day period. Supplementation resulted in a 9–11-fold increase in plasma β-carotene, with no change seen in either vitamin E or vitamin C levels during this period. To avoid any contamination from cigarette smoke, BPO was analysed 12 h after smoking. The smokers started the study with significantly higher levels of BPO than the non-smokers, and supplementation resulted in a significant decrease in BPO, bringing the levels to those of the non-smokers. Interestingly, the non-smoker group did not show any change in BPO, despite the 9-fold increase in plasma β-carotene.

Meydani *et al.* [45] also carried out a double-blind, placebo-controlled study of β-carotene supplementation in a group of older women. The level of phosphatidylcholine hydroperoxide (PC-OOH) was determined as a marker of antioxidant status. The supplementation period was 21 days, and the women were given 90 mg of synthetic β-carotene/day. This dose of β-carotene increased plasma levels 9-fold, but did not affect basal levels of PC-OOH. However, in response to AAPH-treatment of plasma, there was a significant change in the lag phase in the supplemented group, increasing from 2.4 h to 5.4 h.

Summary

The evidence for an antioxidant role of β-carotene, and presumably other plant carotenoids, has been described above. Because of the potential importance of the hypothesis that oxidized LDL is a major player in the development of atherosclerosis [46], much attention has focused on the role of β-carotene in LDL. The *in vitro* experiments, where β-carotene is added to LDL or to plasma, with the subsequent isolation of LDL, remain controversial (Table 1), presumably due to the uncertainty of whether added β-carotene is merely adsorbed on to or incorporated into LDL. And if it is in the LDL, is it really in the same compartment as the material secreted from the liver?

One would hope that LDL isolated from individuals supplemented with β-carotene would provide more useful information, but even these results are controversial (Table 2). What appears to be a more promising approach to evaluating the efficacy of dietary carotenoids on antioxidant status comes from the studies evaluating various parameters of lipid peroxidation in supplemented individuals [41,43,45]. In all of these studies, supplementary β-carotene is shown to act as an antioxidant when the system is subject to an external oxidant stress. What is still lacking is some evidence that under 'normal' oxidative stress, β-carotene and other carotenoids act as part of the antioxidant defence system.

References

1. Krinsky, N.I. (1989) Free Radical Biol. Med. **7**, 617–635
2. Krinsky, N.I. (1992) Proc. Soc. Exp. Biol. Med. **200**, 248–254
3. Palozza, P. and Krinsky, N.I. (1992) Methods Enzymol. **213**, 403–420

4. Rousseau, E.J., Davison, A.J. and Dunn, B. (1992) Free Radical Biol. Med. **12**, 407–433

5. Krinsky, N.I. (1993) Annu. Rev. Nutr. **13**, 561–587

6. Peto, R., Doll, R.J., Buckley, J.D. and Sporn, M.B. (1981) Nature (London) **290**, 201–208

7. Hennekens, C.H., Mayrent, S.L. and Willett, W. (1986) Cancer **58**, 1837–1841

8. Ito, N. and Hirose, M. (1989) Adv. Cancer Res. **53**, 247–302

9. Gerster, H. (1993) Int. J. Vit. Nutr. Res. **63**, 93–121

10. Gey, K.F. (1990) Biochem. Soc. Trans. **18**, 1041–1045

11. Kritchevsky, D. (1992) Nutr. Today **27**, 30–33

12. Seelert, K. (1992) Internist. Prax. **32**, 191–199

13. Krinsky, N.I. (1994) Pure Appl. Chem. **66**, 1003–1010

14. Terao, J. (1989) Lipids **24**, 659–661

15. Jørgensen, K. and Skibsted, L.H. (1993) Z. Lebensm. Unters. Forsch. **196**, 423–429

16. Burton, G.W. (1989) J. Nutr. **119**, 109–111

17. Levin, G. and Mokady, S. (1994) Free Radical Biol. Med. **17**, 77–82

18. Pryor, W.A., Cornicelli, J.A., Devall, L.A., Tait, B., Trivedi, B.K., Witiak, D.T. and Wu, M. (1993) J. Org. Chem. **58**, 3521–3532

19. Canfield, L.M. and Valenzuela, J.G. (1993) in Carotenoids in Human Health (Canfield, L.M., Krinsky, N.I. and Olson, J.A., eds.), vol. 691, pp. 192–199, New York Acad. Sci., New York

20. Krinsky, N.I. and Deneke, S.M. (1982) J. Natl. Cancer Inst. **69**, 205–210

21. Tsuchiya, M., Scita, G., Thompson, D.F.T., Kagan, V.E., Livrea, M.A. and Packer, L. (1993) in Retinoids: Progress in Research and Clinical Application (Livrea, M.A. and Packer, L., eds.), pp. 525–536, Marcel Dekker, New York

22. Tsuchiya, M., Kagan, V.E., Freisleben, H.-J., Manabe, M. and Packer, L. (1994) Methods Enzymol. **234**, 371–383

23. Tsuchiya, M., Scita, G., Freisleben, H.-J., Kagan, V.E. and Packer, L. (1992) Methods Enzymol. **213**, 460–472

24. Krinsky, N.I., Cornwell, D.G. and Oncley, J.L. (1958) Arch. Biochem. Biophys. **73**, 233–246

25. Packer, J.E., Mahood, J.S., Mora-Arellano, V.O., Slater, T.F., Willson, R.L. and Wolfenden, B.S. (1981) Biochem. Biophys. Res. Commun. **98**, 901–906

26. Morel, D.W., Hessler, J.R. and Chisolm, G.M. (1983) J. Lipid Res. **24**, 1070–1076

27. Navab, M., Imes, S.S., Hama, S.Y. et al. (1991) J. Clin. Invest. **88**, 2039–2046

28. Gaziano, J.M., Hatta, A., Flynn, M., Johnson, E.J., Krinsky, N.I., Ridker, P.R., Hennekens, C.H. and Frei, B. (1995) Atherosclerosis **112**, 187–195

29. Jialal, I., Norkus, E.P., Cristol, L. and Grundy, S.M. (1991) Biochim. Biophys. Acta **1086**, 134–138

30. Naruszewicz, M., Selinger, E. and Davignon, J. (1992) Metabolism **41**, 1215–1224

31. Lavy, A., Ben Amotz, A. and Aviram, M. (1993) Eur. J. Clin. Chem. Clin. Biochem. **31**, 83–90

32. Princen, H.M.G.H., van Poppel, G., Vogelezang, C., Buytenhek, R. and Kok, F.J. (1992) Arteriosclerosis Thromb. **12**, 554–562

33. Reaven, P.D., Khouw, A., Beltz, W.F., Parthasarathy, S. and Witztum, J.L. (1993) Arteriosclerosis Thromb. **13**, 590–600

34. Abbey, M., Nestel, P.J. and Baghurst, P.A. (1993) Am. J. Clin. Nutr. **58**, 525–532
35. Reaven, P.D., Ferguson, E., Navab, M. and Powell, F.L. (1994) Arteriosclerosis Thromb. **14**, 1162–1169
36. Foote, C.S., Denny, R.W., Weaver, L., Chang, Y. and Peters, J. (1970) Ann. N.Y. Acad. Sci. **171**, 139–148
37. Mathews-Roth, M.M. (1984) Photochem. Photobiol. **40**, 63–67
38. Mathews-Roth, M.M. (1986) Photochem. Photobiol. **43**, 91–93
39. Dixon, Z.R., Burri, B.J., Clifford, A. et al. (1994) Free Radical Biol. Med. **17**, 537–544
40. Winklhofer-Roob, B.M., Puhl, H., Khoschsorur, G., van't Hof, M.A., Esterbauer, H. and Shmerling, D.H. (1995) Free Radical Biol. Med. **18**, 849–859
41. Gottlieb, K., Zarling, E.J., Mobarhan, S., Bowen, P. and Sugarman, S. (1993) Nutr. Cancer **19**, 207–212
42. Mobarhan, S., Bowen, P., Anderson, B., Evans, M., Stacewicz-Sapuntzakis, M., Sugarman, S., Simms, P., Lucchesi, D. and Friedman, H. (1990) Nutr. Cancer **14**, 195–206
43. Allard, J.P., Royall, D., Kurian, R., Muggli, R. and Jeejeebhoy, K.N. (1994) Am. J. Clin. Nutr. **59**, 884–890
44. Chow, C.K., Thacker, R.R., Changchit, C., Bridges, R.B., Rehm, S.R., Humble, J. and Turbek, J. (1986) J. Am. Coll. Nutr. **5**, 305–312
45. Meydani, M., Martin, A., Ribaya-Mercado, J.D., Gong, J., Blumberg, J.B. and Russell, R.M. (1994) J. Nutr. **124**, 2397–2403
46. Steinberg, D., Parthasarathy, S., Carew, T.E., Khoo, J.C. and Witztum, J.L. (1989) N. Engl. J. Med. **320**, 915–924
47. Suzukawa, M., Ishikawa, T., Yoshida, H., Hosoai, K., Nishio, E., Yamashita, T., Nakamura, H., Hashizume, N. and Suzuki, K. (1994) J. Am. Coll. Nutr. **13**, 237–242

Biochem. Soc. Symp. **61**, 127–137
Printed in Great Britain

Therapeutic iron chelators and their potential side-effects

S. Singh, H. Khodr, M.I. Taylor and R.C. Hider

Department of Pharmacy, King's College, University of London, Manresa Road, London SW3 6LX, U.K.

Abstract

A number of iron-chelating agents are currently being considered as orally active alternatives to desferrioxamine (DFO), the therapeutic agent for the treatment of body iron overload that is available at present. These include bidentate hydroxypyridinones (HPO), tridentate desferrithiocin (DFT) analogues and hexadentate aminocarboxylate (HBED) chelators. All chelating agents have the potential to induce toxic effects when iron homoeostasis is affected within the body. This can arise when the absorption, distribution and utilization of iron is affected. Alternatively, chelating agents can induce toxicity by directly interfering with iron-dependent metalloenzymes located within the body. These effects are, however, mainly localized to non-haem enzymes such as ribonucleotide reductase and lipoxygenase. The resultant iron complexes also have the ability to induce toxicity. Depending on the coordination geometry and donor atoms associated with the metal centre, redox cycling of the iron centre with the corresponding generation of free radicals can result.

Redox activity of iron

There is considerable clinical interest in the redox active metals such as iron due to the postulated involvement of hydroxyl radicals in normal physiological responses as well as in a range of disease states [1]. Iron has two important chemical properties which have rendered it a critically important element to virtually all life forms. Iron possesses two oxidation states, iron (II) and iron (III) and the redox potential between these is such that oxidation processes centred on the iron atom can be readily coupled to metabolic reactions. Iron also has a high affinity for oxygen atoms. These two properties are utilized widely by iron-containing proteins, for instance, as electron transfer proteins in the mitochondria, as hydroxylating enzymes and as oxygen transport proteins such as haemoglobin [2]. These important properties also endow iron with the potential of being toxic,

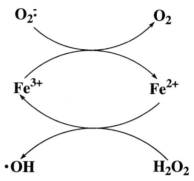

Scheme 1. Iron catalysed Haber–Weiss reaction. Redox cycling of iron between the ferric [Fe(III)] and ferrous [Fe(II)] states and in the process generating toxic hydroxyl radicals.

this being particularly true should the iron be non-specifically bound to the surface of proteins and membranes. Such weakly coordinated iron can redox cycle between the two oxidation states thereby generating a range of oxygen radicals including the hydroxyl radical [3] (Scheme 1). The hydroxyl radical (˙OH) is highly reactive and is capable of interacting with most types of organic molecules, including sugars, lipids, proteins and nucleic acids. Consequently, the production of hydroxyl radicals is undesirable and there are a number of protective measures adopted by cells to protect against its formation, foremost among these is the tight control of iron absorption, transport and storage within multicellular organisms.

β-Thalassaemia major

Several blood diseases require the regular transfusion of red blood cells. One of the most important of these on a worldwide basis is thalassaemia. Thalassaemia is a genetic disorder that is characterized by a defect in the synthesis of haemoglobin, a vital oxygen carrier molecule of the blood [4]. It is estimated that there are up to 200 million carriers of the various forms of the disease worldwide.

The only effective treatment of β-thalassaemia major is to increase haemoglobin levels by regular blood transfusions, without which, the majority of patients die within the first year of life. Repeated blood transfusion will lead inevitably to an excess accumulation of iron in the body due to the inability of man to excrete this metal produced from the breakdown of haemoglobin [5]. The excess iron found in thalassaemic patients is distributed throughout the body but is found in highest concentrations within the liver and other highly perfused organs. The unregulated accumulation of iron causes tissue damage and failure of organs such as the liver and heart, eventually leading to death. Complications associated with the toxicity of iron following blood transfusion can, to a large extent, be alleviated by the use of specific metal-scavenging agents or chelating agents, to trap and allow excretion of excess and potentially toxic forms of iron from the body.

Chelation therapy

Desferrioxamine (DFO) (Fig. 1; 1) has been available for the treatment of iron overload for over 30 years [6]. DFO is highly selective for iron with a stability constant of 10^{31} and only minimal affinity for other metals such as copper, zinc, calcium and magnesium (10^2–10^4). The major limiting factor of DFO is that it is inactive when administered orally and only causes sufficient iron excretion to keep pace with transfusion regimes when given either subcutane-

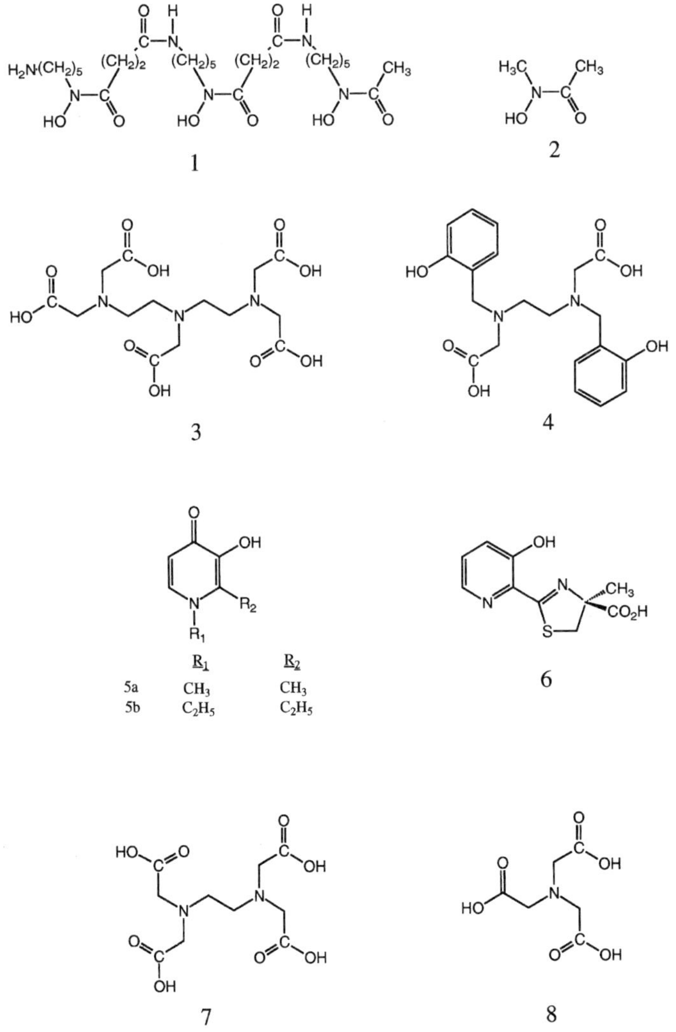

Fig. 1. Chemical structure of various iron chelators. 1, Desferrioxamine (DFO); 2, acetohydroxamic acid (ACH); 3, diethylenetriamine penta-acetic acid (DTPA); 4, hydroxybenzyl ethylenediamine (HBED); 5, 3-hydroxy-pyridine-4-one (HPO); 6, desferrithiocin (DFT); 7, ethylene diamine tetra-acetic acid (EDTA); 8, nitriloacetic acid (NTA).

ously or intravenously over 8–12 h, 5–7 days a week. For this reason, many patients find it difficult to comply with the treatment and some even stop taking the drug altogether. Additionally, DFO and the associated equipment required for treatment such as infusion pumps and syringes are prohibitively expensive to patients in developing countries. There is, therefore, no doubt that an affordable orally active chelating agent is needed to treat patients on lifelong transfusion programmes. The development of an oral iron chelator might also allow the extension of the therapeutic use of red-cell transfusions in sickle-cell anaemia.

Orally active iron-chelating agents

The design of an orally active, non-toxic chelator has been a goal of many medicinal chemists over the past 20 years. Unfortunately, the above goal has not yet been achieved since a wide range of requirements need to be met before such an agent becomes available.

Requirements for selective iron chelation

Iron selectivity

To achieve effective and safe chelation *in vivo*, a compound with a high iron binding constant and a high degree of specificity in relation to other metals is required. Iron exists in two oxidation states, iron (III) or ferric iron, and iron (II) or ferrous iron. Under aerobic conditions, iron (III) is the more stable and chelators with high affinity for this form of iron are therefore of much greater use. Iron (III) forms the most stable bonds with oxygen-containing chelating agents; it is for this reason that the majority of siderophores utilize the dioxo ligands catechol and hydroxamate.

Bidentate versus hexadentate ligands

The stability of the metal complex is also influenced by the number of covalently linked arms on the chelator (Fig. 2). Due to entropy considerations, hexadentate

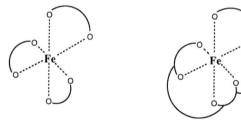

Bidentate ligand 3:1   Hexadentate ligand 1:1

Fig. 2. Bidentate and hexadentate iron complexes. Iron is most stable when bound by six oxygen atoms arranged octahedrally around the metal ion. A bidentate ligand occupies two of the above positions requiring three molecules to totally encompass the iron atom. In contrast, all six coordination positions are occupied by a single hexadentate molecule.

ligands possess a much higher kinetic stability than that of the corresponding bidentate ligands. Thus the affinity constant of iron for the bidentate acetohydroxamic acid (Fig. 1; **2**) and hexadentate desferrioxamine (DFO) (Fig. 1; **1**) are 10^{28} and 10^{33} respectively. Hexadentate ligands also retain appreciable iron-binding power at low concentrations. This is in contrast to bidentate ligands where a third-order concentration dependence applies, as three ligands are required to occupy all co-ordination positions around the iron atom.

As a general rule, oligodentate ligands are kinetically more inert than their bidentate analogues. Thus a potential disadvantage of bidentate ligands which, due to their co-ordination of iron in a stepwise fashion (eqn. 1), can lead partially dissociated (2:1 and 1:1) complexes to form at low concentrations. In principal, these incomplete iron complexes can generate hydroxyl radicals.

$$Fe^{3+} \rightleftharpoons [Fe^{3+}\text{-}L]^{2+} \rightleftharpoons [Fe^{3+}\text{-}L_2]^{+} \rightleftharpoons [Fe^{3+}\text{-}L_3] \qquad (1)$$

Ideally a kinetically inert molecule should be used for chelation therapy, where, once chelated, the iron remains tightly bound to the ligand ensuring minimal redistribution of iron. However, in practice, there is a fine balance as kinetically inert ligands are less able to chelate oligomeric and polymeric forms of iron (for instance haemosiderin and certain forms of non-transferrin-bound iron). Thus hexadentate ligands may be less effective than bidentate compounds when solubilizing aggregate forms of iron. The disadvantage of increased kinetic lability faced by bidentates relative to hexadentates can be minimized by the use of ligands with high affinities for iron (III).

Oral absorption

A key property for an oral iron chelator is its ability to cross biological membranes enabling it to be absorbed from the intestinal tract. Most drugs enter cells by simple diffusion through the hydrophobic region of the cell membrane and consequently uncharged drugs permeate more rapidly than charged molecules. Thus neutral chelators are more likely to cross epithelial cells of the intestine and be orally active than charged molecules. Similarly such chelators should also be able to penetrate into the cytoplasm of cells. Clearly for oral activity to be achieved, the chelator must also be designed to resist the acidity of the stomach and enzymic cleavage.

Oral bioavailability and penetration of biological membranes, in addition to being affected by parameters such as octanol/water partition coefficients and ionic state, are also influenced by molecular size. Generally molecules with molecular masses > 400 Da only poorly penetrate biological membranes by simple diffusion. A major distinguishing feature between bidentate and hexadentate ligands is molecular size; bidentate ligands typically fall in the molecular-mass range 100–250 Da, whereas the larger hexadentate ligands fall in the range 400–1000 Da. Most siderophores, including DFO, have molecular masses between 600 and 900 Da. Diethylenetriamine penta-acetic acid (DTPA) (Fig. 1; **3**) (393 Da) and hydroxybenzylethylene diamine (HBED) (Fig. 1; **4**) (364 Da) are probably close to the minimum size possible for effective hexadentate iron (III) ligands. Thus by virtue of their lower molecular masses, bidentate molecules are likely to have a much higher bioavailability than hexadentate ligands. This is certainly the experience with 3-hydroxypyridin-4-ones such as CP20 (Fig. 1; **5a**) and CP94 (**5b**), which have been studied in man and are efficiently absorbed [7].

Metabolism and pharmacokinetic properties of chelating agents

The metabolism and pharmacokinetics of chelating agents are likely to play a critical role in determining both the efficacy and toxicity of therapeutic agents. It is important to ensure that the chelating agent is not metabolically degraded to metabolites which lack the ability to bind iron. This will inevitably require the use of higher drug levels, increasing the risk of inducing toxic side-effects.

Further therapeutic benefit can be gained by ensuring that the chelating agent is delivered to target sites at an appropriate concentration, rate and duration. Ideally for maximal chelation, a drug must be present within the body at both a reasonable concentration and duration to ensure interception of iron from either extracellular or intracellular iron pools. Compounds with short-plasma half lives are thus likely to be less effective due to the limited pool of chelatable iron present within the body at any one time.

Design of orally active chelating agents

The obvious method of choice is to model novel structures on natural hydroxamate and catechol siderophores [8]. Coordination of iron for both hydroxamates and catechols occurs with oxygen donor atoms which give rise to chelators which possess extremely high affinities for iron(III). Catechol-based ligands are unfortunately prone to oxidation in the intestine as well as generally being poorly absorbed. A further disadvantage of this ligand is that its iron complex has a net negative charge preventing it from efficiently crossing biological membranes. Hydroxamate ligands in contrast form neutral iron complexes but are metabolically labile and only poorly absorbed by the oral route.

A number of iron-chelating agents are currently being considered as orally active alternatives to DFO, the presently available therapeutic agent for the treatment of body iron overload resulting from frequent blood transfusion. These compounds include bidentate hydroxypyridinones (HPOs) (Fig. 1; **5**), tridentate desferrithiocin (DFT) analogues (Fig. 1; **6**) and hexadentate aminocarboxylate chelators, for instance HBED (Fig. 1; **4**) where 3, 2 and 1 of the above ligand(s) are coordinated with ferric iron respectively. The above ligands can also be classified by the donor atoms associated with the metal centre. High-spin tripositive ferric ion, due to its high charge density, forms most stable interactions with weakly polarizable atoms such as oxygen. Ferrous iron, in contrast, has a preference for nitrogen donor atoms. DFT and HBED, unlike HPO and DFO, bind iron via a mixture of oxygen and nitrogen donor atoms and thus are less specific for iron(III).

Potential toxicity of iron chelators

Chelating agents have the potential to induce toxic effects when they affect iron homoeostasis within the body. This can arise when the absorption, distribution and utilization of iron is affected. This safety margin may be increased in the presence of iron overload but as not all cells will be equally iron overloaded, some will be more susceptible to iron deprivation than others. Alternatively, chelating agents can induce side effects by directly interfering with iron-dependent metalloenzymes located within the body. The resultant iron complexes also have the ability to induce toxicity. Under certain circumstances, redox cycling of the iron centre with the corresponding generation of free radicals can result. The affinity constant of the ligand for iron is also important, since the lack of stability of complexes can lead to redistribution of iron from relative non-toxic iron stores to potentially toxic sites in the body, eventually leading to tissue damage.

Lack of iron selectivity

Unfortunately many ligands which possess a high affinity for iron (III) also have high affinities for other metals. Aminocarboxylate ligands such as DTPA, used in patients who develop toxic side-effects with DFO due to its relative lack of selectivity for iron (III), lead to zinc depletion. In an attempt to enhance the selectivity of this class of chelator for iron (III), Martell and co-workers have synthesized several hexadentate analogues which contain both carboxyl and phenolic ligands [9]. A particularly useful compound from this series is HBED which is significantly more effective than DFO when given intramuscularly to iron-overloaded rats. However, HBED is not efficiently absorbed via the oral route and by virtue of its two carboxyl functions, retains a relatively high affinity for zinc.

Another class of chelating agent which has been extensively evaluated over the past decade is DFT, a siderophore isolated from *Streptomyces antibioticus*. This compound is a tridentate molecule which forms a 2:1 complex with iron (III) [10]. DFT, however, retains an appreciable affinity for other metals, particularly copper and shows toxic effects in hepatocytes at high doses [11]. Long-term studies in non-iron-overloaded rodents (20 mg/kg per day) and dogs (30 mg/kg per day) reveal progressive signs of toxicity (reduced body weight gain and food consumption, nephropathy and neurotoxicity) even at relatively low doses. Because of the above toxicity problems, this compound is no longer considered to possess clinical potential as a chelating agent. However, a number of synthetic analogues, where the methyl group on the thiazoline ring has been replaced by a hydrogen atom and which lack some of the toxic effects of the parent drug, are presently being investigated [12]. Unfortunately, the metal selectivity of these new analogues is unlikely to differ significantly from that of the parent compound.

HPOs, which combine favourable aspects of both hydroxamate and catechol groups, give rise to compounds which possess high selectivity for iron (III). Both the free ligand and iron complex remain neutral over the physiological pH range of 5–9 and are hence able to readily cross biological membranes. A range of analogues of these compounds can also be made by varying substituents at positions 1- (R_1) and 2- (R_2) of the molecule. The considerable early promise displayed by HPOs in animal studies has been reflected in preliminary clinical studies conducted both in the U.K. and elsewhere [7,13,14].

Interaction with iron-containing enzymes

Even with a selective chelator for iron (III), toxicity may occur because the compound is capable of interacting with iron-containing enzymes. Iron-containing metalloenzymes can be divided into haem and non-haem types. In general, chelating agents are not effective inhibitors of haem-containing enzymes for two reasons: (i) the avid interaction between the porphyrin nucleus and iron and (ii) that bidentate interaction between the ligand and porphyrin-bound iron is not possible [15]. In contrast many non-haem iron-containing enzymes are extremely susceptible to inhibition by chelators. Iron centres dominated by oxygen and imidazole ligands are particularly susceptible. Such iron centres are found in ribonucleotide reductase, and lipoxygenase family of enzymes and tyrosine hydroxylase. Clearly iron(III) chelators should be designed to possess a low affinity for the active sites of these and other such enzymes.

Selective distribution of chelating agent and its iron complex

A systematic study of Levin [16] clearly indicated that not only is the $K_{part.}$ value of critical importance for the ability of a compound to penetrate the blood–brain barrier (BBB), but also the molecular mass. Thus although there is an excellent linear relationship between partition coefficient and permeability for molecules with molecular mass <300 Da, there is no such relationship with larger molecules (molecular mass >500 Da). Thus, most hexadentate ligands are predicted to penetrate the blood–brain barrier inefficiently, at best. In contrast bidentate ligands will penetrate relatively easily — an undesirable feature for most therapies. However, penetration of low-molecular-mass molecules is strongly dependent on $K_{part.}$ values and molecules with values <0.05 penetrate poorly [17].

Thus the same properties which maximize oral absorption will also endow the molecule with the ability to efficiently penetrate the blood–brain barrier. For this reason, it is important to ensure that chelating agents are directed to target tissue such as the heart and liver while minimizing exposure to critical organs/cells. Once intracellular iron has been chelated by the ligand, the resulting iron complex must also be able to cross cell membranes to remove iron from the cell. Thus both the free ligand and the iron complex should be water soluble and yet possess no charged groups. Consequently the iron complex should also be uncharged. Of the high-affinity iron chelators, only hydroxamate and HPO ligands possess this property.

Minimal redistribution of iron

In principle, the redistribution of iron can occur if both the ligand and its iron complex freely cross biological membranes. The affinity constant of a ligand for iron is also important, since the lack of stability of iron complexes can lead to redistribution from iron stores to potentially toxic sites in the body, eventually leading to tissue damage. Ideally, metal chelate complexes should be excreted rapidly in the faeces or urine with no redistribution of iron from relatively non-toxic sites such as the liver to more harmful ones such as the heart. Complexes formed intracellularly should not accumulate within cells, but should be able to freely permeate from cells. In the case of liver cells, this should result in significant excretion of iron in the bile. Clearly the biliary iron-chelator complex should not then be reabsorbed from the gut.

Toxicity of iron complexes

Depending on the coordination geometry and donor atoms associated with the iron centre, redox cycling of the metal with the corresponding generation of free radicals can result. Iron should be co-ordinated by the chelator in such a manner as to prevent direct access to oxidants and reductants (e.g. hydrogen peroxide and superoxide). If this is achieved, then hydroxyl radical production will be reduced to a minimum. Unfortunately this is not always so readily achieved. The relative ability of different ligands to generate free radicals is highly variable and will depend on a number of parameters [18]. The availability of the free coordination site on the metal is required for catalysis; thus the ability or otherwise of ligands to completely occupy the entire metal cation surface will strongly influence the efficiency of hydroxyl radical generation. The absolute affinity constant (K_1 or β_3) of the ligand for iron can also influence hydroxyl radical generation. A high affinity usually implies reduced access for oxidants/reductants.

Another important property of complexing agents which can influence free radical-generating ability of an iron complex is redox cycling. If the ligating atoms of a complex are mixed, such that some favour the oxidized form of the metal and some the reduced form, then a complex of intermediate redox potential is produced and as such can readily oscillate between oxidized and reduced forms. If the reduced form is readily autoxidized by oxygen then superoxide will be produced. Thus ligands such as DFO, which strongly bind Fe(III) via oxygen donor atoms to form an octahedral iron complex, only poorly generate hydroxyl radicals, in contrast to DFT which binds the metal via a mixture of oxygen and nitrogen donor atoms (Fig. 3).

Iron(III)-EDTA is present in solution as $[Fe(III)EDTA(H_2O)]^-$, EDTA being too small to completely encompass the iron mass [19]. This leads to the generation of a seventh coordination site which is occupied by a water molecule but can be easily displaced by oxidants/reductants, facilitating redox cycling of iron leading to the generation of free radicals. Other aminocarboxylate ligands such as DTPA [20], which bind iron in a 1:1 ratio, and NTA (Fig. 1; 8) [21], which binds in a 2:1 manner, like EDTA form complexes with seven coordination positions around the metal centre. However, unlike EDTA, all ligating atoms are derived from the chelating agents accounting for their reduced hydroxyl radical-generating ability compared with the former (Fig. 3). Although DTPA has a higher affinity for iron compared with NTA, it is significantly more efficient in generating hydroxyl radicals. A possible explanation for this is that the redox potential of the iron atom bound by DTPA differs from that of NTA since three of the seven coordination positions around the metal ion are occupied by nitrogen donor atoms. HBED, in contrast to the other aminocarboxylate ligands, only poorly generates hydroxyl radicals (Fig. 3). Molecular modelling of the HBED iron complex suggests that this ligand, largely due to the presence of two phenolate moieties, is capable of forming a six-coordinate complex. This, coupled with its extremely high affinity for iron ($K_1 = 10^{40}$), dramatically reduces its hydroxyl radical-generating ability (Fig. 3).

A complex with high kinetic stability is also essential to minimize free radical generation. Thus bidentate ligands such as HPOs and, to a lesser extent, tridentate

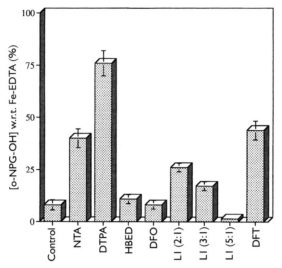

Fig. 3. The hydroxyl radical-generating ability of a range of iron complexes with respect to Fe-EDTA. Xanthine oxidase was used as a source of superoxide and hydrogen peroxide. Incubation conditions: 1 mM hypoxanthine, 0.02 unit/ml xanthine oxidase, 1 mM N,N'-(5-nitro-1,3-phenyl-ene)bisglutaramide (NPG), 0.5 mM iron complexed with various ligands; incubation period, 37 °C for 30 min. Hydroxylated products of NPG were separated and quantified by reversed-phase HPLC.

ligands such as DFT, provide optimal coordination number and stereochemistry, but, due to appreciable dissociation rate of the ligand from the complex, there are short intervals of time (typically 1 ms) when the complex will not be fully coordinated. In such a state, oxidants/reductants such as H_2O_2 and O_2^- can gain access to the metal centre and thereby generate free radicals. This is nicely illustrated by the dramatic decrease in hydroxyl radical generation of bidentate L1 in the presence of excess ligand (5:1) (Fig. 3). Here dissociation of one of the ligands from the metal centre, unlike the case for 3-fold excess of ligand (3:1), is immediately followed by replacement by an identical ligand and prevents oxidants/reductants from gaining access to the metal centre.

Conclusions

The introduction of a safe and effective chelating agent for use in the clinic almost inevitably requires compounds to fulfil most if not all the design criteria outlined in this chapter. Unfortunately this goal has eluded medicinal chemists and clinicians alike for over 20 years. Considerable progress has, however, been made over the last decade and the prospects for the emergence of a suitable iron chelator over the next few years with an acceptable therapeutic index to replace DFO is a realistic objective.

References

1. Halliwell, B. and Gutteridge, J.M.C. (1989) in Free Radicals in Biology and Medicine, 2nd edn., Clarendon Press
2. Wrigglesworth, J.M. and Baum, H. (1980) in Iron Biochemistry and Medicine II, (Jacobs, A. and Worwood, M., eds.), pp. 29–86, Academic Press, London
3. Hider, R.C., Porter, J.B. and Singh, S. (1994) in The Development of Iron Chelators for Clinical Use (Bergeron, R.J. and Britteham, G.M., eds.), pp. 353–371, CRC Press, Boca Raton, FL
4. Weatherall, D.J. and Clegg, J.B. (1981) in The Thalassaemia Syndromes, 3rd edn., Blackwell Scientific Press, London
5. Hider, R.C., Singh, S. and Porter, J.B. (1992) Proc. R. Soc. Edinburgh, **99B**, 137–168
6. Porter, J.B., Huehns, E.R. and Hider, R.C. (1989) in Bailliere's Clinical Haematology, (Hershko, C., ed.), vol. 2, pp. 257–292, Bailliere Tindall, London
7. Olivieri, N.F., Koren, G., Hermann, C., Bentur, Y., Chung, D., Klein, J., St. Louis, P., Freedman, M.H., McClelland, R.A. and Templeton, D.M. (1990) Lancet, **336**, 1275
8. Hider, R.C., Singh, S., Porter, J.B. and Huehns, E.R. (1990) Ann. N.Y. Acad. Sci., **612**, 327–338
9. Martell, A.E., Mortekaitis, R.J. and Clarke, E.T. (1986) Can. J. Chem., **64**, 449–456
10. Hahn, F.E., McMurry, T.J., Hugi, A. and Raymond, K.N. (1990) J. Am. Chem. Soc., **112**, 1845–1860
11. Baker, E., Wong, A., Peter, H. and Jacobs, A. (1992) Br. J. Haematol., **81**, 424–431
12. Bergeron, R.J., Wiegand, J., Dionis, J.B., Egli-Karmakka, M., Frei, J., Huxley-Tencer, A. and Peter, H.H. (1991) J. Med. Chem., **34**, 2072–2078
13. Kontoghiorghes, G.J., Bartlett, A.N., Hoffbrand, A.V., Goddard, J.G., Sheppard, L., Barr, J. and Nortey, P. (1990) Br. J. Haematol., **76**, 295–300
14. Tondury, P., Kontoghiorghes, G.J., Ridolfi-Luthy, A., Hirt, A., Hoffbrand, A.V., Lottenbach, A.M., Sanderegger, T. and Wagner, H.P. (1990) Br. J. Haematol., **76**, 550
15. Singh, S. and Hider, R.C. (1984) in Free Radical Damage and Its Control, (Rice-Evans, C. and Burdon, R.H., eds.), pp. 189–216, Elsevier Press, Amsterdam
16. Levin, V.A. (1980) J. Med. Chem., **23**, 682–687
17. Oldendorf, W.H. (1974) Proc. Soc. Exp. Biol. Med., **147**, 813–817
18. Singh, S. and Hider, R.C. (1988) Anal. Biochem., **171**, 47–54
19. Lind, M.D., Hamor, M.J. and Hoard, J.L. (1964) Inorg. Chem., **3**, 34–44
20. Finnen, D.C., Pinkerton, A.A., Dunham, W.R., Sands, R.H. and Funk-Junion, M.O. (1991) Inorg. Chem., **30**, 3960–3965
21. Clegg, W., Powell, A.K. and Ware, M.J. (1984) Acta Cryst. C. (CR. STR. COMM.), **40**, 1822–1826

Biochem. Soc. Symp. **61**, 139–152
Printed in Great Britain

Oxidative damage by ozone and nitrogen dioxide: synergistic toxicity *in vivo* but no evidence of synergistic oxidative damage in an extracellular fluid

Charles A. O'Neill*, Albert van der Vliet*, Jason P. Eiserich*, Jerold A. Last*, Barry Halliwell† and Carroll E. Cross*‡

*Division of Pulmonary-Critical Care Medicine, UC Davis School of Medicine, University of California, Davis, CA, U.S.A. and †Neurodegenerative Disease Research Centre, King's College, University of London, London, U.K.

Abstract

Inhalation of ozone (O_3) and/or nitrogen dioxide ($^{\bullet}NO_2$) is associated with the development of inflammation in the respiratory tract and various alterations in pulmonary functions. Respiratory tract lining fluids (RTLFs) represent the first biological fluids coming into contact with these inhaled toxicants. Using plasma as a surrogate for RTLFs, we have previously shown that O_3 [Cross, Motchnik, Bruener, Jones, Kaur, Ames and Halliwell (1992) FEBS Lett. **298**, 269–272] and $^{\bullet}NO_2$ [Halliwell, Hu, Louie, Duvall, Tarkington, Motchnik and Cross (1992) FEBS Lett. **313**, 62–66] are both capable of depleting antioxidants and damaging proteins and lipids. O_3 particularly damages proteins, whereas $^{\bullet}NO_2$ induces the peroxidation of lipids and nitrates aromatic amino acids. It has been reported that O_3 and $^{\bullet}NO_2$ cause synergistic toxicity in rodents [Gielzleichter, Witschi and Last (1992) Tox. Appl. Pharmacol. **116**, 1–9]. In the present chapter, we review evidence showing that combined exposure of these two oxidant gases to human plasma fails to exert synergistic oxidative damage to plasma constituents, and in fact, O_3 and $^{\bullet}NO_2$ antagonize each other's actions. We conclude that the potentiating effect of these two gases on morbidity and mortality in rodents represents a complex interactive biological effect rather than a simple synergistic oxidative effect in extracellular fluids.

---

‡To whom correspondence should be addressed.

Introduction

Respiratory tract (RT) defences against toxicity caused by inhalation of the oxidative pollutant gases ozone (O_3) and nitrogen dioxide (NO_2) include the action of antioxidants in both extracellular and cellular compartments. These defences include antioxidants present in the upper and lower respiratory tract lining fluids (RTLFs) [1,2]. Antioxidants present in the RTLFs would be expected to lessen the impact of oxidative stress elicited by both primary pollutants and by the potentially damaging secondary inflammatory-immune processes mediated largely by the recruitment and activation of circulating and resident phagocytes [3,4].

O_3 is a major component of photochemical air pollution and its oxidizing ability is believed to be largely responsible for its adverse biological effects [5–7]. O_3 reacts slowly with water at physiological pH to yield $HO^{\bullet}$ [8,9]. NO_2, like O_3, is an oxidizing gas with established pulmonary toxicity [10,11]. NO_2 is present in high levels in cigarette smoke and burning organic matter (up to 50 p.p.m.) as well as in smog (up to 1 p.p.m.) [12,13]. NO_2 can initiate lipid peroxidation, and end products of this process have been detected in rat lung lining fluids after NO_2 exposure [14,15].

We have investigated the effects of O_3 and NO_2 exposure on human plasma, as a model extracellular fluid [16–18], using an experimental system that approximates conditions whereby environmental oxidants would be presented to the RTLFs upon inhalation. We demonstrated antioxidant depletion and oxidative damage to plasma proteins and lipids during these exposures.

Exposure of rodents to both O_3 and NO_2 simultaneously was found to cause greater tissue damage and mortality than would be expected from the added effects of exposure to the two pollutants individually [19–22]. The authors of these reports have hypothesized that oxidative chemical reaction products generated by O_3 and NO_2 could be responsible for the synergistic toxic effects observed.

In this chapter, we summarize the predominant extracellular antioxidant species present in RTLFs and review our earlier findings with O_3 and NO_2 plasma exposures. We discuss the *in vivo* studies showing synergistic interactions of exposures of O_3 and NO_2 on rodent lungs. Lastly, we present results of *in vitro* experiments in which human plasma was exposed to a combination of O_3 and NO_2, in the exact same chambers as those used in the previously mentioned *in vivo* animal exposures which were performed to investigate whether combined exposure to O_3 and NO_2 results in potentiated respiratory tract damage.

RTLF and plasma antioxidants

The antioxidants in RTLFs include ascorbic acid, uric acid, albumin, mucins and glutathione (GSH), the metal-binding proteins lactoferrin and transferrin, superoxide dismutase and small amounts of other antioxidant enzymes including catalase and glutathione peroxidase [1,2,23]. We and others have quantified the concentrations of selected non-enzymic antioxidants of normal human plasma and

Table 1. Concentrations of some non-enzymic antioxidants in human plasma and peripheral RTLFs (epithelial lining fluid; ELF).

Antioxidant	Plasma (μmol/l)[a]	ELF (μmol/l)
Ascorbic acid	64 ± 8	54 ± 5
Glutathione	1.0 ± 0.2	182 ± 25
Uric acid	379 ± 59	178 ± 3
α-Tocopherol	16 ± 2	1.6 ± 0.2
Albumin	662	50[b]
Mucin	0	Variable

[a]Plasma and ELF values from [48].
[b]ELF albumin from [49].

epithelial lining fluid (ELF; distal RTLFs) obtained through bronchoalveolar lavage. The major antioxidants present in human RTLFs are shown in Table 1 which also provides comparisons with those present in plasma. Important additional aspects of the RTLFs' antioxidant defences include the facts that the fluid depth and antioxidant compositions show considerable variation depending on the anatomical level of the RT being considered. For example, proximal RTLFs are approximately 10 μm in depth [1] and contain large amounts of mucin, which can exert antioxidant effects [24], whereas distal RTLFs are approximately 0.1 μm in depth [1] and contain little mucin.

The difficulty of obtaining undiluted human RTLFs for exposure to O_3 and $\cdot NO_2$ has led us to employ plasma as a model for RTLFs in our exposure systems, due primarily to its easy procurement and well-characterized antioxidant constituents [25–27]. We recognize that plasma does not exactly represent RTLFs since some constituents in the latter are missing in the former, including mucin and surfactant. Furthermore, plasma contains significantly greater concentrations of albumin, which represents an important antioxidant [28]. However, when RT oedema takes place as a result of cigarette smoke exposure, 'neurogenic inflammation' or direct cellular injury, the RTLFs become increasingly plasma-like due to exudation from the vasculature [29,30]. Hence we feel that studies with plasma are an approximate representation of the spectrum of reactions that could occur in RTLFs during interactions with environmental oxidants.

Oxidation of plasma constituents by O_3

In order to assess the effects of O_3 on the human RT we exposed human plasma to this oxidant and determined antioxidant depletions and oxidative modifications to proteins and lipids [16,17]. A concentration of 16 p.p.m. of O_3 was used to accelerate the oxidative changes since the surface:volume ratio in this experimental system is much lower than that of the RT [31] and because, to a major degree, O_3 absorption is believed to be surface area (and reactive solute) dependent [32,33]. As controls, plasma samples were placed in identical chambers and exposed to filtered air. Uric acid and ascorbic acid were quickly oxidized during O_3 exposure, both to approximately 20% of control values at 2 h, and entirely consumed by 4 h (Fig. 1). Quantitatively, more uric acid was consumed during this exposure compared with ascorbic acid, as uric acid is approx. 5 times more concentrated in plasma than ascorbic acid. When plasma was supplemented with ascorbic acid (250 μmol/l) or uric acid (1 mmol/l) before exposure to O_3, similar ascorbic acid and uric acid depletions were observed in percentage terms, but the total oxidation of these antioxidants was larger, illustrating the concept of reactive absorption; a greater amount of oxidizable substance present in the absorbing liquid phase causes increased O_3 absorption via direct reaction with the oxidizable material [33–35]. This illustrates an important point in so far as RT defences against inhaled oxidant pollutants are concerned: the greater the concentrations of antioxidants in the proximal RTLFs, the greater the amount of pollutant that will be absorbed, lessening the amount of pollutant delivered to more sensitive, probably less well protected (decreased RTLF depth), peripheral airway gas-exchanging epithelial surfaces.

We also quantified the effects of O_3 on the lipid and protein constituents of plasma. No significant loss of α-tocopherol was seen after 4 h of 16 p.p.m. O_3 exposure (Fig. 1) [16]. Lipid peroxidation, as measured by the level of lipid hydroperoxides, was observed in only small amounts after a 4 h exposure. Exposure of plasma to 16 p.p.m. O_3 also resulted in loss of protein-SH groups (Fig. 1) [16]. Another index of protein damage, protein carbonyl formation, approximately doubled over a 4 h period [17].

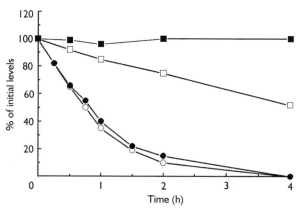

Fig. 1. Depletion of antioxidants and protein thiol groups in human plasma by exposure to 16 p.p.m. O_3. Fresh plasma (4 ml) was placed in Falcon plates (3 cm diameter), inserted into a closed container at 37 °C (5% CO_2/95% air, humidified) and exposed to 16 p.p.m. O_3 for up to 4 h. Results are expressed as a percentage of the antioxidant present (100% at zero time). Ascorbic acid depletions were corrected for the slow loss of ascorbic acid in filtered air-exposed controls. ○, Ascorbic acid; ●, uric acid; □, protein -SH; ■, α-tocopherol.

Oxidation of plasma constituents by $^\bullet NO_2$

We have also investigated the reactions of $^\bullet NO_2$ with plasma antioxidants, proteins and lipids [18]. In order to maintain plasma pH during the $^\bullet NO_2$ exposures it was necessary to buffer fresh human plasma with 500 mmol/l KH_2PO_4/K_2HPO_4 buffer [80:20 (v/v) dilution; pH 7.4]. Plasma buffer solution (4 ml) was placed in Falcon plates and inserted into an environmentally controlled exposure chamber in which a steady concentration of 14 p.p.m. $^\bullet NO_2$ was maintained for up to 6 h. A schematic representation of the exposure chamber setup is shown in Fig. 2.

Exposure of human plasma to $^\bullet NO_2$ leads to a rapid loss of ascorbic acid, uric acid and plasma thiol groups (Fig. 3), with ascorbic acid being lost at the greatest percentage rate and uric acid slightly more slowly [18]. As with O_3 exposure, uric acid was lost in much greater amounts than ascorbic acid and plasma thiol groups. In contrast to our results with O_3 exposure, addition of ascorbic acid (1 mmol/l) to plasma before exposure of the plasma to $^\bullet NO_2$ slowed the loss of uric acid, and the loss of uric acid was faster when plasma ascorbic acid was depleted with ascorbic oxidase. This most likely implies that reaction of $^\bullet NO_2$ (a free radical) with uric acid produces a uric acid radical that can be re-converted into uric acid (recycled) by ascorbic acid [36,37]. Exposure of plasma to $^\bullet NO_2$ induced a significant loss of α-tocopherol at 4 h (Fig. 3) with a concomitant rise in cholesterol ester hydroperoxide formation, to a larger extent than during similar exposure to O_3. The loss of α-tocopherol and formation of cholesteryl ester hydroperoxide was also inhibited by the addition of ascorbic acid, possibly due to the recycling of α-tocopheroxyl radical by ascorbic acid [38,39].

Exposure Chamber

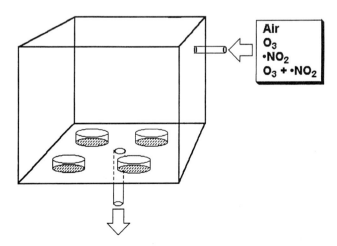

Fig. 2. Schematic representation of the chamber used for the exposures to O_3 and/or $^\bullet NO_2$ in this study.

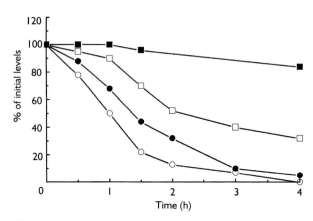

Fig. 3. Depletion of antioxidants and protein thiol groups in human plasma by 14 p.p.m. NO₂ exposure. Results are expressed as a percentage of the antioxidant present (100% at zero time). Ascorbic acid depletions are corrected for the slow loss of ascorbic acid in filtered air-exposed controls. ○, Ascorbic acid; ●, uric acid; □, protein-SH; ■, α-tocopherol.

Effects of combined O₃ and ˙NO₂ exposure *in vivo*: 'synergistic' toxicity

Male adult Sprague–Dawley rats were exposed nocturnally to either 0.8 p.p.m. O₃, 14.4 p.p.m. ˙NO₂, or the combination of 0.8 p.p.m. O₃ and 14.4 p.p.m. ˙NO₂ for 6 h/day 7 days/week in the same exposure chambers as those used for the *in vitro* exposure of plasma to ˙NO₂ (Fig. 2) [19–22]. After approximately 7 to 10 weeks animals demonstrated respiratory insufficiency and weight loss, with half the exposed animals dying between 8 and 11 weeks. No such effects were seen in animals exposed to O₃ alone, ˙NO₂ alone or filtered air. O₃/˙NO₂-exposed animals had increased lung content of DNA, protein, elastin and total collagen (as measured by hydroxyproline analysis) as compared with animals exposed to filtered air. Mature lung collagen, as measured by the content of the tri-functional cross-link hydroxypyridinium, was decreased approximately 40% in animals exposed to O₃/˙NO₂ compared with control animals exposed to filtered air. Histopathological analysis of the O₃/˙NO₂-exposed animals indicated alveolar collapse, increased lung connective-tissue deposition, lung honeycombing, lung macrophage and mast-cell accumulation, and lung vascular smooth-muscle hypertrophy, all indicative of severe progressive centriacinar pulmonary fibrosis and end-stage lung disease [21,22].

Ichinose and Sagai [40] continuously exposed rats and guinea pigs for 2 weeks to O₃ and ˙NO₂, both at 0.4 p.p.m., and found increased lung levels of thiobarbituric acid (TBA)-reactive substances (a putative index of lipid peroxidation) in guinea pigs but not in rats. This increase in TBA-reactive substances was not observed in animals exposed to either ˙NO₂ or O₃ alone. Exposure of rats, but not guinea pigs, to the combination of O₃ and ˙NO₂ caused synergistic increases in non-protein thiol, ascorbic acid and some antioxidant enzyme systems of lung tissue homogenates. The authors concluded that the ability to increase anti-oxidative protective factors following exposure to combined $O_3/\cdot NO_2$ prevents oxidative damage in rats (at least as measured by TBA-reactive substances). Differences in observations between this study and that of Gelzleichter et al. [19,20] may be attributed to the oxidant dose delivered and the duration of exposure.

Modification of plasma constituents by combined exposure to O_3 and $\cdot NO_2$: 'non-synergistic' oxidative damage

To ascertain whether exposure of plasma to the combination of O_3 and $\cdot NO_2$ could produce potentiated oxidative damage, we exposed plasma to the combination of these gases at two levels of O_3 and $\cdot NO_2$: (i) using identical levels as those used in the in vivo studies of Gelzleichter et al. [19]; and (ii) using 6.0 p.p.m. O_3 and 10.0 p.p.m. $\cdot NO_2$ alone and in combination. Freshly obtained human plasma was again buffered with 500 mmol/l phosphate buffer (by 80:20 dilution) to prevent pH changes caused by $\cdot NO_2$ and/or loss of CO_2. Plasma exposed to a combination of O_3 (0.8 p.p.m.) and $\cdot NO_2$ (14.4 p.p.m.) displayed rapid losses of ascorbic acid, uric acid and thiol groups, but these depletions were not increased compared with those in plasma exposed to 14.4 p.p.m. $\cdot NO_2$ alone (Table 2). In fact, depletion of the various antioxidants was slower than expected from the sum of the effects of O_3 and $\cdot NO_2$ alone. Protein carbonyl formation by $O_3/\cdot NO_2$ was less than that observed after exposure to O_3 alone (Fig. 4). α-Tocopherol depletion (Fig. 5) and cholesteryl linoleate hydroperoxide formation (Fig. 6) occurred during exposure to $O_3/\cdot NO_2$ but to a lesser extent than with $\cdot NO_2$ alone.

When plasma was exposed to 6.0 p.p.m. O_3 and 10.0 p.p.m. $\cdot NO_2$, both alone and in combination, similar effects to the 0.8/14.4 $O_3/\cdot NO_2$ exposures were observed. Decreases in plasma ascorbic acid, uric acid, α-tocopherol and protein thiol groups during exposure to $O_3/\cdot NO_2$ were intermediate between those found during exposure to only O_3 or $\cdot NO_2$ (Table 2). Additionally, aromatic hydroxylation by O_3, studied by exposing solutions of phenylalanine in phosphate buffer, and measured by p-, m-, and o-tyrosine (Tyr) formation, was decreased by co-exposure to $\cdot NO_2$. Similarly, nitration of Tyr (in phosphate buffer) by $\cdot NO_2$, as detected by 3-NO_2-Tyr production, was decreased during co-exposure to O_3.

Taken together, we did not observe increased antioxidant depletion or potentiated oxidative damage to plasma proteins or lipids during exposure to both O_3 and $\cdot NO_2$, as compared with exposure to O_3 and $\cdot NO_2$ alone. We conclude that the toxicity seen in vivo with $O_3/\cdot NO_2$ exposure is not due to a synergistic 'oxidizing effect' of these inhaled toxicants (at least in this model system for RTLFs) since we were unable to demonstrate increases in oxidative damage by O_3 and $\cdot NO_2$ combined exposure compared with either O_3 or $\cdot NO_2$ alone. In fact, indices of oxidative damage are decreased during combined O_3 and $\cdot NO_2$ exposure compared with O_3 and $\cdot NO_2$ alone.

Table 2. Depletion of plasma antioxidants following 2 h exposure to O$_3$, ·NO$_2$ or the combination O$_3$ and ·NO$_2$ at different exposure levels. Data represented as a percentage loss of antioxidant (average ±S.E.M., $n \geq 5$) compared with the filtered air-exposed plasma at 2 h. Plasma samples exposed to O$_3$ (0.8 p.p.m.), ·NO$_2$ (14.4 p.p.m.) were diluted 80:20 with 500 μmol/l KH$_2$PO$_4$/K$_2$HPO$_4$, pH 7.4, to maintain pH during exposure.

Plasma	O$_3$ (6 p.p.m.)	·NO$_2$ (10 p.p.m.)	O$_3$ (6 p.p.m.) +NO$_2$ (10 p.p.m.)	O$_3$ (0.8 p.p.m.)	·NO$_2$ (14.4 p.p.m.)	O$_3$ (0.8 p.p.m.) +NO$_2$ (14.4 p.p.m.)
Ascorbic acid	81±10	94±4	92±4	52±14	100	100
Uric acid	91±1	35±7	71±7	34±5	61±3	60±2
Plasma-SH	11±6	33±7	29±9	3±2	49±2	41±3
α-Tocopherol	11±6	7±1	2±4	0±8	23±3	12±5

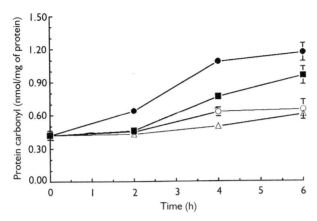

Fig. 4. Formation of plasma protein carbonyls by O₃, ˙NO₂ and combined O₃/˙NO₂ exposure. Results are expressed as nmol/mg of protein (mean±S.E.M., $n = 3$). ●, O₃ (0.8 p.p.m.); ○, ˙NO₂ (14.4 p.p.m.); ■, O₃/˙NO₂ (0.8/14.4 p.p.m.); △, filtered air.

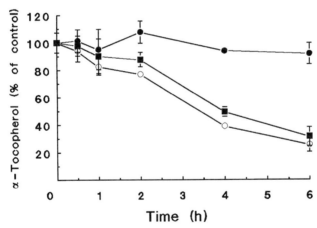

Fig. 5. Depletion of plasma α-tocopherol by O₃, ˙NO₂ and combined O₃/˙NO₂ exposure. Results are expressed as a percentage (mean±S.E.M., $n = 3$) of filtered air-exposed controls. ●, O₃ (0.8 p.p.m.); ○, ˙NO₂ (14.4 p.p.m.); ■, O₃/˙NO₂ (0.8/14.4 p.p.m.).

Possible explanations for increased biological toxicity with O₃ and ˙NO₂ combined exposure

Our results suggest that the observed synergistic toxicity of combined O₃ and ˙NO₂ exposure, *in vivo*, is not due to increased oxidant damage by direct interaction between O₃ and ˙NO₂ in extracellular fluids. Several explanations can be postulated for the *in vivo* synergistic toxicity.

First, either oxidant gas may deplete antioxidants in the upper RT and thereby allow O₃/˙NO₂ to penetrate deeper into the more delicate and less

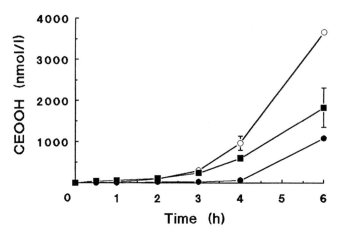

Fig. 6. Formation of plasma cholesteryl linoleate hydroperoxide (CEOOH) by O₃, ˙NO₂ and combined O₃/˙NO₂ exposure. Results are expressed as nmol/l (mean ± S.E.M., $n = 3$). ●, O_3 (0.8 p.p.m.); ○, ˙NO_2 (14.4 p.p.m.); ■, O_3/˙NO_2 (0.8/14.4 p.p.m.).

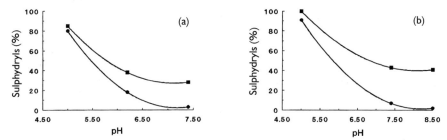

Fig. 7. The effects of pH on sulphydryl depletion of GSH and lipid free BSA by O₃ (a) and ˙NO₂ (b) exposure. (a) GSH and BSA, in 50 mM KH_2PO_4/K_2HPO_4, were exposed to 16 p.p.m. O_3 at the pHs indicated for 2 h. Results are expressed as a percentage of filtered air-exposed control. (b) GSH and BSA, in 50 mM KH_2PO_4/K_2HPO_4, were exposed to 14.4 p.p.m. ˙NO_2 at the pHs indicated for 2 h. Results are expressed as a percentage of filtered air-exposed control.

protected gas-exchanging region of the lung [32,35]. Peden and co-workers [41,42] have shown that uric acid may be a major antioxidant in the upper RT, particularly in the nasal cavity, and our experiments with plasma exposed to O_3 or ˙NO_2 have shown that uric acid is the most important antioxidant, although no quantitative evaluations of the antioxidant contributions that RT mucin could make currently exist in the literature.

Secondly, acidification of the surface upper RTLFs by inhaled high levels of ˙NO_2 will decrease the reactivity of protein and GSH thiol groups towards O_3 and ˙NO_2. *In vitro* studies have shown that oxidation of -SH groups (in GSH, cysteine or albumin) by O_3 or ˙NO_2 strongly depends on pH and is much slower at pH 5 than at neutral pH [43] (Fig. 7). This would imply that reactivity of surface -SH groups in RTLFs (on mucin, albumin, or GSH) could be decreased, resulting in less reactive absorption of O_3 or $\cdot NO_2$ in the upper airways, which in turn would allow for higher concentrations of inhaled O_3 and $\cdot NO_2$ to penetrate to the lower airways and gas-exchanging surfaces. However, a recent short-term study with O_3 exposure in combination with HNO_3 failed to show increased toxicity [44], which is evidence contrary to this suggestion.

The third and most likely explanation is that O_3 and $\cdot NO_2$ react to form higher oxides of nitrogen (either in the gas phase or in the aqueous phase). In the gas phase O_3 is known to react rapidly with $\cdot NO_2$ [45].

$$\cdot NO_2 + O_3 \rightarrow NO_3 \cdot + O_2 \tag{1}$$

The resulting nitrate radical ($NO_3 \cdot$) subsequently reacts extremely fast ($k = 1.2 \times 10^9 \text{ M}^{-1} \cdot \text{s}^{-1}$) with $\cdot NO_2$ [45].

$$NO_3 \cdot + \cdot NO_2 \rightarrow N_2O_5 \tag{2}$$

During the simultaneous exposures to both O_3 and $\cdot NO_2$ these reactions become very significant since O_3 and $\cdot NO_2$ levels were maintained at the same levels as used during simultaneous exposures to $\cdot NO_2$ or O_3 alone. As a consequence, other products are formed (presumably mostly N_2O_5). This is indirectly indicated by stopping the flow of O_3 or $\cdot NO_2$ into the chamber used for the combined exposure to O_3 and $\cdot NO_2$ and measuring the increase in concentration of the other gas (e.g. $\cdot NO_2$ or O_3). As shown in Table 3, when one gas flow was stopped, the measured levels of the other gas (either O_3 or $\cdot NO_2$) increased dramatically, indicating that substantial reaction occurred between O_3 and $\cdot NO_2$ in the exposure chamber. Hence, combined $O_3/\cdot NO_2$ exposures, both *in vivo* and *in vitro*, led to substantial exposure to high amounts of other reaction products (such

Table 3. Actual exposure concentrations of O_3 and $\cdot NO_2$ during combination exposures. During combined exposures to $\cdot NO_2$ and O_3, using either 0.8 p.p.m. O_3/14.4 p.p.m. $\cdot NO_2$ (1) or 6.0 p.p.m. O_3/10 p.p.m. $\cdot NO_2$ (2), significant reaction occurs, as reflected by increased levels of either O_3 or $\cdot NO_2$ when flow of the other oxidant was stopped. O_3* represents the concentration of O_3 in the chamber when O_3 flow into the chamber was maintained and $\cdot NO_2$ flow was stopped; $\cdot NO_2*$ represents the concentrated $\cdot NO_2$ in the chamber when $\cdot NO_2$ flow was maintained while O_3 flow was stopped. These increases (shown between parentheses) indicate that O_3 and $\cdot NO_2$ react stoichiometrically at a 1:2 to 1:3 ratio.

Exposure	1		2	
	O_3 (p.p.m.)	$\cdot NO_2$ (p.p.m.)	O_3 (p.p.m.)	$\cdot NO_2$ (p.p.m.)
$O_3 + \cdot NO_2$	0.8	14.4	5.8	9.7
O_3*	2.3 (+1.5)	—	13.5 (+7.7)	—
$\cdot NO_2*$	—	17.8 (+3.4)	—	31.9 (+22.2)

as N_2O_5). The *in vitro* data suggest that these products are not potent oxidants, as in fact we observed antagonism between O_3 and $\cdot NO_2$ with all of our oxidative endpoints. However, these products may significantly contribute to *in vivo* toxicity. One interesting possibility is that N_2O_5 may decompose to form NO_2^+, a powerful nitrating species. Synthetic chemical studies in organic solvents have shown that O_3 can indeed enhance nitration of aromatic compounds [46]. However, our studies with tyrosine nitration did not confirm this. In the biological aqueous phase N_2O_5 rapidly hydrolyses directly to NO_3^-, decreasing the likelihood that the transient intermediate NO_2^+ is involved in biomolecular damage.

Finally, it could speculatively be suggested that $\cdot NO_2$ could itself scavenge O_3-derived radicals [47], decreasing 'oxidative' damage but forming cytotoxic species. Since $\cdot NO_2$ is in excess of O_3, it could be expected to 'trap' or scavenge O_3-derived radicals that might be present on the surface of biological fluids reacting with O_3.

Suggested future studies

In order to investigate these various possible explanations, reactive absorption of $\cdot NO_2$ or O_3 should be studied during combined exposures and compared with exposures to $\cdot NO_2$ or O_3 alone. It is possible that different products from reactions of O_3 and $\cdot NO_2$ with lipids, for example, may synergistically enhance recruitment of phagocytes and thereby increase the inflammatory immune response. For instance, it is known that O_3 reacts readily with lipids, but does not form high amounts of lipid hydroperoxides (as measured in this study). Instead, O_3 breaks down unsaturated fatty acids to aldehydes, hydrogen peroxide and various radical species [47]. Interactions of the direct effects of $O_3/\cdot NO_2$ with each other, with components of the ensuing inflammatory-immune reaction (e.g. their reactive oxygen and nitrogen species) and/or with reparative responses all need better characterization. As the reactive products between O_3 and $\cdot NO_2$ in the gas phase may contribute to toxicity, studies observing the effect of $O_3/\cdot NO_2$ on various isolated cell systems would yield further insight into the synergistic mechanism of $\cdot NO_2/O_3$ toxicity.

This work was supported by the National Institute of Health Grants HL47628, HL070013, ES 05707 and ES-00628.

References

1. Hatch, G.E. (1992) in Comparative Biology of the Normal Lung (Parent, R.A., ed.), pp. 617–634, CRC Press, Boca Raton, FL
2. Cross, C.E., van der Vliet, A., O'Neill, C.A., Louie, S. and Halliwell, B. (1994) Envir. Health Perspect. **102** (Suppl. 10), 185–192
3. Ward, P.A. (1994) Environ. Health Perspect. **102** (Suppl. 10), 13–16
4. Smith, J.A. (1994) J. Leukoc. Biol. **56**, 672–686
5. Mustafa, M.G. (1990) Free Radical Biol. Med. **9**, 245–265
6. Pryor, W.A. (1992) Free Radical Biol. Med. **12**, 83–88

7. Bhalla, D.K. (1994) Toxicol. Lett. **73**, 91–101
8. Glaze, W.H. (1986) Environ. Health Perspect. **69**, 151–155
9. Kaur, H. and Halliwell, B. (1994) Anal. Biochem. **220**, 11–15
10. Mustafa, M.G. and Tierney, D.F. (1978) Am. Rev. Respir. Dis. **118**, 1061–1068
11. Lai, C.C. and Finlayson-Pitts, B.J. (1991) Lipids **26**, 306–314
12. Pryor, W.A. (1992) Free Radical Biol. Med. **13**, 659–676
13. Cueto, R. and Pryor, W.A. (1994) Vibrat. Spect. **7**, 97–111
14. Cavanagh, D.G. and Morris, J.B. (1987) J. Toxicol. Environ. Health **22**, 313–328
15. Sagai, M. and Ichinose, T. (1991) Toxicology **66**, 121–132
16. Cross, C.E., Motchnik, P.A., Bruener, B.A., Jones, D.A., Kaur, H., Ames, B.N. and Halliwell, B. (1992) FEBS Lett. **298**, 269–272
17. Cross, C.E., Reznick, A.Z., Packer, L., Davis, P.A., Suzuki, Y.J. and Halliwell, B. (1992) Free Radical Res. Commun. **15**, 347–352
18. Halliwell, B., Hu, M.-L., Louie, S., Duvall, T.R., Tarkington, B.K., Motchnick, P. and Cross, C.E. (1992) FEBS Lett. **313**, 62–66
19. Gelzleichter, T.R., Witschi, H. and Last, J.A. (1992) Toxicol. Appl. Pharmacol. **112**, 73–80
20. Gelzleichter, T.R., Witschi, H. and Last, J.A. (1992) Toxicol. Appl. Pharmacol. **116**, 1–9
21. Last, J.A., Gelzleichter, T.R., Pinkerton, K.E., Walker, R.M. and Witschi, H. (1993) Am. Rev. Respir. Dis. **148**, 487–494
22. Last, J.A., Sun, W.-M. and Witschi, H. (1994) Environ. Health Perspect. **102** (Suppl. 10), 179–184
23. Davis, W.B. and Pacht, E.R. (1991) in The Lung: Scientific Foundations, (Crystal, R.G., West, J.B. et al., eds.), pp. 1821–1826, Raven Press, New York
24. Cross, C.E., Halliwell, B. and Allan, A. (1984) Lancet **i**, 1328–1330
25. Halliwell, B. and Gutteridge, J.M.C. (1990) Arch. Biochem. Biophys. **280**, 1–8
26. Stocker, R. and Frei, B. (1991) in Oxidative Stress: Oxidants and Antioxidants (Sies, H., ed.), pp. 213–243, Academic Press, London
27. Sies, H., Stahl, W. and Sundquist, A.R. (1992) Ann. N.Y. Acad. Sci. **669**, 7–20
28. Halliwell, B. (1988) Biochem. Pharmacol. **37**, 569–571
29. Lei, Y.-H., Barnes, P.J. and Rogers, D. (1995) Am. J. Respir. Crit. Care Med. **151**, 1752–1762
30. Greiff, L., Erjefalt, I., Svensson, C., Wollmer, P., Alkner, U., Andersson, M. and Persson, C.G.A. (1993) Clin. Physiol. **13**, 219–233
31. Weibel, E.R. (1987) Annu. Rev. Physiol. **49**, 147–159
32. Postlethwait, E.M., Langford, S.D., Jacobson, L.M. and Bidani, A. (1995) Free Radical Biol. Med. in the press
33. Kanofsky, J.R. and Sima, P.D. (1995) Arch. Biochem. Biophys. **316**, 52–62
34. Postlethwait, E.M. and Bidani, A. (1990) J. Appl. Physiol. **68**, 594–603
35. Postlethwait, E.M. and Bidani, A. (1994) Toxicology **89**, 217–237
36. Maples, K.R. and Mason, R.P. (1988) J. Biol. Chem. **263**, 1709–1712
37. Aruoma, O.I. and Halliwell, B. (1989) FEBS Lett. **244**, 76–80
38. Packer, J.E., Slater, T.F. and Willson, R.L. (1979) Nature (London) **278**, 737–738
39. Packer, L. (1992) Proc. Soc. Exp. Biol. Med. **224**, 271–276
40. Ichinose, T. and Sagai, M. (1989) Toxicology **59**, 259–270
41. Peden, D.B., Hohman, R., Brown, M.E., Mason, R.T., Berkebile, C., Fales, H.M.

and Kaliner, M.A. (1991) Proc. Natl. Acad. Sci. U.S.A. 7, 7638–7642

42. Peden, D.B., Swiersz, M., Ohkubo, K. and Hahn, B. (1993) Am. Rev. Respir. Dis. 148, 455–461

43. O'Neill, C.A., van der Vliet, A., Hu, M.-L., Kaur, H., Cross, C.E., Louie, S. and Halliwell, B. (1993) J. Lab. Clin. Med. 122, 497–505

44. Aris, R., Christian, D., Tager, I., Ngo, L., Finkbeiner, W.E. and Balmes, J.R. (1993) Am. Rev. Respir. Dis. 148, 965–973

45. Huie, R.E. (1994) Toxicology 89, 193–216

46. Suzuki, H., Murashima, T., Kozai, I. and Mori, T. (1993) J. Chem. Soc. Perkin Trans. 1591–1597

47. Pryor, W.A. (1994) Free Radical Biol. Med. 17, 451–465

48. O'Neill, C.A., van der Vliet, A., Wu, R., Cross, C.E., Halliwell, B. and Louie, S. (1994) Respir. Med. 88, 822

49. Rennard, S., Basset, G., Lecossier, D., O'Donnell, K., Martin, P. and Crystal, R.G. (1986) J. Appl. Physiol. 60, 532–538

Biochem. Soc. Symp. **61**, 153–161
Printed in Great Britain

Biological and biochemical effects of air pollutants: synergistic effects of sulphite

Susanne Hippeli and Erich F. Elstner

Lehrstuhl für Phytopathologie, Labor für angewandte Biochemie, Technische Universität München, 85350 Weihenstephan, Germany

Abstract

Air pollution has become a major public and political concern since the beginning of industrialization, particularly motor exhaust over the past three decades. Epidemiological studies, together with clinical trials and experiments in exposition chambers (including biochemical model reactions), have contributed to our knowledge of potential dangers and increased our understanding of the corresponding mechanisms and dose-response effects. Comparison of the threatening reports that appear almost daily in the press with the digest of over 800 scientific publications allows the statement that the impact of ozone and nitric oxide on the health and performance of plants and animals is widely overestimated and appears to be used as a political instrument. In contrast, the combination of SO_2 with soot or asbestos particles may represent an underestimated toxic potential.

In this communication, we shall concentrate on basic redox mechanisms involving SO_2 and important target molecules, as well as looking at the cooperative effects of sulphite and soot particles.

Introduction

Air pollution research has tremendously increased in the past two decades, accompanied by the publication of a wealth of data. To mention just a few titles: 'Responses of Plants to Air Pollutants' [1], 'Introduction to Environmental Toxicology' [2], 'Air Pollution and Forests' [3], 'Effects of Gaseous Air Pollution in Agriculture and Horticulture' [4], 'Gaseous Air Pollutants and Plant Metabolism' [5], 'Air Pollution by Photochemical Oxidants' [6] and 'Air Pollution and Plant Metabolism' [7]. Several reviews emphasizing the importance of oxygen radicals in air pollution have also appeared recently [8–10].

The role of oxidative processes in air pollution has already been reported in the last century when the production of acid rain was recognized as an oxidation by atmospheric hydrogen peroxide of sulphur dioxide stemming from coal combustion [11].

SO_2 emissions are of special interest as the main component of the acid (London-type) smog and as a monocausal trigger of forest decline ('Waldsterben') in SO_2-polluted areas.

Certain trace gases stemming from industry, traffic and agriculture are a growing threat, especially for the industrialized countries all over the world. In the last few years especially, automobile exhaust has advanced to become a focus of public and political discussions and decisions. Airborne soot particles stemming both from industrial incinerators and diesel engines are discussed as potential carcinogens, allergens and/or inducers of respiratory diseases. The combinations of SO_2 and soot from coal burning have been epidemiologically shown to be responsible for thousands of deaths during several severe smog episodes both in London and in New York not too long ago. Several reports have appeared concentrating on biochemical mechanisms underlying these synergisms [10,12–14].

Significant health-threatening effects brought about by gases or air-borne particles may in the first line be seen in the cooperation of catalytically active particles with SO_2. This will be outlined in more detail below.

Reactions of SO_2 with biomolecules

SO_2 is produced during combustion of organic materials, especially coal. SO_2 is a highly water-soluble gas which is rapidly hydrated forming sulphite (SO_3^{2-}) [15]. Principally, SO_2 or HSO_3^- preferentially reacts with the following types of molecules: (a) aldehydes and ketones, where hydroxysulphonates are formed, which in turn are inhibitors of several enzymes; (b) olefines, where sulphonic acids are formed and the double bond is lost; (c) pyrimidines under formation of dihydrosulphonates, which may have mutagenic effects; (d) disulphides during formation of S-sulphonates, where the S–S bridge is split; and (e) superoxide ($O_2^{\cdot-}$) under formation of the very reactive bisulphite radical:

$$O_2^{\cdot-} + SO_3^{2-} + 2H^+ \Leftrightarrow SO_3^{\cdot-} + H_2O_2$$

In this reaction, superoxide may be substituted by transition metal ions:

$$M^{n+} + SO_3^{2-} \rightarrow M^{(n-1)+} + SO_3^{\cdot-}$$

$SO_3^{\cdot-}$ is a powerful initiator of several radical chain processes such as lipid peroxidation (see below). Sulphite modifies the cellular energy metabolism in mammalian tissues by decreasing the cellular ATP pool; this may be due to changing the function of pyridine and flavin nucleotides [16]. Sulphite oxidase, an enzyme absent in human lung tissue, oxidizes sulphite. Thus, if sulphite is not metabolized, it may be oxidized via radical chain mechanisms.

Plant damage by SO_2

Plant damage, caused by SO_2, is oxygen and light dependent. Typical SO_2 effects are the rapid inhibition of photosynthesis before direct symptoms such as bleaching of chlorophyll can be observed. The bleaching of chlorophyll is the most prominent effect of SO_2. SO_2, or its aqueous solution sulphite, can be oxidized in the presence of superoxide ($O_2^{\cdot-}$) [15]. Limited NAD^+ availability in the stroma of chloroplasts results in the formation of superoxide via 'over'-reduction of the electron transport system and subsequent electron channelling to oxygen. Free radicals generated during sulphite autoxidation attack cellular membranes via lipid (L) peroxidation and subsequent chlorophyll (Chl) bleaching:

$$SO_3^{2-} + O_2^{\cdot-} + 2H^+ \rightarrow SO_3^{\cdot-} + H_2O_2$$

$$SO_3^{\cdot-} + LH \rightarrow HSO_3^- + L^\cdot$$

$$L^\cdot + O_2 \rightarrow LOO^\cdot$$

$$LOO^\cdot + LH \rightarrow LOOH + L^\cdot$$

$$LOOH \xrightarrow{Me} LO^\cdot + OH^-$$

$$LO^\cdot + Chl_{red} \rightarrow LOH + Chl_{ox}$$

The bleaching of chlorophyll by lipid peroxidation is only observed if SO_3^{2-} is simultaneously present. Neither LOOH nor SO_3^{2-} alone can destroy the green colour of chlorophyll.

The generated H_2O_2 is thought to be responsible for the inactivation of ascorbate peroxidase, glutathione reductase and enzymes of the Calvin cycle, such as phosphatases [17,18]. Uncoupling of oxidative phosphorylation results in insufficient reoxidation of $NADPH_2$ and thus causes inhibition of photosynthesis in the light due to a lack of ATP.

Cooperative effects of sulphite and soot particles

The discussion on the potential toxicity of diesel exhaust is of growing importance, especially due to the increasing truck traffic in Middle Europe since the opening of the East. Much of the threat of Otto-engine exhaust has been taken away by the introduction of the three-way catalytic converter. Such a redox converter is not applicable for diesel engines due to the different incineration concept: only oxidative reactions are relevant for the diesel catalyst. Of special importance, however, are the particulate emissions which are 30–70 times higher than those from catalyst-equipped spark ignition engines [19,20], rising to approximately 1 g/km [19]. The soot particles are small in size (less than 0.5 μm), easily respirable, and have carbon cores with a very large surface area on to which a variety of organic compounds (polycyclic aromatic compounds, nitro aromatics and quinones) are adsorbed. The number and structure of these compounds depend on the type of engine and the mode of its operation, and may thus be extremely variable [21]. The adsorbed compounds of diesel soot are subject to atmospheric conversions, which make them even more toxic [22–27].

Soot particles have been shown to exhibit mutagenic and carcinogenic properties in certain cell and animal models [28–35]. This is also evident from epidemiological studies concerning indoor coal burning in China [36].

There is also growing evidence that respiratory diseases and allergic reactions may be induced and/or enhanced by particle inhalation. Model experiments have shown that diesel soot particles (DPs), enhanced by aqueous SO_2 solutions (bisulphite), exhibit a considerable destructive potential concerning vital biomolecules such as SH compounds, polyenes, linolenic acid and certain enzymic properties [12]. The cooperative mechanism observed in the presence of DPs and sulphite indicates monovalent oxygen reduction and subsequent lipid peroxidation in the presence of an unsaturated fatty acid. In this process, sulphite is supposed to function both as electron donor and radical propagating agent:

$$SO_3^{2-} + O_2 \overset{DP}{\rightarrow} SO_3^{\bullet-} + O_2^{\bullet-} \qquad \text{(a)}$$

$$SO_3^{\bullet-} + O_2 + H_2O \rightarrow SO_4^{2-} + O_2^{\bullet-} + 2H^+ \qquad \text{(b)}$$

$$O_2^{\bullet-} + DP \rightarrow DP^{\bullet} + O_2 \qquad \text{(c)}$$

$$DP^{\bullet} + SO_3^{2-} \rightarrow DP^- + SO_3^{\bullet-} \qquad \text{(d)}$$

$$DP^- + O_2 \rightarrow DP^{\bullet} + O_2^{\bullet-} \qquad \text{(e)}$$

$$2DP^{\bullet} \rightarrow DP + DP^- \qquad \text{(f)}$$

$$DP^{\bullet} + O_2^{\bullet-} + H^+ \overset{SOD}{\rightarrow} DPH + O_2 \qquad \text{(g)}$$

$$O_2^{\bullet-} + O_2^{\bullet-} + 2H^+ \overset{SOD}{\rightarrow} H_2O_2 + O_2 \qquad \text{(h)}$$

As activating principles of DPs in reaction (a) both nitroaromatics and naphthoquinones have to be considered, since both classes of compounds have been shown to undergo redox cycling, thus driving oxidative destruction in the presence of appropriate electron donor molecules. Reactions (b)–(e) may operate as propagators of the synergistic radical chain reaction observed in the presence of both DPs and sulphite. Superoxide plays an important role as mediator between the DP-redox factors and different sulphur oxidation states. Disproportionation of DPs (f) and superoxide dismutase (SOD)-catalysed dismutations [(g) and (h)] represent chain-terminating events, where reaction (g) would be in agreement with the function of SOD as a superoxide-semiquinone-oxidoreductase [37].

Beside nitroaromatics and naphthoquinones iron may play an important role as an activating principle, as is well documented for asbestos fibres [38,39]. Asbestos fibres are able to generate $OH^{\bullet}$ radicals and $O_2^{\bullet-}$ from H_2O_2 via the catalysis of iron as an integral part of the asbestos complex. Pulmonary epithelial cell injury is mediated by H_2O_2 release from asbestos-activated polymorphonuclear neutrophils (PMNs) [40]. Asbestos alone has less cytotoxic effect on epithelial cells in leucocyte-free media; however, asbestos in combination with PMNs causes significant damage dependent on asbestos dose. As summarized by Mossman et al. [41] several studies support 'the concept of a cause and effect relation between activated oxygen species and the development of asbestosis'. Therefore asbestos fibres, in addition to their mechanical properties, may act as immobilized catalysts for Fenton- or Haber–Weiss-type reactions.

Using simple biochemical model reactions, simulating activated PMNs, the iron-mediated formation of strong oxidants in the presence of asbestos could be demonstrated. The free radical indicator ketomethylthiobutyrate (KMB) is fragmented in the presence of certain strong oxidants such as the OH˙ radical yielding ethylene, which can be sensitively monitored by gas chromatography.

The oxidoreductase of PMNs, responsible for the respiratory burst occurring after activation of these phagocytes, was simulated using a diaphorase (from pig heart), which is able to reduce molecular oxygen at the expense of NADH. As shown in Fig. 1 crocidolite stimulates ethylene release from KMB, triggered by the NADH/diaphorase-system. The chelator ethylenedinitrilotetra-acetic acid (EDTA) strongly enhances certain oxidative processes by facilitating Fe^{3+} reduction as well as electron transfer from Fe^{2+} to H_2O_2, thus allowing the formation of OH˙ radicals according to the Haber–Weiss sequence. Addition of EDTA to the asbestos-stimulated NADH/diaphorase system results, as expected, in a strong increase of ethylene release. Both SOD and catalase inhibit the reaction of the model system in the presence of asbestos and EDTA. Desferrioxamine, a chelator forming an unreactive complex with Fe^{3+} ions, supresses the crocidolite-stimulated ethylene release of the enzyme system. These results clearly indicate an iron-mediated formation of reactive oxygen species via the Haber–Weiss-type reaction.

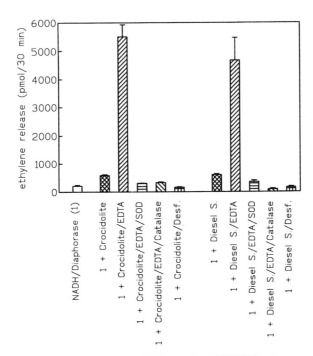

Fig. 1. Ethylene release from KMB in the NADH/diaphorase system. Reaction mixtures contained in a total volume of 2 ml: 2.5 mM KMB; 2.2 units of diaphorase; 75 μM NADH; 400 μg crocidolite or DPs; 0.5 mM EDTA or desferrioxamine (Desf); 100 units of SOD or catalase; 0.1 M phosphate buffer. The reactions were done at 37 °C in the dark. Standard deviations represent $n = 6$.

As also shown in Fig. 1, crocidolite can be replaced by aqueous diesel soot suspensions, underlining the role of iron in diesel soot toxicity.

In addition, aqueous suspensions of soot particles from domestic fuel burners are able to function as catalysts for Fenton-type reactions (Fig. 2). In this respect, different oxidative capacities are observed, allowing a differentiation between diverse types of soot. Of special interest is the distinction of soot particles stemming from mobile (traffic) and immobile (heat systems) sources respectively. As demonstrated in Fig. 2 the soot sample derived from the chimney of a wood-charged boiler causes no increase in the ethylene formation in the NADH/diaphorase system.

Also, addition of EDTA shows no effect. In contrast all soot samples derived from fuel oil (diesel soot, soot from the central heating and soot particles from the room oil stove) enhance the NADH/diaphorase reaction and are stimulated by EDTA. (Increasing ethylene release of the NADH/diaphorase system in the presence of EDTA is due to ubiquitary iron impurities.) Desferrioxamine, as well

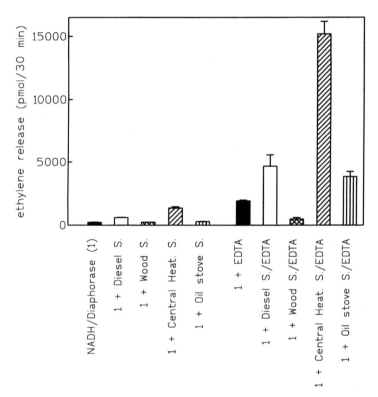

Fig. 2. The oxidative capacities of different soot types. Reaction mixtures are as described for Fig. 1. Soot (S.) samples (400 μg): diesel soot; wood soot (from the chimney of a wood-charged boiler with an efficiency about 730 kW); central heating soot (from the chimney of a fuel oil-fitted boiler for central heating, efficiency 35 kW); oil stove soot (from the stovepipe of a room oil stove, efficiency 8 kW).

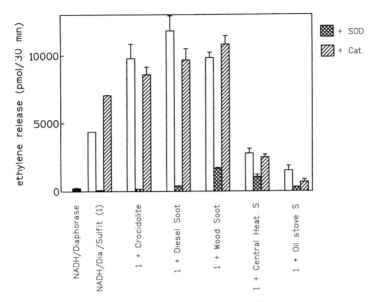

Fig. 3. Cooperative effects of sulphite and different particle types.
Reaction mixtures were as described for Fig. 1. Soot samples were as summarized for Fig. 2.

as SOD and catalase, inhibits the ethylene release in these model systems (data not shown).

As mentioned above, the combination of (diesel) soot particles and sulphite exhibits a remarkably deleterious potential. In Fig. 3 the effects of sulphite on the NADH/diaphorase system are demonstrated. Sulphite alone causes a strong increase in KMB fragmentation. This reaction is strongly inhibited by SOD, but not by catalase. On the contrary this haem-enzyme stimulates the sulphite-modified ethylene release due to the NADH/diaphorase system. In the presence of both sulphite and crocidolite, diesel soot and wood soot respectively, a comparable 2-fold enhancement of ethylene release can be observed. SOD decreases the KMB fragmentation, whereas catalase shows no effect. In contrast the soot samples derived from immobile fuel oil using burners inhibit the sulphite-stimulated generation of reactive oxygen species due to the NADH/diaphorase system. From this model reaction a clear differentiation between fuel oil-derived soot samples from mobile and immobile sources appears to be possible.

In addition vital functions of human PMNs are influenced by aqueous suspensions of soot particles in combination with sulphite *in vitro* ([14]; S. Hippeli and E.F. Elstner, unpublished work).

Since both SO_2 and DPs are present in significant concentrations in urban air pollution (smog) the indicated reactions may contribute to certain respiratory disorders discussed in the context of severe air pollution.

Superoxide, the main radical generated during the interaction of sulphite and asbestos, as well as soot particles, is shown to be also involved during influenza infections [42]. In this connection immune defence against infectious lung diseases in mice is reduced after exposure to diesel exhaust [43]. Thus superoxide-generating systems like soot/sulphite cooperating in the alveolar space, may modify certain immune responses *in vivo*.

References

1. Mudd, J.B. and Kozlowski, T.T. (eds.) (1975) Responses of Plants to Air Pollution, Academic Press, New York, San Francisco, London
2. Guthrie, F.E. and Perry, J.J. (eds.) (1980) Environmental Toxicology, Elsevier, New York
3. Smith, W.H. (ed.) (1981) Air Pollution and Forests, Springer-Verlag, New York, Heidelberg, Berlin
4. Unsworth, M.H. and Ormrod, D.P. (eds.) (1982) Effects of Gaseous Air Pollution in Agriculture and Horticulture, Butterworths, London
5. Koziol, M.J. and Whatley, F.R. (eds.) (1984) Gaseous Air Pollutants and Plant Metabolism, Butterworths, London
6. Guderian, R. (ed.) (1985) Air Pollution by Photochemical Oxidants. Formation, Transport, Control and Effects on Plants, Springer-Verlag, Berlin, Heidelberg, New York, Tokyo
7. Schulte-Hostede, S., Darall, N.M., Blank, L.W. and Wellburn, A.R. (eds.) (1988) Air Pollution and Plant Metabolism, Elsevier Applied Science, London and New York
8. Elstner, E.F. and Osswald, W.F. (1991) Free Radical Res. Commun. **12/13** (Part II), 795–807
9. Hippeli, S. and Elstner, E.F. (1991) in Oxidative Stress: Oxidants and Antioxidants (Sies, H., ed.), pp. 3–55, Academic Press, New York
10. Hippeli, S., Blaurock, B., v. Preen, A. and Elstner, E.F. (1994) in Free Radicals in the Environment, Medicine and Toxicology (Hohl, H., Esterbauer, H. and Rice-Evans, C., eds.), pp. 375–392, Richelieu Press, London
11. Holle, G. (1892) Die Gartenlaube **48**, 795–797
12. Hippeli, S.C. and Elstner, E.F. (1989) Z. Naturforsch. **44c**, 514–523
13. Blaurock, B., Hippeli, S., Metz, N. and Elstner, E.F. (1992) Arch. Toxicol. **66**, 681–687
14. Hippeli, S.C. and Elstner, E.F. (1990) Free Radical Res. Commun. **11**, 29–38
15. Peiser, G.D. and Yang, S.F. (1978) Phytochemistry **17**, 79–84
16. McManus, M.S., Altman, L.C., Koenig, J.Q., Luchtel, D.L., Covert, D.S., Virant, F.S. and Baker, C. (1989) Exp. Lung Res. **15**, 849–865
17. Tanaka, K. (1982) Plant Cell Physiol. **6**, 999–1011
18. Tanaka, K. and Sugahara, K. (1980) Plant Cell Physiol. **21**, 601–611
19. McClellan, R.O. (1986) Am. Ind. Hyg. Assoc. **47**, 1–13
20. Schuetzle, D., Skewes, L.M., Fisher, G.E., Levine, S.P. and Gorse, R.A., Jr. (1981) Anal. Chem. **53**, 837–840
21. Laresgoiti, A., Loos, A.C. and Springer, G.S. (1977) Curr. Res. **11**, 973–978
22. McCoy, E.C., Hyman, J. and Rosenkranz, H.S. (1979) Biochem. Biophys. Res. Commun. **89**, 729–734
23. Staerk, G. and Stauff, J. (1986) Staub – Reinhalt. Luft **46**, 289–291
24. Staerk, G. and Stauff, J. (1986) Staub – Reinhalt. Luft **46**, 396–400

25. Yoshikawa, T., Ruhr, L.P., Flory, W., Giamalva, D., Church, D.F. and Pryor, W.A. (1985) Toxicol. Appl. Pharmacol. **79**, 218–226

26. Pitts, J.N., Jr., Van Cauwenberghe, K.A., Grosjean, D., Schmid, J.P., Fitz, D.R., Belser, W.L., Jr., Knudson, G.B. and Hynds, P.M. (1978) Science **202**, 515–519

27. Apostol, I., Heinstein, P.F. and Low, P.S. (1989) Plant Physiol. **90**, 109–116

28. Claxton, L.D. (1983) Environ. Mutagen. **5**, 609–631

29. Schlipköter, H.W., Brockhaus, A., Einbrodt, H., Königshausen, T., Ohnesorge, F.K., Wichmann, H.E., Wittig, R. and Worth, H. (1987) Zur Frage der krebserzeugenden Wirkung von Dieselmotorabgasen, Gutachten der Arbeitsgruppe 'Immissionswirkung auf den Menschen' im Auftrag des Ministers für Umwelt, Raumordnung und Landwirtschaft des Landes Nordrhein-Westfalen

30. Lewtas, J. (1982) in Toxicological Effects of Emissions from Diesel Engines (Lewtas, J., ed.), pp. 62–82, Elsevier, New York

31. Mitchell, C.E. (1988) Toxicol. Lett. **42**, 159–166

32. McClellan, R.O. (1987) Annu. Rev. Pharmacol. Toxicol. **27**, 279–300

33. Bond, J.A., Mauderly, J.L. and Wolff, R.K. (1990) Toxicology **60**, 127–135

34. Handa, T., Yamauchi, T., Ohnishi, M., Hisamatsu, Y. and Ishii, T. (1983) Environ. Int. **9**, 335–341

35. Henderson, T.R., Li, A.P., Royer, R.E. and Clark, R.C. (1981) Environ. Mutagen. **3**, 211–220

36. Mumford, J.L., He, X.Z., Chapman, R.S., et al. (1987) Science **235**, 217

37. Cadenas, E. (1989) Annu. Rev. Biochem. **58**, 79–110

38. Mossman, B.T. and Landesman, J.M. (1983) Chest **83**, 503–515

39. Weitzman, S.A. and Graceffa, P. (1984) Arch. Biochem. Biophys. **228**, 373–376

40. Kamp, D.W., Dunne, M., Weitzman, S.A. and Dunn, M.M. (1989) J. Lab. Clin. Med. **114**, 604–612

41. Mossman, B.T., Bignon, J., Seaton, A. and Lee, J.B.L. (1990) Science **247**, 294–301

42. Oda, T., Akaike, T., Hamamoto, T., Suzuki, F., Hirano, T. and Maeda, H. (1989) Science **244**, 974–976

43. Lewis, T.R., Green, F.H.Y., Moorman, W.J., Burg, J.R. and Lynch, D.W. (1989) J. Am. Coll. Toxicol. **8**, 345–373

Biochem. Soc. Symp. **61**, 163–170
Printed in Great Britain

Myeloperoxidase as a generator of drug free radicals

Jack P. Uetrecht

Faculties of Pharmacy and Medicine, Drug Safety Research Group,
University of Toronto and Sunnybrook Health Science Centre,
Toronto, Canada

Abstract

Reactive metabolites are believed to be responsible for many types of toxicity, including idiosyncratic drug reactions. Bone marrow is a frequent target of idiosyncratic reactions, and, since these reactions have characteristics that suggest involvement of the immune system, the formation of reactive metabolites by leucocytes could also play a role in the aetiology of idiosyncratic drug reactions.

The major oxidation system in neutrophils and monocytes is a combination of NADPH oxidase and myeloperoxidase. This system oxidizes primary arylamines, such as sulphonamides, to reactive metabolites and these drugs are also associated with a high incidence of agranulocytosis, generalized idiosyncratic reactions and/or drug-induced lupus. Clozapine is oxidized by this system to a relatively stable nitrenium ion; clozapine is also associated with a high incidence of agranulocytosis. Arylamines that have an oxygen or nitrogen in the *para* position, such as amodiaquine, vesnarinone and 5-aminosalicylic acid, are oxidized to quinone-like reactive intermediates. Aminopyrine is oxidized to a very reactive dication. Such reactive metabolites could also inhibit neutrophil function and mediate some of the therapeutic effects of these drugs: for example, the use of dapsone for dermatitis herpetiformis and the use of 5-aminosalicylic acid for inflammatory bowel disease.

Reactive metabolites

Reactive metabolites are believed to be responsible for many types of toxicity [1,2]. The evidence is strongest for chemicals that react with DNA and cause cancer; however, there is evidence that other types of toxicity, such as hepato-

Address for correspondence: Faculty of Pharmacy, University of Toronto, 19 Russell Street, Toronto, Canada M5S 2S2

toxicity, can also involve reactive metabolites. It appears that this can either involve direct cytotoxicity, such as in the case of acetaminophen, or an immune-medicated reaction such as halothane-induced hepatic necrosis. Despite the general acceptance of the involvement of reactive metabolites in adverse drug reactions, in most cases their involvement has not been demonstrated.

There are several types of reactive metabolites. Some metabolites are reactive because they are electron-deficient, i.e. electrophiles, while others are reactive because they possess an unpaired electron, i.e. free radicals. In general electrophiles react with nucleophiles. In biological systems the major nucleophiles are nitrogen-based, such as the ε-amino group of lysine, or sulphur-based, such as the thiol group of cysteine. In contrast, free radicals usually abstract a hydrogen atom from other molecules rather than undergo covalent binding; however, free radicals can add to double bonds and, in addition to being free radicals, they can also be electrophilic, e.g. cation radicals. Abstraction of a hydrogen atom from a lipid can initiate a chain reaction leading to lipid peroxidation. There is a considerable amount of controversy as to whether specific adverse reactions are due to covalent modification of macromolecules by electrophiles or due to lipid peroxidation, oxidative 'stress' or other types of modification of biological molecules by free radicals [3,4].

The myeloperoxidase (MPO) system

Most drug and xenobiotic metabolism occurs in the liver, and although the liver is often involved in adverse drug reactions the incidence of adverse reactions involving other organs can be comparable. The incidence of adverse reactions involving the skin is higher than that of the liver and involvement of bone marrow and kidney is almost as high [5]. Although some reactive species, such as acyl glucuronides [6], can easily reach the circulation, most are probably too reactive to escape from the organ in which they were formed. Therefore it is likely that if reactive metabolites are involved in bone-marrow toxicity, they would be formed in the bone marrow [7,8]. Although leucocytes appear to contain cytochromes P-450 [9], the amount is very small and we have been unable to detect metabolism in leucocytes catalysed by cytochromes P-450 [10]. The major oxidant system of leucocytes, specifically neutrophils and monocytes, is a combination of NADPH oxidase and MPO [11,12]. NADPH oxidase converts oxygen into superoxide which is in turn converted into hydrogen peroxide. Hydrogen peroxide oxidizes MPO to a form of the enzyme referred to as compound I, which is a general term for the two-electron oxidation product of a peroxidase. Although compound I can probably oxidize drugs and xenobiotics directly, the major substrate is the chloride ion. Chloride ion is oxidized to hypochlorite, which is known to be a powerful oxidant and can oxidize other compounds. However, recent kinetic evidence suggests that the free hypochlorite is not the oxidizing species, at least in the oxidation of taurine, but instead the chlorine atom remains attached to the enzyme until it is transferred to the product [13]. The distinction may not be very important since the products formed by the combination of $MPO/H_2O_2/Cl^-$ appear to be the same as those formed by hypochlorite [14]. In addition to this oxidation pathway, there is recent evidence for the reaction of superoxide with MPO to form an oxidant which results in products similar to those expected for reaction with hydroxy radical [15].

The NADPH oxidase/MPO system can generate a large amount of oxidant. Presumably the major function of this oxidant system is to kill bacteria and other pathogens; however, there is evidence that it is also involved in the regulation of proteolytic enzymes and may have other functions as well [12,16]. An important characteristic of this system is that it requires activation of the cells by a stimulus like bacteria in order to activate the NADPH oxidase and for release of the MPO from granules. If reactive metabolites formed by this system are responsible for idiosyncratic drug reactions, it would follow that an infection or other inflammatory condition would be one risk factor of the development of the adverse reaction.

Other oxidizing systems exist in leucocytes. Nitric oxide is produced by murine neutrophils but it appears that human neutrophils produce little or no nitric oxide [17–19]. Leucocytes also contain prostaglandin synthase; however, this is quantitatively less important than the MPO system and we have been unable to detect evidence of drug oxidation by this pathway [20].

Oxidation of specific drugs by the MPO system

Most of the products formed by the MPO system are the same as would be expected for a drug with hypochlorite [14]. The reaction presumably involves the reaction of an electrophilic chlorine with an electron-rich atom such as nitrogen or sulphur. Unlike oxidation by cytochromes *P*-450, oxidation of carbon by MPO is uncommon but it can occur. One example is the hydroxylation and chlorination of phenylbutazone [21]. Similar products are also observed on incubation of a drug with activated neutrophils or monocytes as with hypochlorite.

Oxidation of primary arylamines leads to hydroxylamines and chloramines (Fig. 1). The hydroxylamine is further oxidized to a nitroso derivative and in some cases a nitro derivative. The nitroso derivative appears to be responsible for much of the covalent binding. The chloramine appears to be more active as a chlorinating agent rather than leading to covalent binding of the drug to biological molecules. We have not observed free-radical intermediates in these reactions but we have not looked for them carefully. Examples of drugs which are primary amines and are oxidized in this manner include dapsone [20], sulphonamides [22] and procainamide [23].

Although not a primary arylamine, clozapine contains a nitrogen which is easily oxidized, presumably to an N-chloro derivative that rapidly looses a chloride ion to form a nitrenium ion [24]. The putative nitrenium ion of clozapine is red in colour and reacts rapidly with glutathione to form several conjugates, at least some of which have the glutathione bound to one or both of the aromatic rings. Fischer *et al.* also have indirect evidence for the formation of a clozapine free radical which could also be responsible for the formation of the glutathione adducts [25].

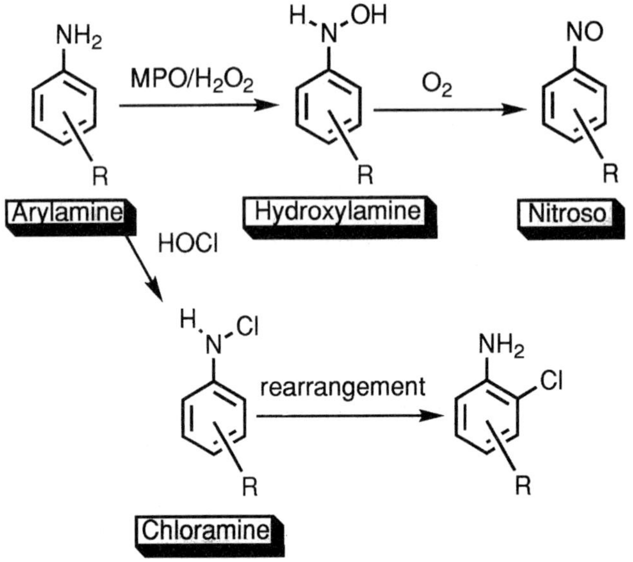

Fig. 1. Metabolic pathways leading to reactive metabolites of arylamines.

Arylamines which have a hetero atom such as oxygen or nitrogen in the *para* position can be oxidized to analogues of quinones. Examples include amodiaquine [26], vesnarinone [27] and 5-aminosalicylic acid [28]. The intermediate of vesnarinone is also in equilibrium with a reddish-purple cation radical (Fig. 2). From the structures of the products, it appears that it is the quinone analogue rather than the cation radical that is responsible for reaction with nucleophiles such as glutathione. By use of radiolabelled drug it appears that almost 5% of vesnarinone incubated with activated neutrophils becomes covalently bound to the neutrophils.

Another type of compound containing more than one nitrogen is aminopyrine. It has been known for some time to be oxidized to a cation radical by peroxidases including MPO. More recently we produced spectral and kinetic evidence that oxidation of aminopyrine to a cation radical by hypochlorite involves a reactive dication intermediate with a half-life of about 15 ms [29] (Fig. 3). As with vesnarinone, either the electrophilic dication or the cation radical could be responsible for the toxicity of aminopyrine, specifically agranulocytosis.

Drugs that contain nitrogen in the form of a hydrazine are also readily oxidized to reactive intermediates by hypochlorite, $MPO/H_2O_2/Cl^-$, or activated neutrophils [30–32]. In this case reactive diazines and diazonium ions appear to be involved, but free radicals are also possible.

Drugs that contain a sulphur such as a sulphydryl group are also easily oxidized. Propylthiouracil is oxidized all the way to a sulphonic acid [33,34]. The sulphonic acid is reactive and reacts with glutathione. In addition, we presume that formation of a reactive sulphenyl chloride is the first step in the reaction but we have not been able to prove this. The only evidence for the sulphenyl chloride is that the first product observed is a disulphide, which is presumably due to the reaction of the sulphenyl chloride with another molecule of the drug.

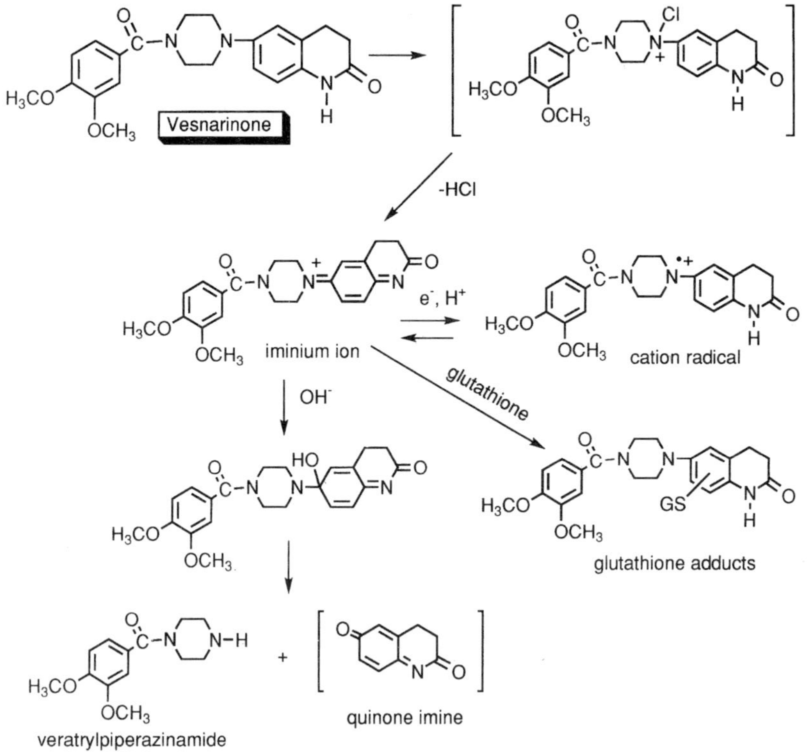

Fig. 2. Oxidation of vesnarinone by HOCl or the MPO system to a reactive iminium ion and cation radical.

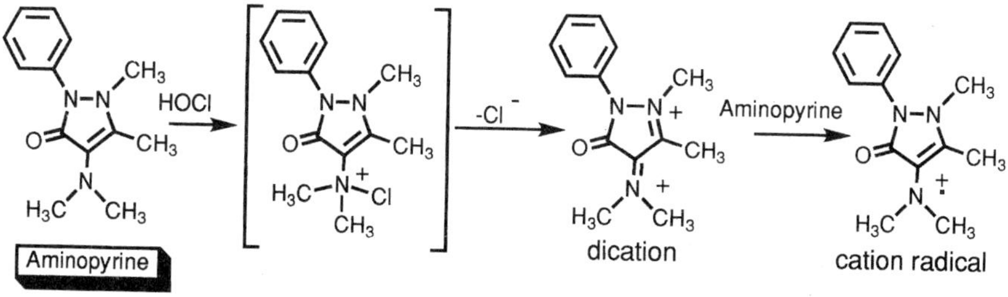

Fig. 3. Oxidation of aminopyrine by hypochlorite to a reactive dication and cation radical.

Association of MPO-mediated reactive metabolite formation with adverse drug reactions

It is relatively easy to demonstrate that specific drugs are oxidized by the MPO/H$_2$O$_2$/Cl$^-$ system to reactive intermediates, but it is much more difficult to demonstrate the significance of these products in adverse drug reactions. In general, use of the drugs described above is associated with a relatively high incidence of idiosyncratic drug reactions, especially agranulocytosis, drug-induced lupus and generalized reactions involving the skin and other organs [7,8]. For example, clozapine, aminopyrine, vesnarinone, propylthiouracil, dapsone and procainamide are all associated with a high incidence of agranulocytosis. It is reasonable to speculate that reactive metabolites produced by the MPO system are responsible for many of these reactions, especially reactions, such as agranulocytosis, that involve the bone marrow; however, proof of this hypothesis is difficult to obtain. There appears to be a higher incidence of agranulocytosis in patients taking vesnarinone who also received influenza vaccine. This also fits the hypothesis because influenza vaccine is capable of activating neutrophils which would lead to the formation of reactive metabolite. In several cases both electrophiles and free radicals are produced and there is no evidence to indicate which may be responsible for the observed toxicity.

The pathological mechanism for most of these adverse reactions is also unknown. The unpredictable nature of idiosyncratic reactions suggests involvement of the immune system, yet with few exceptions this has not been proven. Of the idiosyncratic reactions caused by the drugs described above, certainly drug-induced lupus must involve the immune system because lupus is an autoimmune disease. There is good evidence that aminopyrine-induced agranulocytosis is due to an antibody against mature neutrophils [35,36]. Covalent binding of a reactive metabolite to a biological macromolecule could convert the metabolite into a hapten which could induce either an antibody or cell-mediated response. However, the mechanism of drug-induced agranulocytosis associated with the other drugs discussed is less clear. Although antibodies have been described in association with other drug-induced agranulocytosis, especially amodiaquine [37], propylthiouracil [38] and procainamide [39], the target appears to be the bone marrow rather than mature neutrophils. In addition, the time course of recurrence on re-exposure to the drug, an average of 14 weeks for clozapine [40], would be extremely unusual for an amnestic response of the immune system. There is evidence that direct toxicity may be involved in some cases [41], but then it is difficult to explain the idiosyncratic nature of the toxicity and the lack of toxicity to animals at high dose. Much work remains to be done before it will be possible to say with a reasonable degree of certainty that MPO-mediated reactive-metabolite formation is responsible for a significant number of adverse drug reactions.

Mechanisms by which MPO-generated reactive intermediates may mediate therapeutic effects of drugs

The generation of reactive oxygen species by activated neutrophils and monocytes is believed to be responsible for, or contribute to, many serious illnesses. Many of the same drugs that are metabolized by the MPO system and cause toxicity also have anti-inflammatory effects [42]. This could be due to inhibition of neutrophil and macrophage function by the reactive metabolites produced. Examples include the use of dapsone for the treatment of dermatitis herpetiformis (a vesicular disease associated with an infiltration of neutrophils in the skin) and rheumatoid arthritis; the use of propylthiouracil for the treatment of thyroid disease (in this case because of the inhibition of thyroid peroxidase which is similar to MPO) and alcoholic liver disease [43]; the use of aminopyrine for the treatment of pain, fever and inflammation and the use of 5-aminosalicylic acid for the treatment of inflammatory bowel disease. There is even evidence that patients who are on chronic dapsone therapy for leprosy have a lower incidence of Alzheimer's disease [44]. It has been hypothesized that this is due to inhibition of microglial cells which are the macrophages of the brain and may be responsible for the death of neurons in Alzheimer's disease.

Summary

The MPO system of neutrophils and monocytes can oxidize a large number of drugs to chemically reactive metabolites. Circumstantial evidence suggests that these reactive metabolites may be responsible for idiosyncratic drug reactions, especially those involving leucocytes, such as agranulocytosis and lupus. The same reactive metabolites may also be responsible for some of the therapeutic effects of drugs if they inhibit leucocyte function during an inflammatory reaction.

This work was supported by grants from the Medical Research Council of Canada.

References

1. Pohl, L.R., Satoh, H., Christ, D.D. and Kenna, J.G. (1988) Annu. Rev. Pharmacol. **28**, 367–387
2. Hinson, J.A. and Roberts, D.W. (1992) Annu. Rev. Pharmacol. Toxicol. **32**, 471–510
3. Halliwell, B. (1994) Lancet **344**, 721–724
4. Kehrer, J.P. (1993) Crit. Rev. Toxicol. **23**, 21–48
5. Davies, D.M. (1985) Textbook of Adverse Drug Reactions, Oxford University Press, Oxford
6. Hyneck, M.L., Smith, P.C., Munafo, A., McDonagh, A.F. and Benet, L.Z. (1988) Clin. Pharmacol. Ther. **44**, 107–114
7. Uetrecht, J.P. (1990) CRC Crit. Rev. Toxicol. **20**, 213–235
8. Uetrecht, J.P. (1992) Drug Metab. Rev. **24**, 299–366
9. Robie-Suh, K., Robinson, R. and Gelboin, H.V. (1980) Science **208**, 1031–1033
10. Uetrecht, J. and Sokoluk, B. (1992) Drug Metab. Dispos. **20**, 120–123
11. Klebanoff, S.J. (1968) J. Bacteriol. **95**, 2131–2138
12. Weiss, S.J. (1989) N. Engl. J. Med. **320**, 365–376
13. Marquez, L.A. and Dunford, H.B. (1994) J. Biol. Chem. **269**, 7950–7956
14. Winterbourn, C. (1985) Biochim. Biophys. Acta **840**, 204–210
15. Kettle, A.J. and Winterbourn, C.C. (1994) J. Biol. Chem. **269**, 17146–17151
16. Theron, A. and Anderson, R. (1985) Am. Rev. Respir. Dis. **132**, 1049–1054
17. Schneemann, M., Schoedon, G., Hofer, S., Blau, N., Guerrero, L., et al. (1993) J. Infect. Dis. **167**, 1358–1363
18. Yan, L., Vandivier, R. W., Suffredini, A.F. and Danner, R.L. (1994) J. Immunol. **153**, 1825–1834

19. Denis, M. (1994) J. Leukocyte Biol. **55**, 682–684
20. Uetrecht, J., Zahid, N., Shear, N.H. and Biggar, W.D. (1988) J. Pharmacol. Exp. Ther. **245**, 274–279
21. Ichihara, S., Tomisawa, H., Fukazawa, H., Tateishi, M., Joly, R., et al. (1986) Biochem. Pharmacol. **35**, 3935–3939
22. Cribb, A.E., Miller, M., Tesoro, A. and Spielberg, S.P. (1990) Mol. Pharmacol. **38**, 744–751
23. Uetrecht, J., Zahid, N. and Rubin, R. (1988) Chem. Res. Toxicol. **1**, 74–78
24. Uetrecht, J.P. (1992) Drug Safety **7** (Suppl. 1), 51–56
25. Fischer, V., Haar, J.A., Greiner, L., Loyd, R.V. and Mason, R.P. (1991) Mol. Pharmacol. **40**, 846–853
26. Clarke, J.B., Maggs, J.L., Kitteringham, N.R. and Park, B.K. (1990) Int. Arch. Allergy Appl. Immunol. **91**, 335–342
27. Uetrecht, J.P., Zahid, N. and Whitfield, D. (1994) J. Pharmacol. Exp. Ther. **270**, 865–872
28. Liu, Z.C., McClelland, R.A. and Uetrecht, J.P. (1995) Drug Metab. Dispos. **23**, 246–250
29. Uetrecht, J.P., Ma, H.M., MacKnight, E. and McClelland, R. (1995) Chem. Res. Toxicol. **8**, 226–233
30. Hofstra, A.H., Matassa, L.C. and Uetrecht, J.P. (1991) J. Rheumatol. **18**, 1673–1680
31. Hofstra, A.H., Li-Muller, A.S.M. and Uetrecht, J.P. (1992) Drug Metab. Dispos. **20**, 205–210
32. Hofstra, A. and Uetrecht, J.P. (1993) Chemico-Biol. Interact. **89**, 183–196
33. Lee, E., Miki, Y., Hosokawa, M., Sayo, H. and Kariya, K. (1988) Xenobiotica **18**, 1135–1142
34. Waldhauser, L. and Uetrecht, J. (1991) Drug Metab. Dispos. **19**, 354–359
35. Madison, F.W. and Squier, T.L. (1934) J. Am. Med. Assoc. **102**, 755–759
36. Moeschlin, S. and Wagner, K. (1952) Acta Haemat. **8**, 29–41
37. Christie, G. and Park, B.K. (1988) Br. J. Clin. Pharmacol. **26**, 624P
38. Fibbe, W.E., Claas, F.H.J., Van der Star-Dijlstra, W., Schaafsma, M.R., Meyboom, R.H.B., et al. (1986) Br. J. Haematol. **64**, 363–373
39. Azocar, J. (1984) Lancet **1**, 1069–1070
40. Safferman, A.Z., Lieberman, J.A., Alvir, J.J. and Howard, A. (1992) Lancet **339**, 1296–1297
41. Pisciotta, A.V. (1973) Semin. Hematol. **10**, 279–310
42. Uetrecht, J. (1989) Trends Pharmacol. Sci. **10**, 463–467
43. Orrego, H., Blake, J.E., Blendis, L.M., Compton, K.V. and Israel, Y. (1987) N. Engl. J. Med. **317**, 1421–1427
44. Schnabel, J. (1993) Science **260**, 1719–1720

Biochem. Soc. Symp. **61**, 171–194
Printed in Great Britain

Radicals from one-electron reduction of nitro compounds, aromatic *N*-oxides and quinones: the kinetic basis for hypoxia-selective, bioreductive drugs

Peter Wardman*‡, Madeleine F. Dennis*, Steven A. Everett*, Kantilal B. Patel*, Michael R.L. Stratford* and Michael Tracy†

*Gray Laboratory Cancer Research Trust, P.O. Box 100, Mount Vernon Hospital, Northwood, Middlesex HA6 2JR, U.K. and †Bio-Organic Chemistry Laboratory, SRI International, 333 Ravenswood Avenue, Menlo Park, CA 94025, U.S.A.

Abstract

Drugs based on nitroarene, aromatic *N*-oxide or quinone structures are frequently reduced by cellular reductases to toxic products. Reduction often involves free radicals as intermediates which react rapidly with oxygen to form superoxide radicals, inhibiting drug reduction. The elevation of cellular oxidative stress accompanying oxygen inhibition of reduction is generally less damaging than drug reduction to toxic products, so the drugs offer selective toxicity to hypoxic cells. Since such cells are resistant to radiotherapy, these bioreductive drugs offer potential in tumour therapy. The basis for the selectivity of action entails kinetic competition involving the contesting reaction pathways. The reduction potential of the drug, radical pK_a and nature of radical/radical decay kinetics all influence drug activity and selectivity, including the range of oxygen tensions over which the drug offers selective toxicity. These properties may be quantified using generation of radicals by pulse radiolysis, presenting a physico-chemical basis for rational drug design.

Introduction

Nitro compounds, aromatic *N*-oxides and quinones share the common property of being readily reduced by biologically relevant reductants. Para-doxically, reduction of the compounds (S) can stimulate cellular oxidative stress in

‡To whom correspondence should be addressed.

an aerobic environment where reduction involves the generation of radicals $(SH^{\cdot}/S^{\cdot-})$ as obligate intermediates (eqn. 1) or where radicals can be formed by reaction of oxidant (S) with the reduced compound (SH_2) (eqn. 2). This is because superoxide radicals $(O_2^{\cdot-})$ can be formed (eqn. 3), which in turn can produce hydrogen peroxide (eqn. 4) and hydroxyl radicals $(^{\cdot}OH)$ directly via Fenton chemistry (eqn. 5) or through analogous chemistry involving hypochlorous acid:

$$S + reductant \pm enzyme \rightarrow S^{\cdot-} \; (+H^+ \rightleftharpoons SH^{\cdot}) \tag{1}$$

$$S + SH_2 \rightleftharpoons 2SH^{\cdot} \rightleftharpoons 2S^{\cdot-} + 2H^+ \tag{2}$$

$$S^{\cdot-} + O_2 \rightleftharpoons S + O_2^{\cdot-} \tag{3}$$

$$2O_2^{\cdot-} + 2H^+ \rightarrow H_2O_2 + O_2 \tag{4}$$

$$H_2O_2 + reduced\ metal \rightarrow {}^{\cdot}OH + OH^- + oxidized\ metal \tag{5}$$

In the absence of oxygen, reactions (3)–(5) will not be stimulated by the presence of the oxidant S; however, damaging reactions of radicals or other reduction intermediates may occur with biological targets:

$$SH^{\cdot}/S^{\cdot-} + target \rightarrow damage \tag{6}$$

$$SH_2 + target \rightarrow damage \tag{7}$$

The extent of these competing pathways will obviously depend not only on oxygen tension but also on levels of antioxidant enzymes such as superoxide dismutase, catalase and glutathione peroxidase, which can frequently prevent reactions (4) and (5) leading to the formation of highly reactive hydroxyl radicals by removing $O_2^{\cdot-}$ and/or H_2O_2. The outcome of drug reduction in aerobic or hypoxic environments thus depends on which is the greater of two evils: stimulating cellular oxidative stress or forming reactive drug-reduction intermediates. This competition forms the basis for the rational design of hypoxia-selective bioreductive drugs, as outlined in Fig. 1. When drug reduction leads to more toxic pathways than superoxide formation, either because of low oxygen tension or chemical reactivity, then selective toxicity towards hypoxic cells or organisms will occur. Reactions (1) and (3) together constitute a redox cycling or futile cycling role for the drug, in that it can stimulate cellular oxidative stress without the drug being consumed in the process [1].

Although the prototypical bioreductive drug, metronidazole (Flagyl), is widely used in medicine, there is much current interest in targeting hypoxic cells in tumours. This arises in part from the radioresistance of hypoxic cells. Up to three times higher radiation dose may be required to kill hypoxic cells compared with well-oxygenated cells; if non-cycling, such cells may also be resistant to some chemotherapeutic drugs [2].

This article outlines the chemical kinetic basis for drug selectivity of bioreductive drugs, the majority of which involve nitroarene, aromatic N-oxide or quinone structures. The properties of radical intermediates in drug action are discussed, stressing the similarities between the three groups of compounds and noting key differences where they occur. Overviews of some of the kinetic aspects

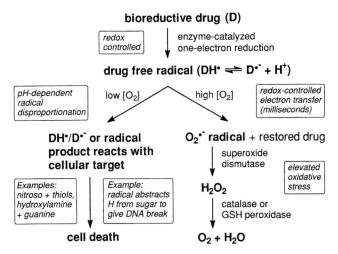

Fig. 1. Activation of a bioreductive drug (D) to a radical intermediate and competing pathways dependent upon the oxygen concentration, drug redox properties and pH.

of radical reactions involving nitroarenes [3] or quinones [4] were presented some time ago. More detailed reviews of the radical chemistry and mechanisms of toxicity of quinones, in particular, have been published [5–7] and the applications of EPR spectroscopy to detect redox cycling radical intermediates have been described [1,8]. Damage to DNA by redox-cycling drugs has been discussed [9]. Recently, emphasis on the design of bioreductive drugs has focused on enzyme-directed drug development [10] and N-oxides have attracted increasing attention [11–13]. However, the nitroarene moiety remains an important basis for bioreductive drugs [14–16].

We do not attempt to present here a comprehensive review of bioreductive drug mechanisms. Rather, we seek simply to present a framework for the logical discussion of chemical pathways based on known or accessible kinetic and thermodynamic information.

Prototypical compounds

Metronidazole (Fig. 2; 1) is probably the nitroarene most widely used in medicine. It is closely related to the hypoxic cell radiosensitizer, misonidazole (2) [2,17]. The dinitrobenzene, CB 1954 (3), has been considered recently as a candidate for antibody-directed enzyme-prodrug therapy [18]. The related dinitrobenzene (4) has higher specificity for hypoxic cells than CB 1954 [19]. Nitrofurans such as nitrofurantoin (5) are used as urinary antibacterials. Nitroquinolines such as 6 are currently being studied in detail as hypoxic cell cytotoxins [20,21].

2-Methyl-1,4-naphthoquinone (menadione, 7) is an analogue of vitamin K, but the 2,3-dimethoxy analogue differs in its biological reactivity because the rapid

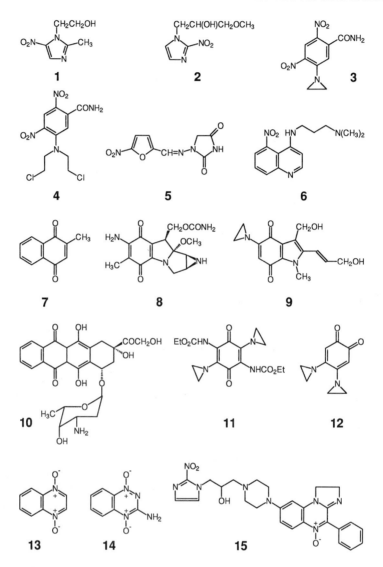

Fig. 2. Typical bioreductive drugs under experimental or clinical evaluation, based on nitroarene, quinone or aromatic N-oxide moieties.

conjugation/reduction characteristic of menadione and glutathione is blocked by the two methoxy substituents [6,22,23]. Mitomycin *c* (**8**) might be viewed as a model quinonoid bioreductive drug, although its oxic/hypoxic differential toxicity is smaller than that of some newer drugs [24,25]. Recent interest in related structures has focused on EO9 (**9**). Hydroxy substituents capable of hydrogen bonding to the quinone oxygens is a feature of the chemotherapeutic drug, doxorubicin (adriamycin, **10**). Whether the latter is a bioreductive drug in the conventional sense is unlikely; although this possibility remains a matter of some dispute [26], redox cycling to stimulate oxidative stress may be associated with the dose-limiting cardiotoxicity [9,27,28]. Substituted benzoquinones of interest include diazaquone (AZQ; 11) and recently reported 1,2-benzoquinone analogues such as 12 [29].

Quinoxaline-di-N-oxides such as quindoxin (13) were used as poultry feed additives many years ago and radical intermediates were implicated in their mode of action [30]. Most current interest in aromatic N-oxides focuses on the benzotriazine, tirapazamine (SR 4233, 14), which is selectively toxic towards hypoxic mammalian cells [31–33]. Although the mono-N-oxide analogue of tirapazamine, SR 4317 (the 1-oxide), has low toxicity, some mono-N-oxides, including bifunctional compounds such as 15 (with both N-oxide and nitroarene moieties), are of current interest as hypoxia-specific cyotoxins [13]. Aliphatic N-oxides include pro-drugs of DNA-binding agents, activated by reduction, but their mode of action does not appear to involve radical intermediates [34].

Mechanisms of bioreductive drug cytotoxicity

This article concentrates on the kinetics of radical reactions, and a comprehensive survey of mechanisms of cytotoxicity is inappropriate here. Reviews of radical mechanisms, particularly of quinones, were noted in the Introduction. In addition, brief overviews have been presented of some mechanistic aspects in relation to cancer therapy [35] and trichomoniasis [36]. Three distinct pathways to cytotoxicity can be envisaged, and an outline will help set the scene for a discussion of the kinetics of critical free-radical reactions.

Product from disproportionation of drug radicals may be toxic

Drug radicals are generally unstable at physiological pH (see below). Radical–radical reactions in many instances involve disproportionation. Nitroarene radicals provide a typical example; quinone radical disproportionation is the reverse of eqn. (2), but there have been no reports of radical generation on mixing the di-N-oxide, tirapazamine (Fig. 2; 14), with the two-electron reduced product, the mono-N-oxide. Nitroarene radicals yield a nitrosoarene (RNO) upon disproportionation (eqn. 8), which is generally reduced further to a hydroxylamine (RNHOH) by e.g. glutathione (eqn. 9) or ascorbate, or nitro radicals:

$$2RNO_2^{\cdot-} + 2H^+ \rightarrow RNO + RNO_2 + H_2O \tag{8}$$

$$RNO + GSH \rightleftharpoons RN(OH)SG\,(+GSH \rightarrow RNHOH + GSSG)\,(or \rightarrow RNHSOG) \tag{9}$$

Reaction with GSH (eqn. 9) is quite complex, as indicated above [37–40], but the half-lives of reaction with, for example, $2\ mmol/dm^3$ GSH and representative nitrosobenzenes are in the range 4–70 ms [38]. A thorough kinetic study has been reported [40]. Free glutathione will be in competition with protein thiols for reaction with nitrosoarenes. 2-Nitrosoimidazoles [41–47] and 5-nitrosoimidazoles [48,49] have been prepared, and their cytoxicity and mutagenicity have been assessed. Hydroxylamines derived from 2-nitroimidazoles are unstable but reactivity of these and other nitroarene reduction products towards nucleophilic bases on DNA (e.g. guanine) has been demonstrated in model systems [44,50–61].

Reduction activates potentially toxic functional groups

Since radical intermediates are not necessarily involved in this route to toxicity, only very brief mention is appropriate here. Nitroarene or quinone moieties effectively deactivate alkylating substituents, and reduction restores the reactivity. Prototypical compounds are CB 1954 (Fig. 2; **3**) [18], mitomycin *c* (**8**) [24,62,63] and diazaquone (**11**) [5]. Another example, not shown, would be the misonidazole (**2**) derivative in which the side-chain terminal methoxy function is replaced by aziridine, RSU 1069, or pro-drugs of this compound [14]. This group of compounds especially is the focus of enzyme-directed bioreductive drug research [10,35], since two-electron reductants such as DT-diaphorase can activate many such drugs, particularly quinones.

Reduction by one-electron, i.e. to the radical, is probably sufficient to activate the alkylating substituents, but whether the radical reacts as an alkylator depends on competing kinetics of radical–radical reactions and alkylation. Quantitative information is lacking.

The drug radical reacts directly with a cellular target

Although nitro radical reactivity towards DNA bases has been deduced from electrochemical measurements and the nature of the damage [51,64–68], quantitative rate data are unavailable, and it remains conjecture whether radical–DNA reactions can occur before other reactions of the radicals in cellular systems. Electrochemical studies of the DNA-damaging reactions of tirapazamine (Fig. 2; **14**) show a pH effect [69] which is consistent with the model for DNA damage via the protonated radical which is discussed below. The main supporting evidence for this mechanism is the lack of cytotoxicity associated with the stable 2- or 4-electron reduction products [70].

Factors controlling bioreductive drug activation

Reduction rate: obligate one-electron reduction

Reaction (1) above is a general expression of one-electron reduction. A representative simple chemical model for enzyme-catalysed reduction is reaction with dihydroflavins, $FMNH_2$, in the absence of oxygen:

$$S + FMNH_2 \rightarrow SH_2 + FMN \tag{10}$$

In the case of nitro compounds (RNO_2), the reaction was found [71] to follow stoichiometry corresponding to reduction to the hydroxylamine, RNHOH:

$$RNO_2 + 2FMNH_2 \rightarrow RNHOH + 2FMN \tag{11}$$

but the initial rate law for reduction of several nitroimidazoles was approximately $k_{11}[RNO_2][FMNH_2]$ and Fig. 3 shows that the rate constant for reduction [71] increased with the reduction potential for adding a single electron [72]. Reduction

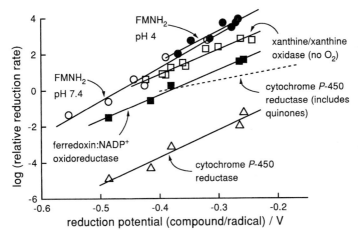

Fig. 3. Redox dependences of relative rates of reduction of nitro-arenes (logarithmic scale). ○, FMNH$_2$+nitroimidazoles; ●, FMNH$_2$+ nitroacridines; □, xanthine/xanthine oxidase+nitroimidazoles; ■, ferredoxin: NADP$^+$ oxidoreductase; △, cytochrome *P*-450 reductase; broken line, cytochrome *P*-450 reductase+nitroarenes and quinones (see text for sources of data).

of nitroacridines by FMNH$_2$ showed a virtually identical redox dependence and absolute reactivity [73], as shown in Fig. 3.

Xanthine oxidase normally catalyses the reduction of oxygen to superoxide with xanthine or hypoxanthine as cofactor, but, in the absence of oxygen, nitro compounds or other bioreductive drugs act as alternative electron acceptors. Clarke *et al.* [74] measured the kinetics of reduction of nitroimidazoles by xanthine/xanthine oxidase and estimated the initial rates at a concentration probably rather less than the Michaelis K_m value. The redox dependence of this flavoenzyme was quite similar to that found with free flavins; the data are shown in Fig. 3.

Probably the most important reductase in mammalian tissues reducing bioreductive drugs to radical intermediates is NADPH-cytochrome *P*-450 reductase, and the enzyme kinetics for oxygen consumption, reflecting reactions (1), (3) and (4) with (1) rate-limiting, was found to have a similar redox dependence to the xanthine oxidase system [75]. The authors estimated the Michaelis parameters $V_{max.}/K_m$; this ratio, in the units used in the report [75], is plotted in Fig. 3. It approximates to the effective rate constant at substrate concentrations much less than K_m. In the same study [75], reduction by ferredoxin:NADP$^+$ oxidoreductase was measured, and the data in Fig. 3 demonstrate a similar redox dependence of reduction rate on catalysis by cytochrome *P*-450 reductase and xanthine oxidase. A later study [76] quantified radical formation using cytochrome *c* reduction as indicator rather than oxygen consumption, and the broken line in Fig. 3 shows the redox dependence for reduction by cytochrome *P*-450 reductase for compounds with reduction potential < -0.15 V. Although the redox dependence was significantly lower than in the earlier studies with this and other enzymes, an important result was that reduction of quinones and nitro compounds followed similar kinetics, depending only on reduction potential. (A recent study [77] measured $K_m = 3$ μmol/dm^3 for 2-methylmethoxy-1,4-naphthoquinone and cytochrome P-450 reductase. Thus the use of a single concentration of 50 μmol/dm^3 in the work of Butler and Hoey [76], higher than the probable K_m for some of the compounds included, may not have been appropriate for the redox analysis. The same criticism may hold partially true for the earlier study with xanthine oxidase [74] for the most electron-affinic compounds.)

None of these investigations measured directly the rate of formation of radical-anions, but from extensive studies using EPR detection of steady-state concentrations of free radicals, it seems likely that the reductases described above (and free, reduced flavins) reduce nitro compounds [78], quinones [5] and aromatic N-oxides [79] by generating radical-anions as obligate intermediates. Radical formation rates are evidently strongly dependent on reduction potential. Cellular reduction, including by mammalian cells, has a redox dependence close to those shown in Fig. 3 [80], as does cytoxicity towards anoxic mammalian cells [81].

Radical formation via two-electron reduction or thiol conjugation

Eqn. (2) implies that if a drug S is reduced by two electrons to SH$_2$, then radicals S$^{\cdot-}$/SH$^{\cdot}$ can still be formed if equilibrium (2) is favourable. In practice, such radical formation has been characterized only for quinones, and does not seem to occur with nitroarenes or aromatic N-oxides at physiological pH. With quinones, equilibrium (2) is pH-sensitive; thus for 2,3,5,6-tetramethyl-1,4-benzoquinone (duroquinone), the semiquinone formation constant, K_f increases from $\sim 10^{-14}$ at pH < 4 to ~ 1 at pH ~ 14 [82]:

$$K_f = K_2 = ([Q^{\cdot-}]_{tot})^2 / ([Q]_{tot}[QH_2]_{tot}) \tag{12}$$

where the subscripts denote total concentrations of the species, summing all prototropic forms. At high pH, the duroquinone radical-anion is produced in high concentration, and is stable, on mixing the quinone and hydroquinone [83]. Factors influencing the magnitude of K_f include the presence of OH substituents where the proton can hydrogen bond to the quinone oxygen, thus stabilizing the radical. This feature is seen in doxorubicin (Fig. 2; **10**), and a particular feature of this drug is that its semiquinone formation constant at pH 7 is about nine orders of magnitude higher than that for duroquinone [84]. Thus doxorubicin reduction, even by enzymes not involving radical intermediates, can potentially stimulate redox cycling via reactions (2) and (3). This may be the basis for the drug's cardiotoxicity [9]. Reducing redox cycling by intentional manipulation of K_f, by varying the substituents to control the pK_a values which influence this parameter, does not seem to have been attempted.

Radical formation via the reduction product SH$_2$ will only occur by this route if SH$_2$ is sufficiently stable to allow significant concentrations to build up to permit the establishment of equilibrium (2). This may not be the case, since with the indoloquinone EO9 (Fig. 2; **9**) the toxicity linked to the obligate two-electron reductant, DT-diaphorase, is not oxygen-sensitive. Indeed, there is an inverse correlation between the levels of DT-diaphorase and hypoxic sensitivity to EO9

[85]. This may imply that reduction activates the aziridine alkylating substituent and this functional group is then so reactive that free hydroquinone cannot build up to generate radicals. This may also explain the fairly low hypoxic/oxic selectivity of mitomycin c (Fig. 2; 8) [24]. Enzyme-directed bioreductive drug therapy [10] and the role of DT-diaphorase in quinone activation [24,25,63,77] are complex topics outside the scope of this article.

The quinone moiety generally represents a highly activated α, β-unsaturated ketone and is particularly sensitive to Michael addition. Thus in menadione (Fig. 2; 7), the unprotected (e.g. by substitution) 3-position is liable to attack by thiolate nucleophiles [86]. The conjugate thioether is a hydroquinone and thus can lead to radical formation via equilibrium (2) [or eqn. (14)]; thiol conjugation is equivalent to reduction:

$$Q + GSH \; (+H^+) \rightarrow Q(SG)H_2 \tag{13}$$

$$Q + Q(SG)H_2 \rightleftharpoons QH^{\bullet} + Q(SG)H^{\bullet} \tag{14}$$

$$Q + Q(SG)H^{\bullet} \rightleftharpoons QH^{\bullet} + Q(SG) \tag{15}$$

The reactions with glutathione are rapid [22,87] and even the fastest examples are accelerated by glutathione S-transferases [88]. Thioether formation has only a small effect on the reduction potential of menadione [89], so the thiol conjugate, when autoxidized, will redox cycle efficiently. Semiquinone radicals may also oxidize thiols to produce thiyl radicals [77], and oxidized glutathione is then produced [77,90]. Glutathione is involved in reductive activation of mitomycin c, involving reactions other than reduction of the quinone (eqn. 13) [91,92].

Direct detection of quinone radicals formed on mixing glutathione and menadione proved unequivocally the potential importance of radical generation via reactions (13)–(15) [93,94]. Which radical predominates at steady state depends on the extent of reaction, on the redox equilibrium (eqn. 15), and on the decay kinetics of the radicals. Pulse radiolysis data [89] yield an estimate of $K_{15} \approx 0.6$.

Factors controlling the rate of reaction of the drug radicals with oxygen

Energetics

Reaction (3) is formally an electron-transfer equilibrium, with a free-energy change, ΔG, given by:

$$\Delta G_3 = -nF \, \Delta E_3 = -RT \ln K_3 \tag{16}$$

where $n = 1$, F is the Faraday constant, R the gas constant, T the absolute temperature and K_3 the equilibrium constant; ΔE_3 is defined by:

$$\Delta E_3 = E_{mi}(O_2/O_2^{\bullet -}) - E_{mi}(S/S^{\bullet -}) \tag{17}$$

where E_{mi} represents the mid-point potentials of the one-electron couples at pH i. The latter are most reliably determined by pulse radiolysis measurements of electron-transfer equilibria before the partners in the equilibrium can decay [72]. These potentials can often be predicted if those of analogues are known [95]. For comparison of electron affinities we use a (non) standard state for O_2 of $1 \, mol \cdot dm^{-3}$, when $E_{m7}(O_2^{\cdot-}) = -0.18$ V versus NHE [96]. Then from eqns. (16) and (17):

$$\log K_3 \approx -3.04 - 16.9 E_{m7}(S/S^{\cdot-}) \tag{18}$$

if potentials are in volts.

The higher the value of $E_{m7}(S/S^{\cdot-})$, the lower the energy 'driving' electron transfer to oxygen, and from Marcus theory, the slower electron transfer is expected to be [97]. Fig. 4 summarizes some rate data for reactions of quinone and nitro radicals with oxygen, which show that the general behaviour is as expected. The quinone data have been presented previously [4], and extend the earlier 'Marcus type' correlation [98]. For quinone radicals with low values of $E_{m7}(S/S^{\cdot-})$, the rate constants are not much lower than the diffusion-controlled limit. In contrast, for similar energetics, nitro radicals react with oxygen around two orders of magnitude more slowly than quinone radicals. The data plotted extend the initial study [99] and include unpublished measurements (P. Wardman and E. D. Clarke, unpublished work).

For both nitro and quinone radicals, over a wide range, the higher the reduction potential, the slower the electron transfer to oxygen This redox relationship is therefore of opposite direction to drug activation to form free radicals, as plotted in Fig. 3. Also shown in Fig. 4 is the value for the rate constant for reaction of the radical from the N-oxide, tirapazamine, with oxygen [100,101]. It is very similar to the value for the metronidazole radical [99].

Kinetics of electron exchange

The main point of Fig. 4 merits reinforcement: reduction potentials influence, but do not in themselves define, electron transfer rates. Equally important are the 'zero energy' electron-exchange rates [97,98]. Nitro compounds are kinetically

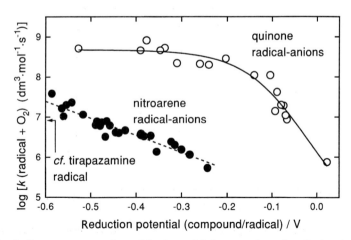

Fig. 4. Rate constants (logarithmic scale) for reaction of radical-anions with oxygen. ○, Nitroarenes (mainly nitroimidazoles); ●, quinones (see text for sources of data).

sluggish in electron transfer reactions generally, and it may well be that reaction of nitro radicals with oxygen involves an intermediate adduct, just as nitro compounds themselves tend to form adducts with reducing radicals [102]. Hence it is worth stressing that the kinetics of reaction (3) may vary over a wide range for different bioreductive drugs, apart from the influence of reduction potential. Fortunately, these reactions are easily characterized by pulse radiolysis.

Factors controlling the stability of radicals in anoxia: radical–radical reactions

Prototropic equilibria of radicals

Radical disproportionation to form a two-electron reduction product is the reverse of eqn. (2) [cf. eqn. (8)]:

$$2S^{\cdot-} \text{ (or SH}^{\cdot}) \, (+2H^+) \rightarrow SH_2 + S \tag{19}$$

and as described above, may represent an important stage in a pathway to toxic reduction products (as with nitroarenes) or a protective step, reducing the lifetime of potentially toxic radicals by forming a non-toxic product, as with tirapazamine. In either case the rates of this radical–radical reaction are important since radical disproportionation, eqn. (19), competes with reaction with oxygen, eqn. (3), or with a target, eqn. (6).

Key factors controlling radical stablity in anoxia are prototropic equilibria of radicals and pH. Fig. 5 illustrates both factors with the well-known superoxide radical [103], the tirapazamine radical [100] and the metronidazole radical [104]. (Note the rate constant is defined by the formalism: $-d[R]/dt = 2k[R]^2$, where [R] is the sum of the concentrations of all the prototropic forms of the radical.)

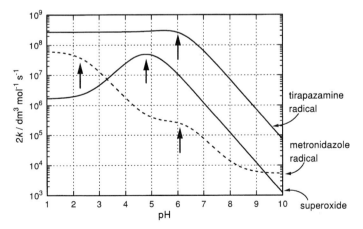

Fig. 5. Rate constants (logarithmic scale) for radical–radical reactions as a function of pH. The pK_a values for dissociation of the protonated conjugates of the radical-anions are marked by the vertical arrows (see text for sources of data).

All three radicals protonate with pK_a values for dissociation of the protonated conjugate which influence the kinetics of radical–radical reaction in the physiological range:

$$SH^{\bullet} \rightleftharpoons S^{\bullet-} + H^+ \tag{20}$$

with values of $pK_{20} = 4.8$ (superoxide [103]), 6.0 (tirapazamine [100]) and 6.1 (metronidazole [104,105]). The form of the curves for superoxide and tirapazamine radicals arises because $k_{21a} > k_{21b}$ and k_{21c} is very low or even zero:

$$SH^{\bullet} + S^{\bullet-} \; (+H^+) \rightarrow SH_2 + S \tag{21a}$$

$$2SH^{\bullet} \rightarrow SH_2 + S \tag{21b}$$

$$2S^{\bullet-}(+2H^+) \rightarrow SH_2 + S \tag{21c}$$

In the case of metronidazole, the radical has two pK_a values, one of which probably represents protonation of the unsubstituted imidazole nitrogen (6.1 in the radical, ~ 2.5 in the ground state [105]). The other:

$$(SH_2^{\bullet})^+ \rightleftharpoons SH^{\bullet} + H^+ \tag{22}$$

has a $pK_{22} = 2.3$ [104] and we ascribe this to protonation of oxygen in the nitro group in the radical. This latter equilibrium has no influence on k_{19} in the physiological pH range.

Quinone radical stability is not illustrated on Fig. 5 because it is not possible to generalize and the effects of pH are less marked. The radical chemistry of quinones has been reviewed [4–6,106,107]. Simpler p- and o-quinone radicals have pK_{20} values around 4–5 and hence the radicals are dissociated (anions) at pH ~ 7. For the p-benzoquinone radical, values of $k_{19} \sim 2 \times 10^8$ and 1×10^9 dm$^3 \cdot$mol$^{-1} \cdot$s^{-1} at neutral pH and pH 2 were reported [108]. For diazaquone (AZQ, Fig. 2, **11**), $2k_{19} \sim 9 \times 10^5$ dm$^3 \cdot$mol$^{-1} \cdot$s^{-1} at pH 7 was measured, 2–3 orders of magnitude lower than for simpler quinone radicals [109].

First-order (concentration-independent) radical decay pathways

Not all nitroarene radicals decay according to rate laws defined by disproportionation, eqns. (8) and (19). The radicals of misonidazole (Fig. 2; **2**) and other 2-nitroimidazoles were found to decay exponentially at low concentrations [110]. Since radical steady-state concentrations are likely to be submicromolar in cellular systems (except perhaps when totally hypoxic), this is an important decay pathway:

$$S^{\bullet-}/SH^{\bullet} \; (+H^+) \rightarrow products \tag{23}$$

At pH 7.3, estimates of $k_{23} \sim 10$ and 5 s^{-1} were made for misonidazole and etanidazole [110]. The reaction rate also decreased with increasing pH (cf. Fig. 5, metronidazole) between pH values of 6.6 and 8.9, with an order of magnitude increase in stability per pH unit. The half-life of reaction (23) ($\sim 0.7/k_{23}$) is about 70 ms for misonidazole at pH 7.3.

The final products of reaction (23) may be the same as disproportionation (8): the important point is that the kinetics are independent of radical concentration. In contrast, the half-lives of 5-nitroimidazole radicals (e.g. metronidazole) were accurately inversely proportional to radical concentration, as expected for a true second-order reaction [eqn. (8)] [110].

Another important group of compounds where unimolecular decay of the radical occurs is nitroarenes substituted with good leaving groups: nitrobenzyl halides are typical. Fig. 6 shows reaction schemes (a) by Teicher and Sartorelli [111] and (b) from the studies of Neta and colleagues [112–115]. In the example from the latter work which is illustrated (dehalogenation of o-nitrobenzyl chloride radical-anion), the formation of a carbon-centred radical occurs with a half-life of ~60 μs at 37 °C; the rates vary according to structure and leaving group. From Fig. 4 we expect these short-lived nitro radical-anions to react with oxygen with rate constants, k_3, no greater than about 10^7 dm$^3 \cdot$mol$^{-1} \cdot$s^{-1}. The half-life of this 'protective' electron transfer to oxygen $\{\sim 0.7/(k_3[O_2])\}$ will thus be at least ~2 ms in well-oxygenated tissue with $[O_2] \sim 40$ μmol$\cdot$dm^{-3}. Hence there will be many instances in this group of compounds where peroxyl radicals, rather than alkylating reduced nitro compounds, are formed (the carbon-centred radical will react very rapidly with O_2). The leaving group will often, but not always, be lost before reaction of nitro radical-anions with oxygen (or with themselves) occurs. These competing pathways are consistent with EPR observations [116].

Shown as an inset to Fig. 6 is an example from recent work [117] which seeks to exploit this chemistry to release a mustard derivative rather than rely on reactive nitroreduction intermediates. It thus seems possible to overcome the kinetic constraints of simpler nitrobenzyl derivatives.

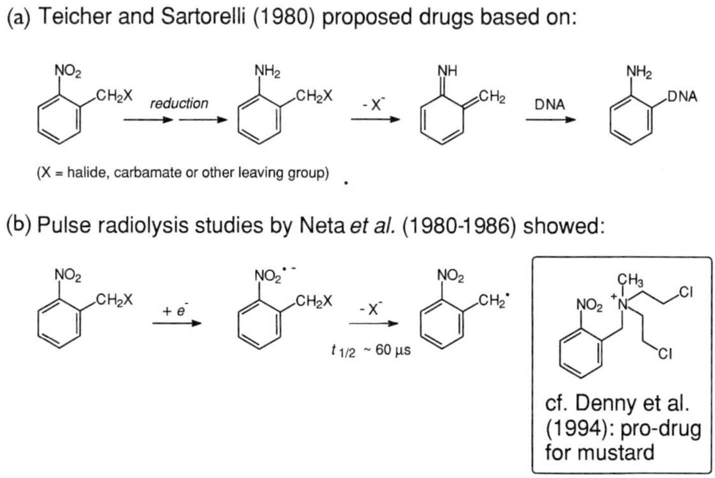

Fig. 6. (a) Hypothetical basis for alkylating DNA following reduction of a nitrobenzyl halide; (b) radical chemistry of o-nitrobenzyl chloride (half-life shown for 37 °C). Inset: compound being evaluated as a bioreductive drug, relying on 'leaving group' chemistry of the radical-anion (see text for references).

Ketyl character

The radical of 4-nitroacetophenone has $2k_{19} \sim 10^7 \, dm^3 \cdot mol^{-1} \cdot s^{-1}$ invariant with pH for pH > 6 [3], presumably because some unpaired spin is delocalized on to the ketone function, and the radical has then partial ketyl character. Hence a nitro radical can be made to disproportionate much faster by substitution of an acetyl or similar function. This could be an important consideration in drug design (see below).

Reaction of the initial radical with a target as the mode of action

Evidence for radicals as damaging species

The possible involvement of 'secondary' radicals in drug metabolism [subsequent to the initial formation of $S^{\cdot-}$ in eqn. (1)] has been noted above. An illustration is nitroxide radicals formed upon reduction of nitrosoarenes [39]. These radicals may be damaging. Mention has also been made of electrochemical studies indicating interaction of the primary radical-anions, or protonated conjugates, with DNA. However, the simplest evidence for a mechanism of cytoxicity involving the initial radical as a damaging species arises when the stable 2- and 4-electron reduction products are non-toxic, particularly if reduction stops essentially at the 2-electron step. Then the drug radical, $S^{\cdot-}/SH^{\cdot}$ is a prime candidate for the toxic intermediate, reaction (6).

This appears to be the case for the di-N-oxide, tirapazamine (Fig. 2; **14**) [11,70]. Fig. 7 outlines the reduction chemistry of tirapazamine and a possible basis for its action [70,100,118]. The damage leading to cytotoxicity has been identified as DNA double-strand breaks which are particularly difficult to repair, perhaps comparable with the clustered damage from densely ionizing radiation [119]. Models for the mechanism of action are discussed below.

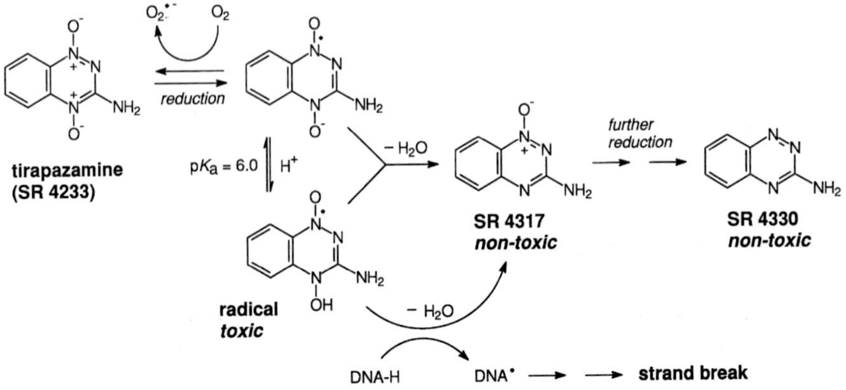

Fig. 7. Reduction chemistry of tirapazamine and possible mode of action.

Clustered damage from a single radical

This could arise from a reductase present in the nucleus 'concentrating' radical attack on DNA [119]. However, we are testing an alternative, novel hypothesis. This involves a single radical initiating a chain reaction which results in multiple strand breaks: (i) a reductase produces a radical, possibly but not necessarily, in the nucleus; (ii) the radical abstracts H from a sugar residue on DNA to give a strand break, much like ˙OH radicals but probably several orders of magnitude slower; (iii) a radical centre remains on the sugar which has reducing properties and produces another drug radical from unreduced tirapazamine; (iv) this radical attacks DNA near the site of generation to give a second strand break and damage which is much more clustered than, for example, that from hydrogen peroxide/iron(II).

Although this latter hypothesis is speculative, experimental evidence using a very simple model system suggests further work to explore the possibility is justified. Fig. 8 shows our measurements of the initial rate of loss of tirapazamine obtained when tirapazamine radicals are generated at a constant rate of $55 \ nmol \cdot dm^{-3} \cdot s^{-1}$ by radiolysis of an N_2-saturated solution containing tirapazamine ($0.5 \ mmol \cdot dm^{-3}$) and deoxyribose ($50 \ mmol \cdot dm^{-3}$). Tirapazamine radicals are produced by reaction of hydrated electrons with tirapazamine and also via ˙OH radicals reacting with deoxyribose to produce a reducing radical. The concentration differential ensures no direct reaction of ˙OH with tirapazamine.

The radical yield was calibrated by irradiating a similar solution but replacing tirapazamine with ferricyanide and measuring conversion into ferrocyanide; the expected yield was obtained. If there were no chain reaction, then one might expect tirapazamine to be lost by reduction to the 2-electron product at the rate of 0.5 molecules of product per radical input. However, as Fig. 8 shows, the loss was well above 0.5 molecules/radical, and at low pH was some 5-fold higher than expected. The pH dependence is probably associated with protonation of the tirapazamine radical ($pK_a = 6.0$ [100]). We suggest that the results point to a chain reaction in which the propagation step is abstraction of H from the sugar to give

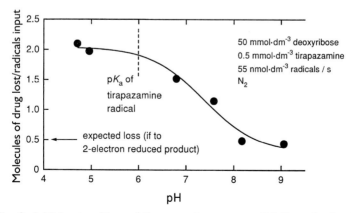

Fig. 8. Initial rate of loss of tirapazamine upon radiolytic reduction in the presence of deoxyribose.

a radical which reduces tirapazamine; the termination steps are radical–radical reactions. The protonated radical evidently abstracts H much faster than the anion-radical. The chain length varies with pH, deoxyribose concentration and dose rate (radical input rate), as would be expected from this model. Qualitatively similar results were obtained with either 2-propanol or formate replacing deoxyribose as H-donor. In addition, preliminary pulse-radiolysis experiments have provided supporting evidence for the model. Full details will be reported elsewhere, but even such a simple model system provides a method of comparing the H-abstracting abilities of radicals from analogues of tirapazamine, to which we plan to extend these studies.

An unusual dependence of tirapazamine-associated cytotoxicity upon oxygen concentration has been reported [120]. This cannot be explained simply on the basis of reactions (3) and (19) competing with reaction (6). If our hypothesis is correct, however, oxygen will also compete by reacting with sugar radicals in an addition/elimination reaction, and the involvement of peroxyl radicals is a possibility. The kinetics of oxygen interaction in our model of tirapazamine reduction involving sugar radicals will be discussed in more detail elsewhere, when pulse radiolysis measurements of such possible competing reactions are complete.

Implications of the rate constants for competing reactions

A model in which the radical reacts with oxygen in competition with disproportionation resulting in toxicity

In this model, radicals are produced in reaction (1) and can react with oxygen in reaction (3). In competition, radicals can react by disproportionation, reaction (19) [cf. reaction (8)], a pathway which leads to toxicity. By setting the expression for the rate of change of radical concentration with time, $-d[S^{\cdot-}]/dt = 0$ (the steady-state approximation), it is easily shown that when the rate of reaction (3) equals the rate of reaction (19):

$$[O_2] = (k_1 k_{19}[S])^{1/2}/k_3 \tag{24}$$

This will be the oxygen concentration when the toxic pathway is balanced by the non-toxic pathway, i.e. at which the 'switch-over' from oxic protection to anoxic cytotoxicity occurs (radiobiologists sometimes call this the 'K value'). In this expression k_1 is a first-order rate constant (zero-order formalism could have been used, omitting [S]). So far as the use of bioreductive drugs in radiotherapy goes, the oxygen concentration of the critical radioresistant cells is of the order of a few micromolar. Few human tumour cells exist at submicromolar oxygen concentrations [121].

To evaluate this expression, the rate of drug reduction (or radical formation) needs to be measured. This can be readily achieved, e.g. with cells in suspension, measuring loss of drug by HPLC, or measuring oxygen consumption reflecting redox cycling, eqns. (3),(4), etc. However, the measurements indicate radicals produced per cell per unit time, and to derive k_1 we need an estimate of the reaction volume. Siim et al. [21] have argued that the chemistry should be integrated over the total volume of cell suspension, around 1000-fold higher than the cellular volume in typical experiments. With this assumption, their measured oxygen sensitivity for toxicity of a nitroquinoline agreed with eqn. (24). In support of this assumption, EPR evidence for nitro radicals outside the cellular space in hepatocytes was noted [122]. However, in these latter experiments the cultures would have become anoxic by the time of measurement, and we question whether the assumption of radicals distributed homogeneously throughout the experimental system is valid in the presence of even submicromolar oxygen concentrations. We must consider the question of mean diffusion distance of the radicals.

What is the reaction volume?

It can be shown that the mean diffusion distance, x, of a radical in time t is:

$$x = (2Dt)^{1/2} \tag{25}$$

where D is the diffusion coefficient. For a typical radical in water this will be about 10^{-9} $m^2 \cdot s^{-1}$, but the cytoplasm is more viscous [122], and a value of about 1.5×10^{-10} $m^2 \cdot s^{-1}$ is probably appropriate. The mean lifetime of the radical will depend on oxygen concentration, reductase activity and appropriate rate constants, but if we focus on the important, partially hypoxic range and take the lifetime as about half that of the 'oxic decay' pathway, i.e.

$$t \approx (2k_3[O_2])^{-1} \tag{26}$$

then we can estimate the (very approximate) mean radical diffusion distance:

$$x \approx \{D/(k_3[O_2])\}^{1/2} \approx 12/(k_3[O_2])^{1/2} \ \mu m \tag{27}$$

For the nitroquinoline studied by Siim et al. [21], $k_3 \sim 2.5 \times 10^6$ $dm^3 \cdot mol^{-1} \cdot s^{-1}$ and even if $[O_2]$ is as low as 0.5 $\mu mol \cdot dm^{-3}$, then the mean diffusion distance is only about 11 μm, i.e. of cellular dimensions. This approach ignores the time taken for an anion to permeate the cytoplasmic membrane. We conclude that most of the chemistry we are considering occurs inside the cell except in essentially anoxic cultures. (Diffusion processes should obviously be included in our model of a radical exerting clustered damage which is discussed above; too low a radical reactivity with DNA might permit diffusion away from the target. However, non-homogeneous kinetics are outside the scope of this article.)

The diffusion distance of an intermediate such as a nitrosoarene may also be estimated using the same approach. Since the rate constants for reactions of nitroarene radicals with oxygen are around 1000-fold higher than those for reactions of nitroso intermediates with glutathione, but the concentration of oxygen in hypoxic cells is around 1000-fold lower than glutathione, then the above conclusion concerning the diffusion distances of nitro radicals will also apply, very broadly, to nitrosoarene intermediates produced in cells.

A model in which the radical reacts with oxygen in competition with a first-order pathway resulting in toxicity

We noted above examples, such as 2-nitroimidazoles, where radicals decay by first-order (concentration-independent) pathways, e.g. eqn. (23). If this occurs in competition with reaction with oxygen, eqn. (3), then we do not need to know the steady-state radical concentration or the reaction volume to estimate the oxygen concentration at which the 'oxic' pathway (3) is balanced by the 'anoxic' pathway (23). When the rates of these two reactions are equal:

$$[O_2] = k_{23}/k_3 \tag{28}$$

and if, for example, $k_{23} \sim 10 \text{ s}^{-1}$ and $k_3 \sim 5 \times 10^6 \text{ dm}^3 \cdot \text{mol}^{-1} \cdot \text{s}^{-1}$ (typical of a 2-nitroimidazole), we might expect a 'K value' [when eqns. (3) and (23) are balanced] of around $2 \text{ } \mu\text{mol} \cdot \text{dm}^{-3} \text{ O}_2$.

Implications of first-order versus second-order 'anoxic pathways'

The key difference between the two simple models outlined above is that the first-order 'anoxic pathway' implies the oxygen sensitivity of bioreduction is independent of reduction rate, eqn. (28), in contrast to the consequence of a radical–radical reaction being involved and reduction rate being important in influencing steady-state concentrations of radicals and hence the rate of reaction (19), eqn. (24).

Rauth et al. [123] measured the oxygen inhibition of reduction of a 5-nitro-imidazole, metronidazole (the radical of which decays by a second-order pathway), or a 2-nitroimidazole, misonidazole (first-order decay) (see [110]). Reduction involved radiolytic radical generation at a rate of $\sim 10 \text{ nmol} \cdot \text{dm}^{-3} \cdot \text{s}^{-1}$ ($= k_1[\text{S}]$). Using the known rate data, k_3, k_{19}, k_{23} for the two compounds [99,110] and eqns. (24) and (28) we can estimate that oxygen should significantly inhibit reduction of metronidazole at a concentration as low as a few nanomolar with the reduction rate used here, but in contrast, inhibiting misonidazole reduction should require ~ 1000-fold higher concentrations of oxygen. Experimental results were broadly in line with expectation [123].

Siim et al. [21] found reduction of a nitroquinoline by mammalian cells in suspension to be inhibited at oxygen tensions of about $0.2 \text{ } \mu\text{mol} \cdot \text{dm}^{-3}$. The majority of radioresistant, hypoxic cells in tumours exist at oxygen tensions an order of magnitude higher than this value [121,124]. We have questioned above their assumption in their theoretical treatment that the radicals diffuse throughout the experimental volume, but this high sensitivity to oxygen is characteristic of a nitroarene bioreductive drug exhibiting second-order radical–radical decay, eqn. (19). Although a sweeping generalization should be treated with caution, in general it appears that such compounds might be less useful in cancer therapy than, for example, bioreductive drugs based on the 2-nitroimidazole moiety, such as RSU 1069 or its pro-drug, RBU 6145 [125], because of the kinetic factors which distinguish these groups of compounds.

Many quinone radicals disproportionate up to four orders of magnitude faster than nitroarene radicals, but the oxygen sensitivity in eqn. (24) is dependent on the square root of this rate constant, and the difference between the two classes of compound is offset by the ~ 100 times higher rate constants for reaction of quinone radicals with oxygen compared with nitro radicals (Fig. 4). Hence the kinetic basis for the use of nitroarene or quinone compounds as bioreductive drugs in cancer therapy has evident parallels even though the absolute rate constants for individual reactions may differ by orders of magnitude.

Conclusions

Bioreductive drugs rely on free radical reactions for their activation and selectivity. Each step in the process can be investigated in model systems. Although the details have not been discussed here, radiolysis methods [101,126] have played a pivotal role in the quantitative understanding of the kinetic factors which control drug efficacy. Redox properties control drug activation and the rates of 'protective' electron transfer to oxygen; pH is important in controlling the rate of radical decay, whether this involves radical–radical reactions or unimolecular processes rate-determining in the decay of some nitroarenes. The effects of pH reflect prototropic equilibria involving radicals, readily quantified by radiolysis methods [100,104,105]. Substituents in aromatic structures will influence both redox properties and radical pK_a. Thus an electron-donating substituent will generally decrease reduction potential [95] and increase radical pK_a. In eqn. (24), k_1 will be reduced and k_{19} could well be increased by such a substituent. In the tirapazamine model described above, a protonated radical is more reactive than the radical-anion, and hence a high radical pK_a may increase the effectiveness of radical damage at $pH > pK_a$. The sensitivity of these parameters to substituent effects could form the basis for rational drug design.

We conclude that reaction kinetics are of central importance in considering the mechanisms of action of bioreductive drugs, and that further work to develop the framework outlined here is desirable. A fuller description of numerical models of the reaction kinetics and oxygen sensitivities of bioreductive drug cytotoxicity will be presented elsewhere.

This work is supported by the Cancer Research Campaign.

References

1. Mason, R.P. (1990) Environ. Health Perspect. **87**, 237–243
2. Adams, G.E. (1981) Cancer **48**, 696–707
3. Wardman, P. (1985) Environ. Health Perspect. **63**, 101–112
4. Wardman, P. (1990) Free Radical Res. Commun. **8**, 219–229
5. Powis, G. (1989) Free. Radical Biol. Med. **6**, 63–101
6. Brunmark, A. and Cadenas, E. (1989) Free. Radical Biol. Med. **7**, 435–477
7. O'Brien, P.J. (1991) Chem. Biol. Interact. **80**, 1–41
8. Mason, R.P. (1992) in Biological Consequences of Oxidative Stress. Implications for Cardiovascular Disease and Carcinogenesis (Spatz, L. and Bloom, A.D., eds.), pp. 23–49, Oxford University Press, New York
9. Butler, J. and Hoey, B.M. (1993) in DNA and Free Radicals (Halliwell, B. and Aruoma, O.I., eds.), pp. 243–273, Ellis Horwood, Chichester
10. Workman, P. and Stratford, I.J. (1993) Cancer Metastasis Rev. **12**, 73–82
11. Zeman, E.M., Baker, M.A., Lemmon, M.J., Pearson, C.I., Adams, J.A., Brown, J.M., Lee, W.W. and Tracy, M. (1989) Int. J. Radiat. Oncol. Biol. Phys. **16**, 977–981
12. Wang, J., Biedermann, K.A., Wolf, C.R. and Brown, J.M. (1993) Br. J. Cancer **67**, 321–325
13. Naylor, M.A., Stevens, M.A., Nolan, J., Sutton, B., Tocher, J.H., Fielden, E.M.,

Adams, G.E. and Stratford, I.J. (1993) Anti-Cancer Drug. Des. **8**, 439–461

14. Jenkins, T.C., Naylor, M.A., O'Neill, P., Threadgill, M.D., Cole, S., Stratford, I.J., Adams, G.E., Fielden, E.M., Suto, M.J. and Steir, M.A. (1990) J. Med. Chem. **33**, 2603–2610

15. Wilson, W.R. (1992) in Cancer Biology and Medicine. (Waring, M.J. and Ponder, B.A.J., eds.), vol. 3, pp. 87–131, Kluver Academic Publishers, Lancaster

16. Mulcahy, R.T., Gipp, J.J., Schmidt, J.P., Joswig, C. and Borch, R.F. (1994) J. Med. Chem. **37**, 1610–1615

17. Adams, G.E. (1992) Radiat. Res. **132**, 129–139

18. Knox, R.J., Friedlos, F. and Boland, M.P. (1993) Cancer Metastasis Rev. **12**, 195–212

19. Palmer, B.D., Wilson, W.R., Atwell, G.J., Schultz, D., Xu, X.Z. and Denny, W.A. (1994) J. Med. Chem. **37**, 2175–2184

20. Denny, W.A. and Wilson, W.R. (1993) Cancer Metastasis Rev. **12**, 135–151

21. Siim, B.G., Atwell, G.J. and Wilson, W.R. (1994) Br. J. Cancer **70**, 596–603

22. Wilson, I., Wardman, P., Lin, T.-S. and Sartorelli, A.C. (1987) Chem. Biol. Interact. **61**, 229–240

23. Goin, J., Gibson, D.D., McCay, P.B. and Cadenas, E. (1991) Arch. Biochem. Biophys. **288**, 386–396

24. Rockwell, S., Sartorelli, A.C., Tomasz, M. and Kennedy, K.A. (1993) Cancer Metastasis Rev. **12**, 165–176

25. Rauth, A.M., Marshall, R.S. and Kuehl, B.L. (1993) Cancer Metastasis Rev. **12**, 153–164

26. Feinstein, E., Canaani, E. and Weiner, L.M. (1993) Biochemistry **32**, 13156–13161

27. Ubezio, P. and Civoli, F. (1994) Free. Radical Biol. Med. **16**, 509–516

28. Milei, J. (1993) in Vitamin E in Health and Disease (Packer, L. and Fuchs, J., eds.), pp. 417–431, Marcel Dekker, New York

29. Huang, Z.-D., Chen, Y.-N., Menon, K. and Teicher, B.A. (1993) J. Med. Chem. **36**, 1797–1801

30. Suter, W., Rosselet, A. and KnÅsel, F. (1978) Antimicrob. Agents Chemother. **13**, 770–783

31. Baker, M.A., Zeman, E.M., Hirst, V.K. and Brown, J.M. (1988) Cancer Res. **48**, 5947–5952

32. Walton, M.I. and Workman, P. (1990) Biochem. Pharmacol. **39**, 1735–1742

33. Silva, J.M. and O'Brien, P.J. (1993) Br. J. Cancer **68**, 484–491

34. Patterson, L.H. (1993) Cancer Metastasis Rev. **12**, 119–134

35. Workman, P. (1992) Int. J. Radiat. Oncol. Biol. Phys. **22**, 631–637

36. Moreno, S.N.J. and Docampo, R. (1985) Environ. Health Perspec. **64**, 199–208

37. Eyer, P. (1979) Chem. Biol. Interact. **24**, 227–239

38. Diepold, C., Eyer, P., Kampffmeyer, H. and Reinhardt, K. (1982) in Biological Reactive Intermediates - II. Chemical Mechanisms and Biological Effects (Snyder, R., Jollow, D.J., Parke, D.V., Gibson, C.G., Kocsis, J.J. and Witmer, C.M., eds.), pp. 1173–1181, Plenum Press, New York

39. Fischer, V. and Mason, R.P. (1986) Chem. Biol. Interact. **57**, 129–142

40. Kazanis, S. and McClelland, R.A. (1992) J. Am. Chem. Soc. **114**, 3052–3059

41. Noss, M.B., Panicucci, R., McClelland, R.A. and Rauth, A.M. (1988) Biochem.

Pharmacol. **37**, 2585–2593

42. Noss, M.B., Panicucci, R., McClelland, R.A. and Rauth, A.M. (1989) Int. J. Radiat. Oncol. Biol. Phys. **16**, 1015–1019

43. Mulcahy, R.T., Gipp, J.J., Ublacker, G.A., Panicucci, R. and McClelland, R.A. (1989) Biochem. Pharmacol. **38**, 1667–1671

44. McClelland, R.A. (1990) in Selective Activation of Drugs by Redox Processes (Adams, G.E., Breccia, A., Fielden, E.M. and Wardman, P., eds.), pp. 125–136, Plenum Press, New York

45. Gipp, J.J., McClelland, R.A. and Mulcahy, R.T. (1991) Biochem. Pharmacol. **42** (Suppl.), S127–S133

46. Bérubé, L.R., Farah, S., McClelland, R.A. and Rauth, A.M. (1991) Biochem. Pharmacol. **42**, 2153–2161

47. Bérubé, L.R., Farah, S., McClelland, R.A. and Rauth, A.M. (1992) Int. J. Radiat. Oncol. Biol. Phys. **22**, 817–820

48. Ehlhardt, W.J., Beaulieu, B.B., Jr. and Goldman, P. (1988) Biochem. Pharmacol. **37**, 2603–2606

49. Ehlhardt, W.J. and Beaulieu, B.B., Jr. (1988) J. Med. Chem. **31**, 323–329

50. Floyd, R.A. (1981) Radiat. Res. **86**, 243–263

51. Knox, R.J., Knight, R.C. and Edwards, D.I. (1983) Biochem. Pharmacol. **32**, 2149–2156

52. McClelland, R.A., Fuller, J.R., Seaman, N.E., Rauth, A.M. and Battistella, R. (1984) Biochem. Pharmacol. **33**, 303–309

53. Varghese, A.J. and Whitmore, G.F. (1984) Radiat. Res. **97**, 262–271

54. Varghese, A.J. and Whitmore, G.F. (1985) Chem. Biol. Interact. **56**, 269–287

55. Whitmore, G.F. and Varghese, A.J. (1986) Biochem. Pharmacol. **35**, 97–103

56. McClelland, R.A., Panicucci, R. and Rauth, A.M. (1987) J. Am. Chem. Soc. **109**, 4308–4314

57. Bolton, J.L. and McClelland, R.A. (1989) J. Am. Chem. Soc. **111**, 8172–8181

58. Tocher, J.H., Edwards, D.I. and Thomas, A. (1994) Int. J. Radiat. Oncol. Biol. Phys. **29**, 307–310

59. Herreno-Saenz, D., Evans, F.E. and Fu, P.P. (1994) Chem. Res. Toxicol. **7**, 806–814

60. Malia, S.A. and Basu, A.K. (1994) Chem. Res. Toxicol. **7**, 823–828

61. Upadhyaya, P., von Tungeln, L.S., Fu, P.P. and El-Bayoumy, K. (1994) Chem. Res. Toxicol. **7**, 690–695

62. Sartorelli, A.C. (1988) Cancer Res. **48**, 775–778

63. Ross, D., Siegel, D., Beall, H., Prakash, A.S., Mulcahy, R.T. and Gibson, N.W. (1993) Cancer Metastasis Rev. **12**, 83–101

64. Knight, R.C., Skolimowski, I.M. and Edwards, D.I. (1978) Biochem. Pharmacol. **27**, 2089–2093

65. Rowley, D.A., Knight, R.C., Skolimowski, I.M. and Edwards, D.I. (1980) Biochem. Pharmacol. **29**, 2095–2098

66. Rowley, D.A., Knight, R.C., Skolimowski, I.M. and Edwards, D.I. (1979) Biochem. Pharmacol. **28**, 3009–3013

67. Zahoor, A., Lafleur, M.C.M., Knight, R.C., Loman, H. and Edwards, D.I. (1987) Biochem. Pharmacol. **36**, 3299–3304

68. Dale, L.D., Tocher, J.H. and Edwards, D.I. (1988) Anti-Cancer Drug. Des. **3**,

169–175

69. Tocher, J.H., Virk, N.S. and Edwards, D.I. (1990) Biochem. Pharmacol. **39**, 781–786
70. Zeman, E.M., Brown, J.M., Lemmon, M.J., Hirst, V.K. and Lee, W.W. (1986) Int. J. Radiat. Oncol. Biol. Phys. **12**, 1239–1242
71. Clarke, E.D., Wardman, P. and Goulding, K.H. (1980) Biochem. Pharmacol. **29**, 2684–2687
72. Wardman, P. (1989) J. Phys. Chem. Ref. Data **18**, 1637–1755
73. O'Connor, C.J., McLennan, D.J., Sutton, B.M., Denny, W.A. and Wilson, W.R. (1991) J. Chem. Soc., Perkin Trans. 2 951–954
74. Clarke, E.D., Goulding, K.H. and Wardman, P. (1982) Biochem. Pharmacol. **31**, 3237–3242
75. Orna, M.V. and Mason, R.P. (1989) J. Biol. Chem. **264**, 12379–12384
76. Butler, J. and Hoey, B.M. (1993) Biochim. Biophys. Acta **1161**, 73–78
77. Giulivi, C. and Cadenas, E. (1994) Biochem. J. **301**, 21–30
78. Mason, R.P. and Josephy, P.D. (1985) in Toxicity of Nitroaromatic Compounds (Rickert, D.E., eds.), pp. 121–140, Hemisphere Pub. Corp., Washington
79. Lloyd, R.V., Duling, D.R., Rumyantseva, G.V., Mason, R.P. and Bridson, P.K. (1991) Mol. Pharmacol. **40**, 440–445
80. Olive, P.L. (1979) Cancer Res. **39**, 4512–4515
81. Adams, G.E., Ahmed, I., Clarke, E.D., O'Neill, P., Parrick, J., Stratford, I.J., Wallace, R.G., Wardman, P. and Watts, M.E. (1980) Int. J. Radiat. Biol. **38**, 613–626
82. Wardman, P. (1987) in Radiation Chemistry. Principles and Applications (Farhataziz and Rodgers, M.A.J., eds.), pp. 565–599, VCH Publishers, Deerfield Beach
83. Baxendale, J.H. and Hardy, H.R. (1953) Trans. Faraday Soc. **49**, 1433–1437
84. Mukherjee, T., Land, E.J., Swallow, A.J. and Bruce, J.M. (1989) Arch. Biochem. Biophys. **272**, 450–458
85. Plumb, J.A., Gerritsen, M. and Workman, P. (1994) Br. J. Cancer **70**, 1136–1143
86. Nickerson, W.J., Falcone, G. and Strauss, G. (1963) Biochemistry **2**, 537–543
87. Butler, J. and Hoey, B.M. (1992) Free. Radical Biol. Med. **12**, 337–345
88. Coles, B., Wilson, I., Wardman, P., Hinson, J.A., Nelson, S.D. and Ketterer, B. (1988) Arch. Biochem. Biophys. **264**, 253–280
89. Wilson, I., Wardman, P., Lin, T.-S. and Sartorelli, A.C. (1986) J. Med. Chem. **29**, 1381–1384
90. Ross, D., Thor, H., Orrenius, S. and Moldeus, P. (1985) Chem. Biol. Interact. **55**, 177–184
91. Sharma, M., He, Q.-Y. and Tomasz, M. (1994) Chem. Res. Toxicol. **7**, 401–407
92. Sharma, M. and Tomasz, M. (1994) Chem. Res. Toxicol. **7**, 390–400
93. Gant, T.W., d'Arcy Doherty, M., Odowole, D., Sales, K.D. and Cohen, G.M. (1986) FEBS Lett. **201**, 296–300
94. Takahashi, N., Schreiber, J., Fischer, V. and Mason, R.P. (1987) Arch. Biochem. Biophys. **252**, 41–48
95. Wardman, P. (1990) in Selective Activation of Drugs by Redox Processes (Adams, G.E., Breccia, A., Fielden, E.M. and Wardman, P., eds.), pp. 11–24, Plenum Press, New York

96. Wardman, P. (1991) Free Radical Res. Commun. **14**, 57–67
97. Marcus, R.A. (1993) Angew. Chem. Int. Ed. Engl. **32**, 1111–1121
98. Meisel, D. (1975) Chem. Phys. Lett. **34**, 263–266
99. Wardman, P. and Clarke, E.D. (1976) Biochem. Biophys. Res. Commun. **69**, 942–949
100. Laderoute, K., Wardman, P. and Rauth, A.M. (1988) Biochem. Pharmacol. **37**, 1487–1495
101. Wardman, P., Candeias, L.P., Everett, S.A. and Tracy, M. (1994) Int. J. Radiat. Biol. **65**, 35–41
102. Wardman, P. and Clarke, E.D. (1985) in New Chemo and Radiosensitizing Drugs (Breccia, A. and Fowler, J.F., eds.), pp. 21–38, Lo Scarabeo, Bologna
103. Bielski, B.H.J., Cabelli, D.E. and Arudi, R.L. (1985) J. Phys. Chem. Ref. Data **14**, 1041–1100
104. Henry, Y., Guissani, A. and Hickel, B. (1987) Int. J. Radiat. Biol. **51**, 797–809
105. Wardman, P. (1975) Int. J. Radiat. Biol. **28**, 585–588
106. Swallow, A.J. (1982) in Functions of Quinones in Energy Conserving Systems (Trumpower, B.L., eds.), pp. 59–72, Academic Press, New York
107. Neta, P. (1988) in The Chemistry of Quinonoid Compounds. Vol. II. (Patai, S. and Rappopport, Z., eds.), pp. 879–898, John Wiley, Chichester
108. Adams, G.E. and Michael, B.D. (1967) Trans. Faraday Soc. **63**, 1171–1180
109. Butler, J., Hoey, B.M. and Lea, J.S. (1987) Biochim. Biophys. Acta **925**, 144–149
110. Wardman, P. (1985) Life Chem. Rep. **3**, 22–28
111. Teicher, B.A. and Sartorelli, A. (1980) J. Med. Chem. **23**, 955–960
112. Behar, D. and Neta, P. (1981) J. Phys. Chem. **85**, 690–693
113. Bays, J.P., Blumer, S.T., Baral-Tosh, S., Behar, D. and Neta, P. (1983) J. Am. Chem. Soc. **105**, 320–324
114. Norris, R.K., Barker, S.D. and Neta, P. (1984) J. Am. Chem. Soc. **106**, 3140–3144
115. Meot-Ner (Mautner), M., Neta, P., Norris, R.K. and Wilson, K. (1986) J. Phys. Chem. **90**, 168–173
116. Moreno, S.N.J., Schreiber, J. and Mason, R.P. (1986) J. Biol. Chem. **261**, 7811–7815
117. Denny, W.A., Wilson, W.R., Tercel, M., Van Zijl, P. and Pullen, S.M. (1994) Int. J. Radiat. Oncol. Biol. Phys. **29**, 317–321
118. Laderoute, K.R. and Rauth, A.M. (1986) Biochem. Pharmacol. **35**, 3417–3420
119. Wang, J., Biedermann, K.A. and Brown, J.M. (1992) Cancer Res. **52**, 4473–4477
120. Koch, C.J. (1993) Cancer Res. **53**, 3992–3997
121. Gatenby, R.A., Kessler, H.B., Rosenblum, J.S., Coia, L.R., Moldofsky, P.J. and Al, E.T. (1988) Int. J. Radiat. Oncol. Biol. Phys. **14**, 831–838
122. Rao, D.N.R., Jordan, S. and Mason, R.P. (1988) Biochem. Pharmacol. **37**, 2907–2913
123. Rauth, A.M., McClelland, R.A., Michaels, H.B. and Battistella, R. (1984) Int. J. Radiat. Oncol. Biol. Phys. **10**, 1323–1326
124. Vaupel, P., Schlenger, K.-H., Hoeckel, M. and Okunieff, P. (1992) in Oxygen Transport to Tissue XIII (Goldstick, T.K., McCabe, M. and Maguire, D.J., eds.), pp. 361–371, Plenum, New York

125. Adams, G.E. and Stratford, I.J. (1994) Int. J. Radiat. Oncol. Biol. Phys. **29**, 231–238

126. Wardman, P. (1992) in Radiation Science - Of Molecules, Mice and Men (BJR Supplement 24) (Denekamp, J. and Hirst, D.G., eds.), pp. 6–10, British Institute of Radiology, London

Biochem. Soc. Symp. **61**, 195–207
Printed in Great Britain

Side-effects of drugs used in the treatment of rheumatoid arthritis

P.J. Evans* and B. Halliwell

Pharmacology Group, University of London King's College, Chelsea Campus, Manresa Road, London SW3 6LX, U.K.

Abstract

A number of anti-inflammatory and other drugs used in the treatment of rheumatoid arthritis have been screened for their ability to cause oxidative damage to lipids and proteins *in vitro*. Although many drugs exhibited an antioxidant profile, a few drugs tested were pro-oxidant, increasing peroxidation of arachidonic acid by mixtures of haem proteins and H_2O_2. This system may be an appropriate model to use in the inflammatory situation, since microbleeding to release haemoglobin occurs in the inflamed rheumatoid joint, where H_2O_2 is produced by invading neutrophils.

The damaging effects of the pro-oxidant drugs phenylbutazone, meclofenamic acid and flufenamic acid were investigated in some detail using this system. Arachidonic acid peroxidation was accentuated in a dose-dependent manner and in the presence of haem proteins and H_2O_2, phenylbutazone also causes inactivation of α_1-antiproteinase, a major serine proteinase inhibitor in biological fluids.

The above drugs may interact with ferryl haemoglobin, produced by the reaction of H_2O_2 with haemoglobin, to generate drug-derived radicals causing oxidative damage in these systems. If such reactions occur *in vivo*, they could contribute to the side-effects induced by these drugs on administration to certain rheumatoid arthritis patients.

Side-effects of drugs used in the treatment of rheumatoid arthritis

Rheumatoid arthritis is a painful, crippling disease of the joints affecting all age groups both as a chronic and as an acute disorder. The aetiology of the disease is a progressive erosion of the articular cartilage and bone epiphysis within the inflamed joint. During this process the cartilage is invaded by a proliferating

---

*To whom correspondence should be addressed.

overgrowth known as the pannus and the whole joint becomes inflamed and swollen, particularly during acute phases of the disorder when there may be bleeding into the synovial fluid within the joint capsule. As the disease progresses, the joint becomes increasingly immobile and eventually all joint function may be lost with fusion of the bones across the joint. The disease has no identifiable cause, although an autoimmune reaction has long been suspected as the disease does not affect single joints, with most of the major joints affected bilaterally. Treatment for the disease is targeted at both the inflammatory and proliferative aspects of the disorder, consisting of non-steroidal anti-inflammatory drugs (NSAID) and corticosteroids respectively, although recently cytotoxic immuno-suppressants such as methotrexate have been introduced (Table 1). Second-line agents such as gold thiols can also be effective in some patients.

A major limitation on the use of NSAID in the treatment of rheumatoid arthritis (RA) is the incidence of side-effects. For example, phenylbutazone was one of the first NSAID to be introduced in the 1950s. Although it is effective in treating the symptoms of RA [1], it can produce serious side-effects which include fluid retention, aplastic anaemia and agranulocytosis, which have resulted in the withdrawal of this drug from clinical use for RA. Despite this, phenylbutazone is still widely sold 'over the counter' in many countries.

Table 1. Drugs used in the treatment of rheumatoid arthritis.

Agent	Classification
First line agents: to relieve pain and stiffness	
Acetyl salicylate	Non-steroidal anti-inflammatory drugs
Diclofenac	
Ibuprofen	
Indomethacin	
Mefenamic acids	
Naproxen	
Phenylbutazone	
Piroxicam	
Tolmetin	
Second-line agents: aiming to suppress the rheumatic disease process	
Prednisolone	Corticosteroid
Gold thiols	Miscellaneous group
Sulphasalazine	
Penicillamine	
Chloroquine	Anti-malarials
Hydroxychloroquine	
Azothioprine	Immunosuppressants
Methotrexate	
Cyclophosphamide	
Cyclosporin	

There is no doubt that oxidative stress accompanies most human diseases and RA is no exception. Intra-articular injection of agents able to generate H_2O_2 causes severe joint damage in experimental animals [2] and there is much *in vitro* evidence suggesting that reactive oxygen species (ROS) can damage or interfere with joint components including hyaluronic acid [3,4], proteoglycans [5], collagens [6] and tissue and fluid proteinase inhibitors such as α_1-antiproteinase [7]. There is now increasing evidence (summarized in Table 2) that oxidative stress occurs within the inflamed joint *in vivo* and that joint components are probably being damaged by ROS. The inflamed joint is infiltrated by large numbers of activated neutrophils and the pannus contains many macrophage-like cells; both these cell types produce the ROS $O_2^{\cdot-}$ and H_2O_2 [16–18] and perhaps the $NO^{\cdot}$ radical [19]. Neutrophils additionally make HOCl. In the presence of 'free iron ions', $O_2^{\cdot-}$ and H_2O_2 become converted into the highly reactive hydroxyl radical, probably by a mechanism similar to the iron-catalysed Haber–Weiss reaction:

$$Fe^{3+} + O_2^{\cdot-} \rightarrow Fe^{2+} + O_2$$

$$Fe^{2+} + H_2O_2 \rightarrow Fe^{3+} + OH^- + OH^{\cdot}$$

The interaction of $NO^{\cdot}$ and $O_2^{\cdot-}$ can also be dangerous [20]. The product, peroxynitrite, is not only directly toxic, e.g. by oxidizing methionine and protein sulphydryl groups, but also breaks down to generate multiple toxic products including nitrogen dioxide gas ($NO_2^{\cdot}$), $OH^{\cdot}$ and nitronium ion (NO_2^+) [20,21].

Table 2. Evidence consistent with increased oxidative stress in rheumatoid arthritis.

Agent	Classification
1. Increased lipid peroxidation products in serum and synovial fluid.	Rowley et al. [8]
2. Degradation of hyaluronic acid by free radical mechanisms.	Grootveld et al. [4]
3. Formation of fluorescent proteins, presumably due to oxidative damage to proteins.	Lunec et al. [9]
4. Increased levels of protein carbonyls, an end-product of oxidative damage to proteins.	Chapman et al. [10]
5. Increased urinary excretion of 8-hydroxydeoxyguanosine, a product of oxidative damage to DNA.	Blount et al. [11]
6. Depletion and oxidation of ascorbic acid in serum and synovial fluid.	Blake et al. [12]; Situnayake et al. [13]
7. Increased concentrations of oxidation products of uric acid.	Grootveld and Halliwell [14]
8. Formation of 2,3-dihydroxybenzoate from salicylate in increased amounts.	Grootveld and Halliwell [15]

$$O_2{}^{\cdot-} + NO^{\cdot} \rightarrow ONOO^-$$

Synthesis not only of $O_2{}^{\cdot-}$, but also of $NO^{\cdot}$ [19] appears elevated in RA patients. Demonstration of the presence of nitrotyrosines in patients with active RA [22] is consistent with the formation of peroxynitrite *in vivo* [20].

Synovial fluid from RA patients often contains measurable quantities of iron [23] capable of catalysing oxidative damage *in vitro* [24]. The origins of this free iron may be 3-fold. First, small quantities of iron may be released from ferritin in rheumatoid synovial fluid [25], particularly in the presence of reducing agents such as superoxide. Secondly, small amounts of iron might also be released from the intracellular iron pool on cell lysis [26], and finally iron may be released from haemoglobin in the presence of H_2O_2 during microbleeding into the joint [27]. Interestingly, the iron status of RA patients has been shown to influence the disease pathology [28,29] and there is a well-known relationship between disordered iron metabolism and chronic inflammation [30].

The putative ability of anti-inflammatory drugs to diminish oxidative damage by suppressing inflammation and slowing the recruitment of phagocytes to the inflamed joint has often been suggested to be connected with the ability of the drug to scavenge ROS. A few anti-inflammatory drugs might directly scavenge ROS or inhibit phagocytic production of ROS — there are many claims of such effects in the literature, but they are usually based on *in vitro* experiments (e.g. studying drug effects on isolated neutrophils) that employ drug concentrations far higher than those ever achieved *in vivo* [31]. Detailed evaluations carried out in this laboratory have shown that scavenging of ROS, or inhibition of their formation, is an unlikely mode of action of most anti-inflammatory drugs *in vivo* [31–33]. Indeed for several drugs the reverse may be true [32,33]. Myeloperoxidase, haem proteins and prostaglandin synthetase can oxidize many drugs into free radicals, some of which can then exacerbate oxidative damage [34]. Gastric peroxidases may also be capable of oxidizing some drugs into forms which could cause damage [35,36], possibly contributing (in a mechanism additional to that of cyclo-oxygenase inhibition) to NSAID-induced gastric lesions. Some of the side-effects of phenylbutazone [32], indomethacin [36] and penicillamine [33] may be caused by such mechanisms. Thus one could have a paradoxical situation in which a drug might alleviate some of the symptoms of RA (e.g. reducing pain and swelling by inhibiting cyclo-oxygenase in the case of NSAID) but actually exacerbate oxidative damage to the tissues. Such damage could be responsible for, or contribute to, the side effects observed with several drugs used in the treatment of RA.

Effects of drugs on oxidative damage to lipids and proteins

In the inflamed joint, haemoglobin liberated by microbleeding might interact with H_2O_2 formed by activated phagocytes to produce damaging oxidants [37–39]. Addition of H_2O_2 to solutions of oxy-, deoxy- and met-haemoglobin results in the formation of a ferryl species in which the oxidation state of the haem iron is thought to be raised to $+IV$ and a free radical (possibly a tyrosine radical) is generated on the protein [40]. This property is shared by myoglobin, which is more often used in drug oxidation studies as there is less tendency for protein precipitation to occur. Oxidation of the iron in the haem groups of these two proteins by H_2O_2 causes changes in the visible spectrum of the proteins (Fig. 1) and the ferryl derivatives are oxidants which stimulate lipid peroxidation using arachidonic acid as a substrate (Table 3, lines 1 and 2). Although activated haem proteins are not such powerful oxidants as the hydroxyl radical, they are extremely stable and the ferryl spectrum is detectable for several hours. Ferryl-haem species could be present in the inflamed joint and interact with any drugs administered.

As part of our extensive studies on RA, we have determined the influence of drugs used in the treatment of RA upon oxidative damage induced by haem protein/H_2O_2 or ferryl systems. Damage to arachidonic acid was used as a primary screen to detect drugs able to stimulate peroxidative damage. Such drugs were then studied in more detail, with damage to both lipids and proteins investigated. α_1-Antiproteinase was used as a target molecule for protein damage, being an important inhibitor of serine proteinases (especially elastase) in human body fluids, yet highly susceptible to oxidative inactivation, thus accelerating proteolytic damage at sites of injury [41]. We show additionally that the mitochondrial protein cytochrome c can promote oxidative damage to lipids and proteins in the presence of certain drugs; this is a potential mechanism by which drugs could

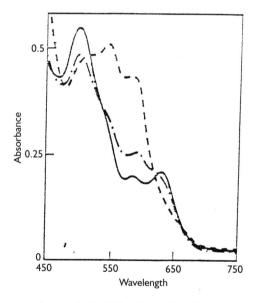

Fig. 1. Spectra of myoglobin (50 μM) in 25 mM phosphate buffer pH 7.4 (———). (— — —) Myoglobin plus H_2O_2 (500 μM, ferryl derivative); and (— · —) myoglobin plus H_2O_2 to which phenylbutazone (500 μM) was added and the spectrum recorded immediately after mixing. A similar result is given on mixing either meclofenamic or flufenamic acid (200 μM) with ferryl-myoglobin (results not shown).

Table 3. Stimulation of myoglobin–H₂O₂-dependent peroxidation of arachidonic acid by certain anti-inflammatory drugs. Reaction mixtures contained in a final volume of 1 ml: 0.5 mM arachidonic acid, 50 μM myoglobin, the drug under investigation and 0.5 mM H_2O_2 in a 25 mM phosphate buffer at pH 7.4. After incubation at 37 °C for 10 min, peroxidation was measured by the TBA test and expressed as absorbance at 532 nm. Drugs were added to give the following final concentrations: phenylbutazone 500 μM, meclofenamic and flufenamic acids 200 μM. Where indicated ascorbic acid was added to a final concentration of 1 mM.

Addition to assay	Extent of peroxidation (A_{532})
Arachidonic acid/myoglobin	0.24
Arachidonic acid/myoglobin/H_2O_2	0.47
Plus phenylbutazone	0.80
Plus meclofenamic acid	0.75
Plus flufenamic acid	0.66
Arachidonic acid/myoglobin/H_2O_2/ascorbic acid	0.27
Plus phenylbutazone	0.39
Plus meclofenamic acid	0.22
Plus flufenamic acid	0.24

cause mitochondrial damage *in vivo*. Cytochrome *c* is also easily released from damaged mitochondria and so could exert pro-oxidant effects at other sites.

Effect of drugs on *in vitro* lipid peroxidation

A wide range of drugs has been screened for their ability to exert pro-oxidant effects on lipid peroxidation using myoglobin/H_2O_2/arachidonic acid as a test system. A mixture of myoglobin and H_2O_2 causes peroxidation of arachidonic acid (Table 3) and this peroxidation may theoretically be accelerated, decreased or unaffected in the presence of drugs. Ability to decrease peroxidation may indicate a beneficial antioxidant action of the drug, whereas drugs which accentuate peroxidation could exacerbate oxidative damage *in vivo*. Drugs were screened at concentrations in the range 50–1000 μM (Table 4). Most had no effect on lipid peroxidation at the concentrations tested and some were inhibitory. However, a significant stimulation of lipid peroxidation was observed with phenylbutazone, flufenamic and meclofenamic acids, which was maximal at about 500 μM concentration for phenylbutazone and around 200 μM for the fenamic acids, diminishing at higher concentrations (data shown in Table 3). Control experiments showed that none of these drugs interfered with the assay used to measure the peroxidation, nor did the drugs themselves generate a chromogen in the assay. The peroxidation induced by phenylbutazone was inhibited by a number of antioxidants, including the iron chelator desferrioxamine and ascorbic acid, and to a lesser

Table 4. Effects of anti-rheumatic drugs on myoglobin-dependent lipid peroxidation. Assays were performed as described in Table 3 with each assay containing arachidonic acid, myoglobin, H_2O_2 and drug. Concentrations of 50 μM to 1 mM were tested for each drug.

Drugs which had no significant effect on lipid peroxidation	
Acetyl salicylate	Non-steroidal anti-inflammatory drugs
Indomethacin	
Naproxen	
Piroxicam	
Tolmetin	
Prednisolone	Corticosteroid
Aurothiomalate	Miscellaneous group
D-Penicillamine disulphide	
Chloroquine	
Azothioprine	Immunosuppressant drugs
Methotrexate	
Drugs which inhibited lipid peroxidation	
Diclofenac	Non-steroidal anti-inflammatory drug
Quinacrine	Anti-malarial drug
D-Penicillamine	Miscellaneous group
Sulphasalazine	
Drugs which accelerated lipid peroxidation	
Flufenamic acid	Non-steroidal anti-inflammatory drugs
Meclofenamic acid	
Phenylbutazone	

extent by cysteine (Table 5). These molecules may be preferentially oxidized by activated haem proteins [42–44]. Peroxidation was not significantly inhibited by addition of superoxide dismutase (SOD) (500 units/ml), but chain-breaking antioxidants such as trolox C and butylated hydroxytoluene were inhibitory. Addition of phenylbutazone or one of the fenamic acids at the optimum concentration causes a loss of the myoglobin ferryl spectrum, confirming that these drugs are interacting with H_2O_2-activated myoglobin (Fig. 1).

Effect of drugs on myoglobin–H_2O_2-dependent inactivation of α_1-antiproteinase

The haem protein–H_2O_2 system can cause oxidative damage not only to lipids but also to proteins. Since protein damage is an important consequence of oxidative stress *in vivo*, we examined the effect of drugs on this process, using α_1-antiproteinase as a model system. The activity of α_1-antiproteinase was measured by its ability to inhibit the serine proteinase elastase [41]. Phenyl-

Table 5. Effect of antioxidants on phenylbutazone-stimulated arachidonic acid peroxidation. Experimental conditions are as described in Table 3. The following concentrations were used in the assays: phenylbutazone (PB) (500 μM), cysteine, butylated hydroxytoluene (BHT) and trolox C (5 mM), ascorbate and desferrioxamine (DFO) (500 μM), and SOD (500 units/ml). Concentrations quoted are the final concentrations in the reaction mixture. PB alone gave no chromogen in the TBA test, nor did it have any effect when added at the end with the TBA reagents.

Reaction mixture	Extent of peroxidation (A_{532})
AA.MB (blank)	0.00
AA.MB.H_2O_2	0.18
AA.MB.H_2O_2.PB	0.54
AA.MB.H_2O_2.PB plus cysteine	0.21
AA.MB.H_2O_2.PB plus ascorbate	0.12
AA.MB.H_2O_2.PB plus DFO	0.05
AA.MB.H_2O_2.PB plus SOD	0.52
AA.MB.H_2O_2.PB plus trolox C	0.04
AA.MB.H_2O_2.PB plus BHT	0.10

butazone had an inhibitory effect on elastase but neither flufenamic nor meclofenamic acid had any significant effect on elastase alone (Table 6, column 1) although flufenamic acid slightly decreased the ability of α_1-antiproteinase to inhibit elastase (Table 6, column 2, line 4). However, mixtures of the three drugs with myoglobin and H_2O_2 caused much greater decreases in the elastase-inhibitory capacity of α_1-antiproteinase, seen as rises in the elastase activity measured. Damage to α_1-antiproteinase could be prevented by adding 1 mM ascorbic acid (Table 6, column 3).

Cytochrome c-dependent lipid peroxidation

Several drugs in therapeutic use induce mitochondrial damage [45], so it was of interest to see whether the abundant mitochondrial haem protein cytochrome c could catalyse the formation of damaging drug-derived species. Cytochrome c plus H_2O_2 induced some peroxidation of arachidonic acid (Table 7), as expected [46,47]. Addition of phenylbutazone or (to a lesser extent) meclofenamic acid, but not flufenamic acid, stimulated the peroxidation caused by cytochrome c. Purification of commercial cytochrome c by gel filtration on a Sephadex G25 column to remove any contaminating haem peptides did not affect its ability to stimulate lipid peroxidation. As a further control, commercial microperoxidase did not cause lipid peroxidation in the presence of H_2O_2. Cytochrome c-dependent peroxidation, with or without drugs present, was inhibited by ascorbic acid.

Cytochrome c could also promote protein damage, in that α_1-antiproteinase was inactivated by mixtures of cytochrome c, H_2O_2 and phenylbutazone

Table 6. Inactivation of α_1-antiproteinase by drug/myoglobin/H_2O_2 mixtures. α_1-Antiproteinase (α_1-AP; 0.06 mg/ml) was preincubated in PBS for 15 min at room temperature with a combination of the following reagents, where indicated: myoglobin (50 μM), H_2O_2 (500 μM), ascorbic acid (1 mM) and meclofenamic or flufenamic acid (200 μM) or phenylbutazone (500 μM). Ascorbic acid has no effect on elastase or α_1-antiproteinase. Porcine pancreatic elastase (30 mg/ml, final concentration) was then added and the residual elastase activity measured after a further 15 min. Activities shown are the mean $\pm$ S.D. of six individual determinations.

Addition to reaction mixture	Elastase activity ($10^3 \times \Delta A$/min)		
	Alone	With α_1-AP present	With α_1-AP and ascorbic acid present
MB.H_2O_2 (Control)	559 ± 38	32 ± 29	15 ± 21
MFA	518 ± 27	49 ± 57	48 ± 28
MB.H_2O_2.MFA	566 ± 42	334 ± 62	37 ± 27
FFA	538 ± 32	126 ± 12	137 ± 33
MB.FFA.H_2O_2	547 ± 26	273 ± 33	172 ± 55
PB	240 ± 16	17 ± 1	16 ± 15
MB.H_2O_2.PB	307 ± 21	302 ± 32	162 ± 11
MB.H_2O_2.PB (100 μM)	550 ± 38	436 ± 25	67 ± 5

(Table 8). Again, ascorbic acid inhibited the damage. By contrast, α_1-antiproteinase was not markedly affected by mixtures of cytochrome c and H_2O_2 with flufenamic or meclofenamic acids.

In the presence of H_2O_2 and haem proteins, meclofenamic acid, flufenamic acid and phenylbutazone are oxidized to species that can accelerate lipid peroxidation and protein damage. Phenylbutazone was the most damaging drug examined, although the concentration required to give the maximum damage (500 μM) is greater than that required for the fenamic acids (200 μM). Damage to arachidonic acid is still, however, observed at lower concentrations. All three drugs are NSAID, and microbleeding which releases haemoglobin often accompanies both acute and chronic inflammation.

Oxidative damage also occurs by interaction of phenylbutazone and meclofenamic acid with mixtures of cytochrome c and H_2O_2. Presumably the activated haem species oxidizes the drug to a radical while the haem iron is reduced. Fig. 1 indicates that the ferryl spectrum of myoglobin reverts to the free metmyoglobin spectrum on addition of the drug. Electron spin resonance (ESR) studies on mixtures of myoglobin, H_2O_2 and phenylbutazone to which has been added the spin trap 5,5-dimethyl-1-pyrroline N-oxide (DMPO) yield complex ESR signals which are probably a mixture of the spectra of the DMPO-adducts of several radical species. No spectra are observed in the absence of the spin trap, presum-

Table 7. Stimulation of cytochrome c–H₂O₂-dependent peroxidation of arachidonic acid by anti-inflammatory drugs. Experimental conditions are as described for Table 3 with cytochrome c replacing myoglobin. Concentrations quoted are the final concentrations in the reaction mixtures, which contained 50 μM cytochrome c. Where indicated, ascorbic acid was added to a final concentration of 1 mM.

Addition to assay	Extent of peroxidation (A_{532})
Arachidonic acid/cytochrome c	0.21
Arachidonic acid/cytochrome c/H₂O₂	0.44
Plus phenylbutazone (0.2 mM)	0.90
Plus phenylbutazone (1.0 mM)	0.92
Plus meclofenamic acid (0.2 mM)	0.54
Plus meclofenamic acid (1.0 mM)	0.57
Plus flufenamic acid (0.2 mM)	0.38
Plus flufenamic acid (1.0 mM)	0.32
Arachidonic acid/cytochrome c/H₂O₂/ascorbic acid	0.32
Plus phenylbutazone (1.0 mM)	0.58
Plus meclofenamic acid (1.0 mM)	0.30

ably since the lifetimes of the radicals are too short. A phenylbutazone radical has been identified spectrophotometrically using pulse radiolysis during which a solution of phenylbutazone was bombarded with hydroxyl radicals (P.J. Evans and O.I. Aruoma, unpublished work). It is therefore likely that these ferryl systems oxidize the drugs to free radical forms which cause the oxidative damage to arachidonic acid and α_1-antiproteinase.

Respiring mitochondria generate both H_2O_2 and $O_2^{\cdot-}$ [45]. Thus cytochrome c-dependent oxidation of drugs could be a mechanism of drug-induced mitochondrial injury. In addition, damaged mitochondria at sites of tissue injury can leak cytochrome c and so could cause extramitochondrial oxidative damage. Damage by these haem protein–H_2O_2 systems to α_1-antiproteinase was used as a model system for ability to cause protein damage in our experiments. It is also clinically relevant since α_1-antiproteinase has an exposed methionine group which is sensitive to oxidative damage and, as a major inhibitor of serine proteinases, has a protective effect on both structural and functional extracellular proteins. Damage to α_1-antiproteinase, apparently by free radicals, has been detected in the rheumatoid joint [48] and the generation of radicals from anti-inflammatory drugs could exacerbate this.

Addition of antioxidants such as ascorbic acid and trolox C to assays of lipid peroxidation and protein damage causes a decrease in the damage, possibly due to the activated haem species being reduced back to the lower oxidation state by ascorbate or trolox C in preference to oxidation of the drug or to scavenging of the protein-derived radicals by these substances. An additional explanation is that

Table 8. Inactivation of α_1-antiproteinase (α_1-AP) by drug/cytochrome c/ H_2O_2 mixtures. Conditions were exactly as described in the legend to Table 6 except that cytochrome c (Cyt c) replaced myoglobin. Phenylbutazone (PB) concentration was 500 μM. Abbreviations: MFA, meclofenamic acid; FFA, flufenamic acid.

Addition to reaction mixture	Elastase activity ($10^3 \times \Delta A$/min)		
	Alone	With α_1-AP present	With α_1-AP and ascorbic acid present
Cyt c.H_2O_2 (Control)	528 ± 49	83 ± 61	42 ± 39
MFA	518 ± 77	94 ± 32	66 ± 44
Cyt c/H_2O_2/MFA	579 ± 14	104 ± 36	72 ± 20
FFA	440 ± 20	131 ± 32	90 ± 46
Cyt c/FFA/H_2O_2	433 ± 24	180 ± 59	127 ± 30
PB	254 ± 21	25 ± 22	29 ± 10
Cyt c/H_2O_2/PB	327 ± 26	283 ± 9	13 ± 12

ascorbate reduces the drug-derived radical. Production of drug-derived radicals by haem proteins and H_2O_2 may contribute to the side-effects observed with certain drugs. Although therapeutically effective [1], phenylbutazone was withdrawn from use in RA patients some years ago on account of adverse side-effects. If drug-derived radicals could be removed by co-administration of an antioxidant such as ascorbic acid, the therapeutic potential of this drug and possibly others could be restored. In this context, it is interesting to note that RA patients are often deficient in ascorbic acid [49] and, unlike ankylosing spondylitis patients who may still receive this drug, are particularly prone to its side-effects.

The financial support of the Arthritis and Rheumatism Council is gratefully acknowledged.

References

1. Brooke, P.M., Kean, W.F. and Buchanan, W.W. (1986) in The Clinical Pharmacology of Anti-Inflammatory Agents, pp. 81–82, Taylor and Francis, London
2. Schalkwijk, J., Van Den Berg, W.B., Van de Putte, L.B.A. and Joosten, L.A.B. (1986) Arthritis Rheum. **29**, 532–538
3. McCord, J.M. (1974) Science **185**, 529–531
4. Grootveld, M., Henderson, E.B., Farrell, A., Blake, D.R., Parkes, H.G. and Haycock, P. (1991) Biochem. J. **273**, 459–467
5. Cooper, B., Creeth, J.M. and Donald, A.S.R. (1985) Biochem. J. **228**, 615–626
6. Davies, J.M.S., Horwitz, D.A. and Davies, K.J.A. (1993) Free Radical Biol. Med. **15**, 637–643
7. Wasil, M., Halliwell, B., Moorhouse, C.P., Hutchison, D.C.S. and Baum, H. (1987) Biochem. Pharmacol. **36**, 3847–3850

8. Rowley, D.A., Gutteridge, J.M.C., Blake, D.R., Farr, M. and Halliwell, B. (1984) Clin. Sci. **66**, 691–695
9. Lunec, J., Blake, D.R., McCleary, S.J., Brailsford, S. and Bacon, P.A. (1985) J. Clin. Invest. **76**, 2084–2090
10. Chapman, M.L., Rubin, B.R. and Gracy, R.W. (1989) J. Rheumatol. **16**, 15–18
11. Bhusate, L.L., Scott, D.L. and Perrett, D. (1992) Ann. Rheum. Dis. **53**, 8–12
12. Blake, D.R, Hall, N.D., Treby, D.A., Halliwell, B. and Gutteridge, J.M.C. (1981) Clin. Sci. **61**, 483–486
13. Situnayake, R.D., Thurnham, D.I., Kootathep, S., Chirico, S., Lunec, J., Davis, M. and McConkey, B. (1991) Ann. Rheum. Dis. **50**, 81–86
14. Grootveld, M. and Halliwell, B. (1987) Biochem. J. **243**, 803–808
15. Grootveld, M. and Halliwell, B. (1986) Biochem. J. **237**, 499–504
16. Nurcombe, H.L., Bucknall, R.C. and Edwards, S.W. (1991) Ann. Rheum. Dis. **50**, 147–153
17. Robinson, J., Watson, F., Bucknall, R.C. and Edwards, S.W. (1992) Biochem. J. **286**, 345–351
18. McCarthy, D.A., Bernhagen, J., Taylor, M.J., Hamblin, A.S., James, I., Thompson, P.W. and Perry, J.D. (1992) Ann. Rheum. Dis. **51**, 13–18
19. Farrell, A.J., Blake, D.R., Palmer, R.M.J. and Moncada, S. (1992) Ann. Rheum. Dis. **51**, 1219–1222
20. Beckman, J.S., Chen, J., Ischiropoulos, H. and Crow, J.P. (1994) Methods Enzymol. **233**, 229–240
21. Van der Vliet, A., Smith, D., O'Neill, C.A., Kaur, H., Darley-Usmar V., Cross, C.E. and Halliwell, B. (1994) Biochem. J. **303**, 295–301
22. Kaur, H. and Halliwell, B. (1994) FEBS Lett. **350**, 9–12
23. Gutteridge, J.M.C. (1987) Biochem. J. **245**, 415–421
24. Gutteridge, J.M.C., Rowley, D.A. and Halliwell, B. (1982) Biochem. J. **206**, 605–609
25. Biemond, P., Swaak, A.J.G., Van Eijk, H.G. and Koster, J.F. (1986) Arthritis Rheum. **29**, 1187–1193
26. Halliwell, B., Aruoma, O.I., Mufti, G. and Bomford, A. (1988) FEBS Lett. **241**, 202–204
27. Blake, D.R., Hall, N.D., Bacon, P.A., Dieppe, P.A., Halliwell, B. and Gutteridge, J.M.C. (1981) Lancet **2**, 1142–1144
28. Trenam, C.W., Winyard, P.G., Morris, C.J. and Blake, D.R. (1992) in Iron and Human Disease (Lauffer, R.B., ed.), pp. 395–417, CRC Press, Boca Raton
29. Halliwell, B., Hoult, J.R.S. and Blake, D.R. (1988) FASEB J. **2**, 2867–2873
30. Means, J.T., Jr. and Krantz, S.B. (1992) Blood **80**, 1639–1647
31. Aruoma, O.I. and Halliwell, B. (1988) Xenobiotica **18**, 459–470
32. Evans, P.J., Cecchini, R. and Halliwell, B. (1992) Biochem. Pharmacol. **44**, 981–984
33. Aruoma, O.I., Halliwell, B., Butler, J. and Hoey, B.M. (1989) Biochem. Pharmacol. **38**, 4353–4357
34. Uetrecht, J. (1990) Crit. Rev. Toxicol **20**, 213–235
35. Bannerjee, R.K. (1990) Biochim. Biophys. Acta **1034**, 275–280
36. Vaananen, P.M., Meddings, J.B. and Wallace, J.L. (1991) Am. J. Physiol. **261**, G470–G475

37. Puppo, A. and Halliwell, B. (1988) Free Radical Res. Commun. **4**, 415–422
38. Davies, M.K. (1990) Free Radical Res. Commun. **10**, 361–370
39. Puppo, A. and Halliwell, B. (1988) Biochem. J. **249**, 185–190
40. McArthur, K.M. and Davies, M.J. (1993) Biochim. Biophys. Acta **1202**, 173–181
41. Wasil, M., Halliwell, B., Hutchison, D.C.S. and Baum, H. (1987) Biochem. J. **243**, 219–223
42. Rice-Evans, C., Okunade, G. and Khan, R. (1989) Free Radical Res. Commun. **7**, 45–54
43. Puppo, A., Cecchini, R., Aruoma, A., Bolli, R. and Halliwell, B. (1990) Free Radical Res. Commun. **10**, 371–381
44. Kanner, J. and Harel, S. (1987) Free Radical Res. Commun. **3**, 309–317
45. Hayes, D.J. (1994) in Mitochondria: DNA, Protein and Disease, (Darley-Usmar, V. and Schapira, A.H.V., eds.), pp. 157–178, Portland Press, London
46. Harel, S., Salan, M.A. and Kanner, J. (1988) Free Radical Res. Commun. **5**, 11–19
47. Radi, R., Turrens, J.F. and Freeman, B.A. (1991) Arch. Biochem. Biophys. **288**, 118–125
48. Chidwick, K., Winyard, P.G., Zhang, Z., Farrell, A.J. and Blake, D.R. (1991) Ann. Rheum. Dis. **50**, 915–916
49. Lunec, J. and Blake, D.R. (1986) Free Radical Res. Commun. **1**, 31–39

Biochem. Soc. Symp. **61**, 209–219
Printed in Great Britain

Tamoxifen as an antioxidant and cardioprotectant

Helen Wiseman

Department of Nutrition and Dietetics, King's College London, Kensington, London W8 7AH, U.K.

Abstract

Tamoxifen is widely used in the treatment of breast cancer and has been proposed as a prophylactic agent in this disease. Tamoxifen is an effective anti-oxidant and protects membranes and low-density lipoprotein (LDL) particles against oxidative damage. This antioxidant action is shared by endogenous and synthetic oestrogens. The ability of tamoxifen to protect LDL particles against the oxidative damage implicated in atherosclerosis may be an important factor in the reported cardioprotective action of tamoxifen in women being treated for breast cancer. In addition, tamoxifen has been found to act in a similar manner to oestrogens to lower plasma cholesterol levels. The cardioprotective action of tamoxifen may be a key factor in predicting the likely risk/benefit ratio for prophylactic tamoxifen treatment in otherwise healthy women, who have been calculated to be genetically predisposed to developing breast cancer. In the future, predisposition to breast cancer may be determined by genetic screening.

Evidence for a cardioprotective action for tamoxifen?

Introduction

Tamoxifen is widely used in the treatment of breast cancer and has now been proposed as a prophylactic agent for this disease [1,2]. Although hormonally related cancers such as breast cancer are the most common causes of mortality in women aged 40–60-years-old, in women over the age of 60 cardiovascular disease becomes the leading cause. Myocardial infarction is the main cause of death in women in this age group and far exceeds all other causes in the later years of life. This makes consideration of the long-term effects of tamoxifen therapy particularly important. Tamoxifen has been reported to have beneficial cardiovascular effects and the benefits of prophylactic tamoxifen therapy, including potential protection against coronary heart disease and osteoporosis, in addition to decreasing the risk of breast cancer should outweigh the risk of deleterious side-effects. However, this high benefit/risk ratio remains to be demonstrated in large-scale trials. The evidence for the cardioprotective action of tamoxifen and its possible mechanisms will now be examined [3]. Retrospective studies on the two randomized arms of the Scottish adjuvant tamoxifen trial have revealed a significant decrease in the incidence of fatal myocardial infarction in breast cancer patients treated with tamoxifen [4]. Tamoxifen therapy for at least 5 years appears to have cardioprotective action in post-menopausal women similar to that of oestrogen. The Stockholm randomized trial of adjuvant tamoxifen therapy in post-menopausal women with early-stage breast cancer reported that even short-term tamoxifen therapy significantly decreased occurrence of coronary heart disease [5]. In addition, tamoxifen therapy for 5 years again produced a significant decrease in coronary heart disease, but had very little effect on thromboembolic disease [5].

Effect on cholesterol and lipoprotein levels

Treatment with tamoxifen as an adjuvant in a group of 123 women with stage-I and -II breast cancer produced a significant decrease in serum cholesterol levels (a known risk factor for coronary heart disease) compared with a control group of 81 women with stage-I and -II breast cancer who were not taking a hormonal treatment or supplement [6]. In this study decreases in serum cholesterol of more than 10 mg/dl were recorded in 73% of tamoxifen-treated patients compared with 35% of controls. Decreases in cholesterol of more than 40 mg/dl were found in 40% of tamoxifen-treated patients compared with 13% of controls. The age of the women and their initial serum cholesterol level were found to be important factors in the magnitude of the decrease in cholesterol levels observed. In a study on 45 post-menopausal Indian women with breast cancer, evaluation after 3 and 6 months showed significantly decreased levels of total cholesterol and low-density lipoprotein (LDL) cholesterol (another important risk factor) and increased levels of high-density lipoprotein (HDL) cholesterol, in patients receiving tamoxifen [7]. A study of 24 patients receiving chemohormonal therapy (tamoxifen alone or in combination with chemotherapy) reported average decreases in total serum cholesterol of 17% and in LDL cholesterol of 27% [8] and these potentially beneficial decreases in cholesterol were observed regardless of whether tamoxifen was administered alone or in combination with cytotoxic chemotherapy [8]. In the Wisconsin Tamoxifen Study, a randomized placebo-controlled double-blind study in disease-free women, tamoxifen treatment was found to lower total cholesterol levels by 26 mg/dl and LDL cholesterol levels by 20% after 3 months of treatment [9,10]. These changes were maintained throughout the 2 years of tamoxifen treatment, and women with greater baseline cholesterol levels showed greater decreases with tamoxifen treatment. Similarly the Royal Marsden Hospital preventative feasibility trial, again in disease-free women, reported a 15% decrease in serum cholesterol levels [11,12].

Effect on fibrinogen and antithrombin III levels

The Wisconsin Tamoxifen Study reported also that fibrinogen levels decreased by 52 mg/dl after 6 months and this may be associated with a decreased risk of arterial thrombosis [10,13]. A small decrease in antithrombin III levels were also found in some women. However, none of the subjects displayed a clinically significant decrease in antithrombin III levels and this small decrease is unlikely to explain the small thrombophlebitis-promoting effect of tamoxifen. Indeed, in a study of post-menopausal women receiving long-term adjuvant therapy with tamoxifen, associated thromboembolism was rare [12,14]. Furthermore, the Royal Marsden Hospital pilot trial reported no adverse effect of tamoxifen on coagulation (fibrinogen/antithrombin III ratio) [11].

Effect on lipoprotein(a) levels

Tamoxifen has been reported to decrease the circulating levels of lipoprotein(a) in post-menopausal women and in breast cancer patients [15,16]. Similar findings have also been reported for oestrogen [15]. This could be of particular importance because lipoprotein(a) levels have been suggested to account for much of the previously unattributable risk for coronary heart disease [17]. Plasma levels of this particular lipoprotein are not influenced by the dietary changes that can lower many of the other risk factors for coronary heart disease. Lipoprotein(a) differs structurally from LDL only by an extra protein molecule, apolipoprotein(a), which resembles plasminogen and is linked to apolipoprotein B-100. The reasons for the extreme atherogenicity of lipoprotein(a) are not yet clear but following oxidative modification it may promote macrophage transformation to foam cells (even more effectively than oxidized LDL [18] — see below) and it may directly promote the growth of atherosclerotic plaques. The apolipoprotein(a) moiety may cause blood clots to persist because its molecular similarity to plasminogen could enable it to compete with, and thus prevent, the normal action of plasminogen [17].

Effect on homocysteine levels

Tamoxifen has been reported to decrease plasma levels of the amino acid homocysteine [19]. This may also contribute to its cardioprotective action because elevated plasma levels of homocysteine is a known risk factor for cardiovascular disease [20]. Premature vascular disease and thrombosis are associated with elevated homocysteine levels and it is of interest that homocysteine can induce tissue factor activity in endothelial cells [21]. In addition, homocysteine can induce oxidative damage to LDL [22], which is implicated in atherosclerosis (see below). The plasma homocysteine level is controlled partly by genetic factors [23]. Various inborn errors of homocysteine metabolism (homocystinuria) can cause elevation of plasma homocysteine and patients with this metabolic disorder frequently suffer from cardiovascular disease in early adolescence, or earlier [24]. Even moderately elevated homocysteine levels have been reported to be associated with an increased risk of premature cardiovascular disease in retrospective case control studies [20,25] and in prospective studies [26,27]. Folate and cobalamin deficiencies can also cause elevated plasma homocysteine levels. Oestrogen status may be another influencing factor and pre-menopausal women have lower plasma homocysteine levels than post-menopausal women and men [28]. Furthermore, pregnancy and oestrogen replacement therapy decrease plasma homocysteine levels [29,30]. In a study of 31 post-menopausal women with breast cancer the plasma homocysteine level was decreased by a mean value of 30% after 9–12 months of tamoxifen treatment [19]. It appears that tamoxifen is acting like oestrogen to produce this beneficial effect on plasma homocysteine levels.

Tamoxifen appears to have significant beneficial effects on some of the risk factors for coronary heart disease. Similarly, post-menopausal oestrogen use is associated with a reduction in the incidence of coronary heart disease as well as in mortality from cardiovascular disease, but does not influence the risk of stroke [31]. Protection against cardiovascular disease could thus be a health benefit of both disease therapy and preventative treatment with tamoxifen.

Contribution of antioxidant action to cardioprotection?

Inhibition of microsomal and liposomal lipid peroxidation

Tamoxifen, its derivatives and 17*β*-oestradiol (structures shown in Fig. 1) are all good inhibitors of lipid peroxidation in microsomal and pre-formed liposomal systems [32–36]. 4-Hydroxytamoxifen was found to be a better inhibitor of microsomal lipid peroxidation in both the Fe(III)-ascorbate and Fe(III)-ADP/NADPH systems and of liposomal peroxidation, than tamoxifen, 3-hydroxytamoxifen (droloxifene) or 17*β*-oestradiol. Time-course studies showed that tamoxifen and related compounds and 17*β*-oestradiol (all at their IC_{50} concentra-

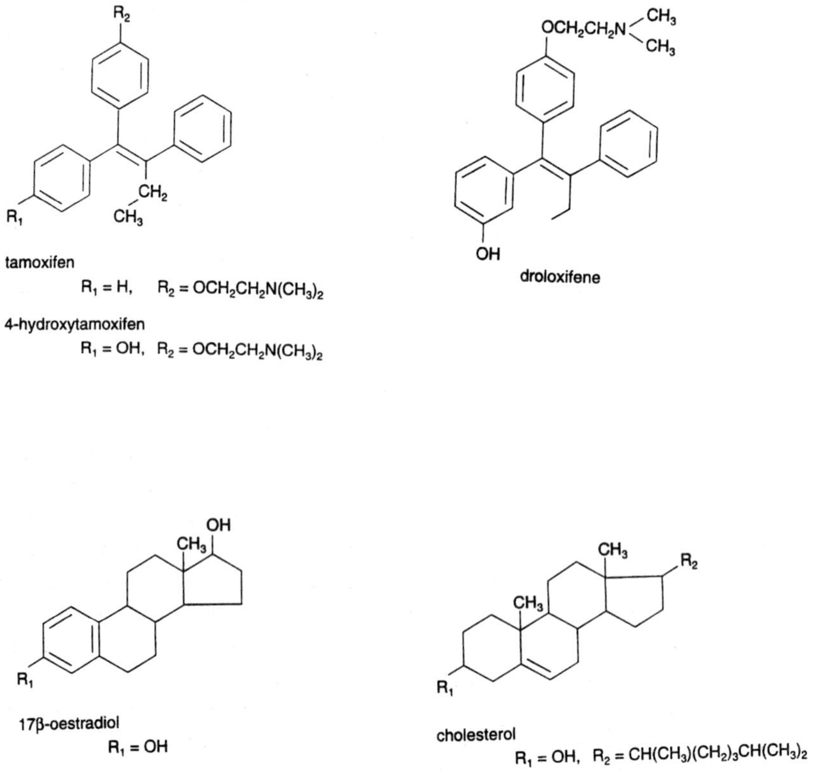
R2
R1
CH2
CH3
tamoxifen
R1 = H, R2 = OCH2CH2N(CH3)2
4-hydroxytamoxifen
R1 = OH, R2 = OCH2CH2N(CH3)2
OCH2CH2N CH3 CH3
OH
droloxifene
OH
CH3
R1
17β-oestradiol
R1 = OH
CH3
R2
CH3
R1
cholesterol
R1 = OH, R2 = CH(CH3)(CH2)3CH(CH3)2

Fig. 1. Structures of tamoxifen and related compounds.

tions) inhibited microsomal and liposomal lipid peroxidation throughout the incubation period and there was no clear evidence of a lag period followed by an acceleration of peroxidation to the control rate. This suggests that these compounds are unlikely to be classical chain-breaking antioxidants, even though hydroxy groups with potentially donatable hydrogen atoms are present in many of these compounds (tamoxifen itself being an exception). It has been suggested that these compounds act in part or in whole by stabilizing membranes against peroxidation via a decrease in membrane fluidity [37,38]. Indeed, such an ability to decrease membrane fluidity has been demonstrated for tamoxifen and related compounds [39,40]. Tamoxifen and 4-hydroxytamoxifen have both been reported to be effective inhibitors of Fe(III)-dependent lipid peroxidation in rat cardiac microsomes [41]. Tamoxifen was also a good inhibitor of lipid peroxidation in liposomes prepared from the phospholipid obtained from rat liver microsomes [41]. The role of lipid peroxidation in cardiovascular injury [42,43] and the development of atherosclerosis is well documented [44–47]. Some of the cardioprotective effect of tamoxifen may therefore be related to its ability to inhibit membrane lipid peroxidation.

When introduced into liposomes during their preparation [37], tamoxifen inhibited lipid peroxidation to a greater extent than cholesterol (it cannot enter pre-formed liposomal membranes and thus has no effect in that system). 4-Hydroxytamoxifen and 17β-oestradiol were approximately equipotent and both were more effective than tamoxifen. These results indicate the superiority of tamoxifen and related compounds over the natural membrane component cholesterol. Cholesterol is vital for cell growth and is taken up as LDL cholesterol at an enhanced rate by rapidly proliferating cancer cells, including breast cancer cells, which increase their expression of the LDL receptor as they become hormone independent and their growth becomes more uncontrolled [48]. This may explain the association between low serum cholesterol levels and cancer [49]. The total-cholesterol- and LDL-cholesterol-lowering abilities of tamoxifen (see above) may thus contribute to its inhibition of breast cancer cell growth (by depriving the cells of cholesterol for growth) as well as contributing to its cardioprotective action.

Protection of LDL against oxidative damage

Tamoxifen and in particular 4-hydroxytamoxifen have been reported to protect isolated human LDL against oxidative modification [50]. This may be of importance because oxidative damage to LDL is considered to be an important stage in the development of atherosclerosis: it is a prerequisite for macrophage uptake and cellular accumulation of cholesterol [18,44]. Lipid peroxidation is thought to start in the polyunsaturated fatty acids of the phospholipids on the surface of LDL and then propagate to core lipids, resulting in modification of the cholesterol, phospholipids and the apolipoprotein B molecule, in addition to the polyunsaturated fatty acids [18,51,52]. In a study on the action of tamoxifen and related compounds on oxidative damage to LDL, isolated human LDL was stimulated to undergo lipid peroxidation by the addition of Cu(II) ions [50]. This is a widely used experimental system [44,47] that is relevant to events occurring within the atherosclerotic lesion [53]. 4-Hydroxytamoxifen was more effective as an inhibitor of Cu(II) ion-dependent lipid peroxidation than tamoxifen and 17β-oestradiol and also prevented peroxidation-induced modifications in the surface charge of the LDL, whereas tamoxifen did not. These alterations in the surface charge of LDL are associated with its recognition and uptake by macrophages in atherosclerotic lesions [44]. This action of the 4-hydroxy metabolite of tamoxifen could be particularly important to the observed beneficial cardiovascular effects of tamoxifen therapy. The lack of effectiveness of tamoxifen itself in preventing alteration of the surface charge of LDL may be because it is a much less effective inhibitor of lipid peroxidation than 4-hydroxytamoxifen. Tamoxifen, over the concentration range tested (5–30 μM), maximally inhibited LDL peroxidation by only approximately 50% compared with approximately 90% achieved by 4-hydroxytamoxifen. In the presence of tamoxifen, therefore, it is likely that sufficient aldehydic breakdown products of lipid peroxidation such as malondialdehyde and 4-hydroxynonenal are produced to modify the ε-amino groups of the lysine residues of the apolipoprotein B molecule and thus the surface charge of LDL [50]. It would also be of interest to determine whether tamoxifen can protect against homocysteine-induced lipid peroxidation of LDL [22] (see above) in addition to its ability to lower plasma homocysteine levels [19]. Tamoxifen and its derivatives are highly lipophilic compounds that are likely to accumulate in the atheromal plaques associated with the damaged arterial wall to achieve the protective concentrations reported [50]. Tamoxifen (and 4-hydroxytamoxifen) may stabilize LDL against lipid peroxidation by interactions between their hydrophobic rings and the polyunsaturated residues of the phospholipid layer of LDL, this suggestion is supported by the inhibition of lipid peroxidation arising from similar interactions in liposomal membranes [3,39,54].

Comparison with oestrogen

Although tamoxifen is often described as an anti-oestrogen anti-cancer drug it can also be a partial or full oestrogen agonist depending on the target organ and tissue. Tamoxifen actually shows considerable structural similarity to sterols including oestrogen (see Fig. 1) and the similar cardioprotective actions observed for both tamoxifen and oestrogens suggest that tamoxifen acts as an oestrogen-mimicking cardioprotectant. Oestrogen is recognized to have a protective effect against coronary atherosclerosis [31] and its ability to protect LDL against oxidative damage [50,55,56] could contribute to the cardiovascular benefits observed on oestrogen administration in post-menopausal women [31], independently of a favourable alteration of the plasma lipid profile. Studies in rabbits and monkeys have shown the anti-atherogenic effect of hormonal replacement to be independent of variations in lipid profiles. Female cholesterol-fed rabbits treated with oestradiol for 33 weeks developed less atheroma in arterial tissue than controls, even though no differences in total cholesterol or lipoproteins were observed [57]. In oophorectomized female monkeys on an atherogenic diet, hormonal replacement with 17β-oestradiol, either alone or with cyclical progesterone for a period of 30 months, significantly decreased the development of coronary artery atherosclerosis independently of lipid profile changes [58].

17β-Oestradiol inhibits the peroxidation of isolated human LDL *in vitro* [50,55,56] and has now been shown to inhibit the oxidation of LDL in post-menopausal women. This was measured by the time of the onset of LDL oxidation (i.e. the lag time in the presence of Cu(II) ions [47]) in LDL isolated from women treated with 17β-oestradiol [59]. Acute intra-arterial infusion of 17β-oestradiol increased serum oestradiol levels from typical post-menopausal levels to physiological concentrations for reproductive-aged women at mid-cycle [60] and significantly prolonged the lag time of the LDL compared with baseline levels, indicating a decrease in susceptibility to oxidation. Transdermal patch administration of oestradiol for 3 weeks again increased serum levels of oestradiol and significantly prolonged the lag time but there were no significant changes in lipid profiles compared with baseline values. One month after discontinuation of treatment the LDL lag time had returned to baseline levels [59], suggesting that prolonged hormonal replacement therapy would be required to maintain the cardioprotective benefits. However, oestrogen hormonal replacement therapy has been indicated to carry similar risks of endometrial cancer to tamoxifen prophylaxis and requires careful monitoring [61]. It is clear that clinical investigations similar to the studies on 17β-oestradiol are required to explore the *in vivo* effects of tamoxifen on LDL oxidation. Clinical evidence for the inhibition of LDL oxidation by tamoxifen would be an important addition to the debate on the use of tamoxifen to prevent breast cancer in post-menopausal women [3,62].

Tamoxifen as a cardioprotective agent: the future

The justification for the routine use of tamoxifen as a protective agent against breast cancer in healthy women could depend not only on its effectiveness as a

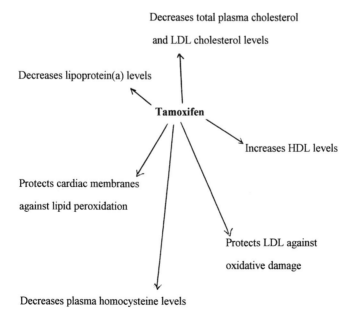

Fig. 2. Cardioprotective actions of tamoxifen.

prophylactic agent but also on its other beneficial health effects such as its possible cardioprotective action. The results of the large prophylactic tamoxifen trials are thus awaited with interest to see if significant cardioprotection is observed. An overview of the cardioprotective actions of tamoxifen is shown in Fig. 2. Alternatives to tamoxifen for breast cancer treatment (and possibly in the future prevention) are being developed including the tamoxifen derivative droloxifene [63] and the pure oestrogen antagonists (derived from 17β-oestradiol) such as ICI 164 384 and ICI 182 780 (structures shown in Fig. 3). Droloxifene has several advantages over tamoxifen, including a shorter terminal elimination half-life, lower accumulation, improved drug tolerance and decreased occurrence of resistant cancer cells and a decreased risk of endometrial cancer, and is currently being used in a trial with women with advanced breast cancer [63]. Furthermore, droloxifene has an effective antioxidant action [33]. ICI 182 780 is being investigated for use with breast cancer patients [64] particularly those who have suffered a relapse following onset of resistance to tamoxifen therapy [65]. However, it is

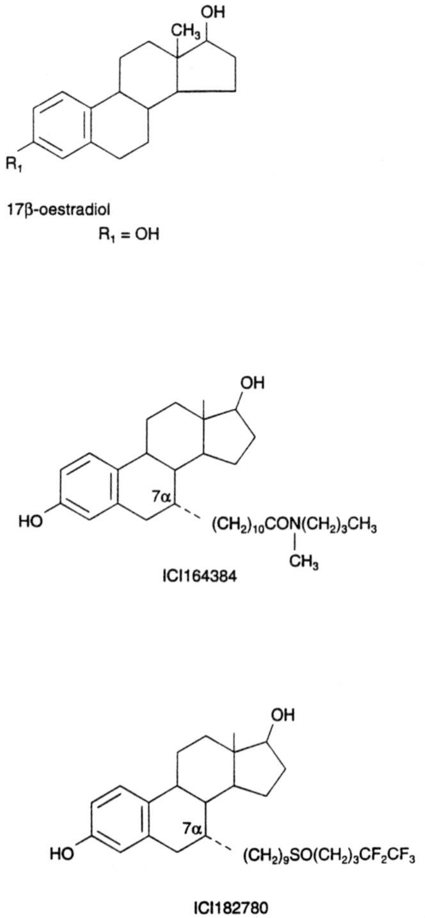

17β-oestradiol

R$_1$ = OH

ICI164384

ICI182780

Fig. 3. Structures of pure oestrogen antagonists.

important to note that the cardioprotective plasma cholesterol-lowering action of tamoxifen arises from its partial oestrogen antagonist action. Pure anti-oestrogens may still achieve a cardioprotective action similar to that of tamoxifen providing they possess a good antioxidant ability because it is likely that protection of LDL against oxidative damage is an important component of the cardioprotective action of tamoxifen. It is of considerable interest, therefore, that ICI 164 384 has been reported to be a good inhibitor of lipid peroxidation in both microsomal and liposomal systems [36]. The order of effectiveness in the microsomal system was 4-hydroxytamoxifen > 17β-oestradiol > tamoxifen > ICI 164 384 and in the liposomal system 4-hydroxytamoxifen > 17β-oestradiol > ICI 164 384 > tamoxifen. This indicates that this pure anti-oestrogen was overall of comparable effectiveness with tamoxifen, although not as effective as 4-hydroxytamoxifen and 17β-oestradiol. The ability of these new pure oestrogen antagonists to protect LDL against oxidative damage also requires urgent investigation to provide a more relevant indicator of possible antioxidant cardioprotective action.

References

1. Jordan, V.C. (1993) Br. J. Pharmacol. **110**, 507–517
2. Chlebowski, R.J., Butler, J., Nelson, A. and Lillington, L. (1993) Cancer **72**, 1032–1037
3. Wiseman, H. (1994) Tamoxifen: Molecular Basis of Use in Cancer Treatment and Prevention, John Wiley & Sons, Chichester
4. McDonald, C.C. and Stewart, H.J. (1991) Br. Med. J. **303**, 435–437
5. Rutqvist, L.E. and Mattsson, A. (1993) J. Natl. Cancer Inst. **85**, 1398–1406
6. Schapira, D.V., Kumar, N.B. and Lyman, G.H. (1990) Breast Cancer Res. Treat. **17**, 3–7
7. Thangaraju, M., Kumar, K., Gandhirajan, R. and Schdanandam, P. (1994) Cancer **73**, 659–663
8. Dnistrian, A.M., Schwartz, M.K., Greenberg, E.J., Smith, C.A. and Schwartz, D.C. (1993) Clin. Chim. Acta **223**, 43–52
9. Love, R.R., Wiebe, D.A., Newcombe, P.A., Cameron, L., Leventhal, H., Jordan, V.C., Feyzi, J. and DeMets, D.L. (1991) Ann. Intern. Med. **115**, 860–864
10. Love, R.R. (1992) in Introducing New Treatments for Cancer: Practical, Ethical and Legal Problems (Williams, C.J., ed.), pp. 342–356, John Wiley & Sons, Chichester
11. Powles, T.J., Tillyer, C.R., Jones, A.L., Treleavan, J., Davey, J.B. and McKinna, J.A. (1990) Eur. J. Cancer **6**, 680–684
12. Jones, A.L. and Powles, T.J. (1992) in Introducing New Treatments for Cancer: Practical, Ethical and Legal Problems (Williams, C.J., ed.), pp. 323–339, John Wiley & Sons, Chichester
13. Love, R.R., Surawicz, T.S. and Williams, E.C. (1992) Arch. Int. Med. **152**, 317–320
14. Henderson, B.E., Ross, R.K. and Pike, M.C. (1993) Science **259**, 633–638
15. Shewmon, D.A., Stock, J.L., Rosen, C.J., Heiniluoma, K.M., Hogue, M.M., Morrison, A., Doyle, E.M., Ukena, T., Weale, V. and Baker, S. (1994) Arteriosclerosis Thromb. **14**, 1586–1593
16. Shewmon, D.A., Stock, J.L., Abusamra, L.C., Kristan, M.A., Baker, S. and

Heiniluoma, K.M. (1994) Metabolism **43**, 531–532

17. Hayden, M.R. and Reidy, M. (1995) Nat. Med. (NY) **1**, 22–23
18. Witztum, J.L. (1994) Lancet **344**, 793–795
19. Anker, G., Lonning, P.E., Ueland, P.M., Refsum, H. and Lien, E.A. (1995) Int. J. Cancer **60**, 365–368
20. Ueland, P.M., Refsum, H. and Brattstrom, L. (1992) in Plasma Homocysteine and Cardiovascular Disease (Francis, R.B., ed.), pp. 183–236, Marcel Dekker Inc., New York
21. Fryer, R.H., Wilson, B.D., Gubler, D.M., Fitzgerald, L.A. and Rogers, G.M. (1993) Arteriosclerosis Thromb. **13**, 1327–1333
22. Hirano, K., Ogihara, T., Miki, M., Yauda, H., Tamai, H., Kawamura, N. and Mino, M. (1994) Free Radical Res. **21**, 267–276
23. Reed, T., Manilow, M.R., Christian, J.C. and Upson, B. (1991) Clin. Genetics **39**, 425–428
24. Mudd, S.H., Levy, H.L. and Skovby, F. (1989) in The Metabolic Basis of Inherited Disease (Scriver, C.R., Beadet, A.L., Sly, W.S. and Vale, D., eds.), pp. 639–734, McGraw-Hill, New York
25. Kang, S.-S., Wong, P.W.K., Zhou, J. and Cook, H.Y. (1986) Metabolism **35**, 889–891
26. Stampfer, M.J., Manilow, M.R., Willet, W.C., Newcomer, L.M., Upson, B., Ullmann, D., Tishler, P.V. and Hennekens, C.H. (1992) J. Am. Med. Assoc. **268**, 877–881
27. Arnesen, E., Resfum, H., Bonaa, K.H., Ueland, P.M., Forde, O.H. and Nordrehaug, J.E. (1995) Int. J. Epidemiol., in the press
28. Andersson, A., Brattstrom, L., Israelsson, B., Isaksson, A., Hamfelt, A. and Hultberg, B. (1992) Eur. J. Clin. Invest. **22**, 79–87
29. Andersson, A., Hultberg, B., Brattstrom, L. and Isakson, A. (1992) Eur. J. Clin. Chem. Biochem. **30**, 377–379
30. Van der Mooren, M.J.,Woulters, M.G.A., Blom, H.J., Schellekens, L.A., Eskes, T.K.A.B. and Rolland, R. (1993) 7th Int. Congr. on the Menopause, Abstr. 26
31. Stampfer, M.J., Colditz, G.A., Willett, W.C., Manson, J.E., Rosner, B., Speizer, F.E. and Hennekens, C.H. (1991) N. Engl. J. Med. **325**, 756–762
32. Wiseman, H., Laughton, M.J., Arnstein, H.R.V., Cannon, M. and Halliwell, B. (1990) FEBS Lett. **263**, 192–194
33. Wiseman, H., Smith, C., Halliwell, B., Cannon, M., Arnstein, H.R.V. and Lennard, M.S. (1992) Cancer Lett. **66**, 61–68
34. Wiseman, H. and Halliwell, B. (1993) FEBS Lett. **332**, 159–163
35. Wiseman, H. and Halliwell, B. (1994) Free Radical Biol. Med. **17**, 485–488
36. Wiseman, H. (1994) Biochem. Pharmacol. **47**, 493–498
37. Wiseman, H., Arnstein, H.R.V., Cannon, M. and Halliwell, B. (1990) FEBS Lett. **274**, 107–110
38. Wiseman, H., Cannon, M., Arnstein, H.R.V. and Barlow, D.J. (1992) Biochim. Biophys. Acta **1138**, 197–202
39. Wiseman, H., Quinn, P. and Halliwell, B. (1993) FEBS Lett. **330**, 53–56
40. Wiseman, H. and Quinn, P. (1994) Free Radical Res. **21**, 187–194
41. Wiseman, H., Cannon, M., Arnstein, H.R.V. and Halliwell, B. (1993) Biochem. Pharmacol. **45**, 1851–1855

42. Niki, E., Yamamoto, Y., Komuro, E. and Sato, K. (1991) Am. J. Clin. Nutr. **53**, S201–S205
43. Kukreja, R.C. and Hess, M.L. (1992) Cardiovasc. Res. **26**, 641–655
44. Steinberg, D., Parthasarathy, S., Carew, T.E., Khoo, J.C. and Witztum, J.L. (1989) N. Engl. J. Med. **320**, 915–924
45. Rimersma, R.A., Wood, D.A., MacIntyre, C.C.A., Elton, R.A., Grey, K.F. and Oliver, M.F. (1991) Lancet **337**, 677
46. Regenstrom, J., Nilsson, J., Tornvall, P., Landou, C. and Hamsten, A. (1992) Lancet **339**, 1183–1186
47. Esterbauer, H., Gebicki, J., Puhl, H. and Jurgens, G. (1992) Free Radical Biol. Med. **13**, 341–390
48. Guerrin, M., Prats, H., Mazars, P. and Valette, A. (1992) Biochim. Biophys. Acta **1137**, 116–120
49. Manninger, F. (1983) Cancer Res. **43**, 2503s–2507s
50. Wiseman, H., Paganga, G., Rice-Evans, C. and Halliwell, B. (1993) Biochem. J. **292**, 635–638
51. Steinbrecher, U.P., Zhang, H.F. and Lougheed, M. (1990) Free Radical Biol. Med. **9**, 155–168
52. Witztum, J.L. (1993) Br. Heart J. **69**, S12–S18
53. Smith, C., Mitchinson, M.J., Aruoma, O.I. and Halliwell, B. (1992) Biochem. J. **286**, 901–905
54. Wiseman, H. (1994) Trends Pharmacol. Sci. **15**, 83–89
55. Huber, L.A., Scheffler, E., Poll, T., Ziegler, R. and Dresel, H.A. (1990) Free Radical Biol. Med. **8**, 167–173
56. Rifici, V.A. and Khachadurian, A.K. (1992) Metabolism **41**, 1110–1114
57. Hough, J.L. and Zilversmit, D.B. (1986) Arteriosclerosis **6**, 57–63
58. Adams, M.R., Kaplan, J.R. and Manrick, S.B. (1990) Arteriosclerosis **10**, 1051–1057
59. Sack, M.N., Rader, D.J. and Cannon, R.O. (1994) Lancet **343**, 269–270
60. Carr, B.R. (1992) in Williams Textbook of Endocrinology (Wilson, J.D. and Foster, D.W., eds.), pp. 733–798, Saunders, Philadelphia
61. Gelety, T.J. and Judd, H.L. (1992) Curr. Opin. Obstet. Gynecol. **4**, 346–353
62. Wiseman, H. (1994) Lancet **343**, 598
63. Bruning, P.E. (1992) Eur. J. Cancer **28A**, 1404–1407
64. De Friend, D.J., Howell, A., Nicholson, R.I., Anderson, E., Dowsett, M., Mansel, R.E., Blamey, R.W., Bundred, N.J., Robertson, J.F., Saunders, C., Baum, M., Walton, P., Sutcliffe, F. and Wakeling, A.E. (1994) Cancer Res. **54**, 408–414
65. Wakeling, A.E. (1993) Breast Cancer Res. Treat. **25**, 1–10

Biochem. Soc. Symp. **61**, 221–234
Printed in Great Britain

Antioxidant agents in raw materials and processed foods

Caj E. Eriksson* and An Na†

*LMC, Centre for Advanced Food Studies, Rolighedsvej 30, DK-1958, Frederiksberg C, Denmark and †Chalmers University of Technology, Department of Food Science, c/o SIK, P.O. Box 5401, S-402 29 Göteborg, Sweden

Abstract

Many food raw materials contain natural antioxidants which exert control of oxidative processes in the living cells. Among antioxidative agents are found enzymes such as superoxide dismutase, glutathione peroxidase and glucose oxidase-catalase. Among naturally occurring non-enzymic antioxidants are carotenoids, especially astaxanthin (e.g. in fish), tocopherols in oils and other phenolic compounds in plant material. Enzymic antioxidants are mostly inactivated in food processing but the non-enzymic ones can be active also in heat-treated food and might also be active after consumption of the food, as is claimed with β-carotene, and vitamins A and E. Vitamin C is a generally reducing substance which acts synergistically with other antioxidants.

Processing of food can result in the formation of antioxidative compounds, e.g. by protein hydrolysis, Maillard reaction and fermentation by lactic acid bacteria. Curing of meat yields nitrosylhaem pigments which can act as radical scavengers and protect both the meat pigment and the lipids from oxidation.

Two or more antioxidants together can act synergistically, i.e. affect lipid oxidation to a higher extent than the sum of the contributions from each single antioxidant.

Introduction

Lipids and some lipid-soluble substances in foods (including fats, oils, mono- and di-acylglycerols, sterols, fat-soluble vitamins, phospholipids, flavours, aromas, etc.) may spontaneously react with atmospheric oxygen and lead to deterioration of foods. The autoxidation of lipids, which exist in most foods derived from plants or animals, may be the primary cause of reduction in food quality, affecting colour, aroma, taste, nutritive value, texture, consistency and functionality [1].

Antioxidation is consequently of decisive importance to the storage and shelf-life of foods, and antioxidants are the most effective inhibitors of autoxidation of fats and fatty foods. This paper emphasizes the mechanisms of antioxidant activity and antioxidant systems in raw materials and food processing.

The mechanism of lipid autoxidation

Free radicals and radical reactions

A free radical is defined as any compound containing one or more unpaired electrons. Therefore, it can donate its unpaired electron to another molecule or take one electron from another molecule. A free radical reaction is usually a chain reaction; one radical begets another radical and so on. Most biological molecules are non-radicals containing only paired electrons [2,3].

Autoxidation of lipids

A lipid molecule is usually not a radical. The reaction between lipids and molecular oxygen is induced by the intervention of initiators which can convert lipid molecules to active species. Some important initiators are listed in Table 1 [4–6].

The autoxidation process can be divided into three stages: initiation, propagation and termination. The primary products of autoxidation, hydroperoxides formed in the initiation reaction, readily undergo further decomposition and convert into various free radicals, which results in a variety of possible reactions and products. Therefore, lipid autoxidation is part of the radical chain reaction. When radical species are converted into non-radicals, the reactions may terminate.

The primary oxidation products, hydroperoxides, have no objectionable effect on the flavour and quality of foods, but the secondary oxidation products of the propagation reactions cause food rancidity [1,3,7–9].

Factors that affect autoxidation of lipids

Lipid oxidation is affected by many promoting and inhibiting factors (Table 2) [1,10–13].

Lipid autoxidation in raw materials or processed foods is largely dependent on the composition of the lipid, particularly on the proportion of unsaturated fatty acids, which are much more susceptible to oxidation than their saturated analogues [1].

Table 1. Important initiators of lipid autoxidation [4].

Initiator	Reaction products
Lipoxygenase	Lipid hydroperoxides
Light + photosensitizer	Lipid hydroperoxides
Ozone	Lipid ozonides
Nitroxides	Nitrous acids

Table 2. Factors that affect lipid oxidation [1].

Type of lipid	Non-polar/polar, fatty acids, sterols, terpenes
Fatty acids	Chain length, unsaturation, *cis–trans* isomers, free or bound
Catalysts	Enzymes, haem compounds, trace metals
State and access of oxygen	Triplet, singlet or radical, package
Light	Frequency, intensity, sensitizers
Temperature	Denaturing, non-denaturing
pH	Dissociation, denaturing
Inhibitors	Antioxidants, chelators, enzymes, enzyme inhibition or inactivation

To reduce lipid autoxidation, it is necessary to control conditions and substances that promote oxidation. This can be done in the following ways:

(1) Eliminating oxygen as far as possible and keeping oxygen uptake at a low level during manufacture and storage of foods. For example, the selection of appropriate containers and packing materials, and the use of vacuum packaging techniques can reduce the oxygen uptake of processed foods [14,15].

(2) Eliminating endogenous oxidative activators. Metal ions (such as Cu, Fe, Mn, Co, etc.) are catalysts of lipid oxidation via enzymic or non-enzymic pathways. Most foods generally contain trace amounts of these metals from refining equipment, metal containers or processes such as hydrogenation [16]. Photosensitizers (such as phytin pigments, FD & C red No. 3) may convert the triplet oxygen usually found in the substrate to singlet oxygen, the reaction rate of which is about 1000 times greater [17,18]. In order to eliminate these oxidation activators, good quality raw materials, packaging materials and appropriate processing techniques should be selected in the manufacture of foods.

(3) Minimizing exogenous promoting factors. At an elevated temperature, the rate of oxidative decomposition of lipids (particularly unsaturated lipids) rapidly increases. Light, especially UV radiation, is another major promoter of lipid autoxidation. Thus, food storage under cool, dark conditions is necessary for the prevention of food rancidity [19].

(4) Utilizing antioxidants. Antioxidants play a major role in inhibiting auto-xidation of lipids in foods. Their role is detailed in the following section.

Mechanisms of antioxidant action

Antioxidants are those substances which can delay, retard or prevent the oxidation process in storage of raw materials or in food processing. Antioxidants are classified into two groups, according to the mechanism by which they prevent or retard oxidation: primary (chain-breaking) antioxidants and secondary (preventive) antioxidants. Some antioxidants may exhibit more than one mechanism of antioxidation and are therefore called multiple-function antioxidants [5].

Primary antioxidants

Primary antioxidants interrupt autoxidation by reacting with lipid radicals as electron donors and converting the free radicals into more stable species. Thus, no further reactions can occur and the chain reaction is broken. Phenolic anti-oxidants such as tocopherols (vitamin E), propylgallate (PG), butylated hydroxy-anisole (BHA), butylated hydroxytoluene (BHT) and tertiary butylhydroquinone (TBHQ) belong to this group [20–27].

Secondary antioxidants

Secondary antioxidants inhibit the autoxidation of lipids by delaying and retarding the rate of oxidation rather than by breaking the radical chain reaction. Secondary autoxidants may act by a variety of mechanisms such as binding metal ions, scavenging oxygen, decomposing hydroperoxides to non-radical species, absorbing UV radiation or deactivating singlet oxygen [5].

Chelating (sequestering agents)

Compounds such as citric acid, amino acids, ethylenediaminetetra-acetic acid (EDTA) and certain phosphoric acid derivatives can chelate metallic ions, which catalyse lipid oxidation, and thus retard the oxidative decomposition of lipids. These compounds are called chelating agents [28–30].

Chelating agents are often referred to as synergists, since most of them (except amino acids) exhibit little or no antioxidant activity when used alone. They can, however, greatly enhance the activities of other antioxidants such as phenolic antioxidants.

Oxygen scavengers

Oxygen scavengers are those compounds which can react with oxygen and thus remove oxygen from a system. Ascorbic acid (vitamin C), ascorbyl palmitate, sulphites, erythorbic acid and sodium erythorbate are the oxygen scavengers most commonly used as antioxidants [5,30,31].

Singlet oxygen quenchers

It is known that the reaction rate of singlet oxygen with unsaturated fatty acids is over 1000 times greater than that of triplet oxygen [12]. Some compounds can convert singlet oxygen into more stable triplet oxygen and are therefore called singlet oxygen quenchers. For example, β-carotene can react with singlet oxygen according to the formula below [5,32–34]:

$$^1O_2 + {}^1\beta\text{-carotene} \rightarrow {}^3O_2 + {}^3\beta\text{-carotene}$$

Antioxidative enzymes

Some enzymes can catalyse the reaction of certain substances with oxygen and thus remove oxygen from a system or catalyse highly oxidative species to more stable species. For example, glucose oxidase catalyses the reaction between glucose and oxygen, yielding D-gluconic acid and hydrogen peroxide [30]. Superoxide dismutase (SOD) can catalyse superoxide radicals $O_2^{\cdot-}$ produced from hydrogen peroxide to triplet oxygen according to the reaction:

$$2O_2^{\cdot -} + 2H^+ \rightarrow H_2O_2 + {}^3O_2$$

Catalase further catalyses the conversion of hydrogen peroxide into water and triplet oxygen [5,35,36]:

$$2H_2O_2 \rightarrow 2H_2O + {}^3O_2$$

Cholesterol oxidation *in vitro* was strongly inhibited in the presence of SOD isolated from yeast [37].

Radical scavengers

Different carotenoids were shown to suppress oxidation of methyl linoleate in the order astaxanthin > canthaxanthin > β-carotene > zeaxanthin. The stability of the four carotenoids followed the same order, i.e. the more stable the more efficient as antioxidant (Fig. 1) [38].

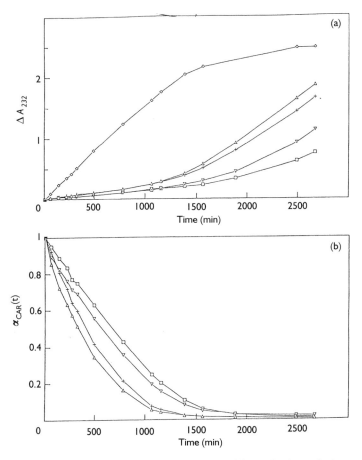

Fig. I. Formation of conjugated dienes (a) and degradation of carotenoids (b) in oxidation of methyl linoleate [38]. ◇, Control without added carotenoid; △, zeaxanthin; +, β-carotene; ▽, canthaxanthin; □, astaxanthin.

Other secondary antioxidants

Thiodipropionic acid and dilauryl thiodipropionate can decompose the hydrogen peroxide produced during lipid oxidation into stable end products [30,31]. Sterols (such as Δ^5-avenasterol, fucosterol and citrostadienol) may be oxidized and inhibit the propagation of free radical chains [31,39–41].

Antioxidants with multiple functions

Some antioxidants, such as phospholipids and Maillard-reaction products (MRPs) inhibit autoxidation of lipids by more than one mechanism. The antioxidant activity of phospholipids may arise from their ability to chelate metallic ions and from their capacity to release protons to bring about the rapid decomposition of hydroperoxides without the formation of free radicals. Moreover, synergistic phospholipids can promote the regeneration of primary antioxidants [5,42–45].

Maillard products come from the Maillard reaction, which is a complex reaction between reducing sugar and amino acids, peptides or proteins. Maillard-reaction products such as intermediate reductone compounds and high-molecular-mass melanoidins exhibit antioxidant activity. They have been proved to have metal-chelating properties and to be effective in reducing hydroperoxides to non-radical products [46,47].

Antioxidant systems in raw materials and processed foods

An antioxidant system in raw materials and processed foods may include: (i) endogenous antioxidants which are their natural constituents; (ii) substances formed during food processing; and (iii) exogenous antioxidants from natural sources or from chemical syntheses.

Endogenous antioxidants

Numerous substances in plant and animal tissues, including vitamins, amino acids, peptides, proteins, nucleotides, pigments, etc., have been demonstrated to have antioxidant properties. They exist as endogenous antioxidants in raw materials and processed foods [4,14].

Antioxidants formed during food processing

Antioxidant substances are known to form during heat-processing of foods and microbial fermentation. Several examples are listed in Table 3.

MRPs have the most attention, since the Maillard reaction occurs often in food storage and processing, especially in heat-processing of foods rich in proteins. The major reactants and factors which influence the reaction are listed in Table 4. The substances with antioxidant activity in MRPs are mainly reductones, melaniodins and heterocyclic compounds such as pyrroles and pyridines [47–49].

MRPs from some combinations of amino acids and sugars, e.g. histidine–glucose and arginine–xylose, have stronger antioxidant properties than other combinations. These MRPs were also shown to act as antioxidants in bakery and meat products [46].

Table 3. Antioxidants formed during heat-processing and fermentation.

Antioxidant	References
MRPs	[14, 46–49]
Volatile compounds formed from heated foods	[49–50]
Soy protein hydrolysates	[51]
Tempeh	[52]
Microbial fermentation	[30, 37]
Nitrosylmyoglobin	[53]

Table 4. Reactants involved in the Maillard reaction and contributory factors [47].

Reactant
Amino acids, peptides, proteins, amines, ammonia + reducing sugar, carbonyl compounds (from oxidation of fatty acid, ascorbic acid and polyphenol)
Contributory factors
pH, temperature, moisture content, heavy metal ions, oxygen, light, sulphite and other constituents

It has been found that some volatile antioxidant substances are formed in heated foodstuffs such as cooked meats, roasted beans and nuts, and baked goods. Further studies identified those substances as 1-alkylpyrroles and their 2-alkyl homologues [49,50]. Soy and other vegetable protein hydrolysates include a number of low-molecular-mass phenolic compounds and thus show an antioxidant capacity [51]. Many antioxidants can be formed during microbial fermentation; for example, the fermentation of beer, sherry and tea produces certain antioxidants [49]. Tempeh (a fermented soybean product) contains isoflavones and genistein, which have been known to inhibit oxidation [52].

The improved oxidative stability of cured meat products is a result of reduction of nitrite to yield the free radical nitric oxide, which is stored in several 'chemical reservoirs' in the product. The cured meat pigment nitrosylmyoglobin is such a free radical buffer, which may provide nitric oxide to terminate free radical processes during lipid oxidation [53].

Some commercial antioxidant enzymes, such as glucose oxidase, catalase and SOD, are produced by microbial fermentation [30,37].

Exogenous antioxidants

Commercial antioxidants used in foods

The most common antioxidants used in foods and their customary applications are listed in Table 5.

The more important natural antioxidants used in foods are tocopherols and ascorbic acid (including its derivatives). Tocopherols include two families, tocols and tocotrienols. Each family includes α, β, Γ, and δ, four homologues depending on the number and position of methyl groups attached to a chromane ring [14]. Their antioxidant activity increases from α to δ [54]. Tocopherols are mainly present in plant tissues. Cereals, oil-seeds and vegetables such as peas, beans and

Table 5. The most common antioxidants used in foods and their customary applications [31].

Antioxidant (common abbreviation)	'E' number[a]	Typical applications
L-Ascorbate	E300	Fruit juices, drinks, mayonnaise, cured meat, fish products, butter, etc.
Sodium L-ascorbate	E301	Meat products
Calcium L-ascorbate	E302	
Palmitoyl L-ascorbic acid (ascorbylpalmitate)	E304	Scotch eggs, sausages, milk fat
Mixed natural tocopherols concentrate	E306	Vegetable oils, milk fat, mayonnaise
Synthetic α-tocopherol (α-T)	E307	Infant foods, milk fat, mayonnaise
Synthetic β-tocopherol (γ-T)	E308	
Synthetic δ-tocopherol (δ-T)	E309	
Propyl gallate (PG)	E310	Chewing gum, vegetable oils
Octyl gallate (OG)	E311	
Dodecyl gallate (DG)	E312	
Butylated hydroxyanisole (BHA)	E320	Animal fat, cheese spread, biscuits, potato flakes, beef stock cubes
Butylated hydroxytoluene (BHT)	E321	Walnuts, chewing gum
Lecithins	E322	Low-fat spread, milk fat, margarine
Citric acid	E330	Vegetable oils, mayonnaise
Others such as:		
Tertiary butylhydroquinone (TBHQ)[b]		Palm oil, frying oils
Ethoxyquin, diphenylamine		Antiscald agents for pears and apples, animal feeds
2,4,5-Trihydroxybutyrophenone (THBP)		
2,6-Di-tert-butyl-4-hydroxymethylphenol (Ionox-100)		
Nordihydroguaiaretic acid (NDGA)[c]		
3-3'-Thiodipropionic acid (TDPA)		
Citrate mixture		

[a]'E' numbers are the European Economic Community (EEC) codes at the time of writing.
[b]Not permitted in EEC countries at the time of writing.
[c]Found to have toxic properties and subsequently removed from the GRAS list by the U.S. Food and Drug Administration (FDA).

carrots are rich sources of tocopherols. They can also be chemically synthesized [14,27]. Ascorbic acid occurs commonly in nature. However, commercial ascorbic acid is usually produced by chemical syntheses [14]. Most of the synthetic anti-oxidants used in foods are phenolic types (Table 5). Their effectiveness and biological impact have been evaluated by many researchers [27,31,55,56], although the toxicology of some synthetic antioxidants such as BHA and BHT has become controversial. Nevertheless, synthetic antioxidants are still the most common antioxidants used in food storage and food processing [54–59].

Commercially exploited natural antioxidants

Although many antioxidant substances have been found to occur naturally, only a limited number of them are actually put to commercial uses as exogenous anti-oxidants. However, these materials have received extensive study as potential sources of natural antioxidants. The more important natural antioxidants from plant and animal tissues are listed in Table 6.

Many plant extracts are also the potential sources of natural antioxidants (Table 7). Antioxidant spices have a special significance, because they are traditionally used in foods as added ingredients and, therefore, could be easily used directly for their antioxidant properties (Table 7).

Rosemary was added to cooked meatballs which were packed under various atmospheric conditions (air, 5% O_2/95% N_2, 3% O_2/97% N_2, 1% O_2/99% N_2, 100% N_2) and stored at 5 °C. Controls without rosemary addition were run parallel. Fig. 2 shows the amount of thiobarbituric acid-reactive substances (TBARS) in all samples, without rosemary along the x-axis and with rosemary

Table 6. Natural antioxidants from plant and animal tissues.

Antioxidants	References
Tocopherols (vitamin E)	[14, 27, 50]
Ascorbic acid (vitamin C)	[30, 50]
β-carotene (vitamin A precursor)	[32, 50, 60, 61]
Riboflavin (vitamin B_2)	[62–64]
Soy bean proteins	[51, 65]
Milk casein	[66]
Maize gluten and zein	[67, 68]
Wheat gliadin	[69, 70]
Plasma	[71, 72]
Egg yolk	[73, 74]
Amino acids	[75–78]
Flavonoids	[79–82]
Sesame-seed oil	[83, 84]
Phenolic acids	[25]
Uric acid	[85, 86]
Ribonucleotides	[87]
Glucoside	[88]

Table 7. Antioxidants present in plant extracts and spices.

Extract	References
Rice and bean hull	[87–90]
Plant leaves	[91–93]
Transhen	[94]
Rosemary	[95–97]
Sage	[95–97]
Labiatae family	[96]
Cloves, cinnamon, black pepper and ginger	[97, 98]

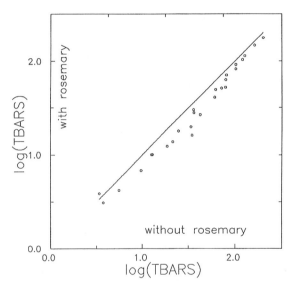

Fig. 2. Log(TBARS) (μmol of malondialdehyde/kg) of reheated pork meatballs with 0.05% added rosemary plotted against samples without rosemary addition [99].

added along the y-axis. The location of all points but one below the identity line means that added rosemary suppressed TBARS formation and development of so-called warmed-over flavour (WOF) in the meatballs [99].

Synergism of antioxidants

When antioxidants with different mechanisms are used together, they often are more active than if used alone. This synergistic effect is very significant for reducing the level of antioxidants added to foods, thereby reducing undesirable side-effects from antioxidants as well as manufacturing costs for foods [14].

Pronounced synergistic effects occur between phenolic compounds and certain acidic substances (such as ascorbic acid, citric acid and phosphoric acid), phospholipids, amino acids and melanoidin [27,43,44,100–104]. In addition, some

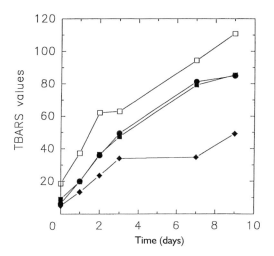

Fig. 3. Increase in TBARS (μmol of malondialdehyde/kg of meat) in stored turkey meatballs packed in 1% O$_2$ [106]. □, Control, no added antioxidant; ■, 200 p.p.m. tocopherols; ●, 200 p.p.m. ascorbyl palmitate; ◆, 200 p.p.m. tocopherol + 200 p.p.m. ascorbyl palmitate.

phenolic antioxidants, such as BHA, BHT and PG, exhibit excellent synergistic effects when used in combination [27,59,105].

Natural tocopherols and ascorbyl palmitate were shown to synergistically depress lipid oxidation in stored turkey meatballs packed in 1% O$_2$. Separate addition of tocopherols or ascorbyl palmitate had both a similar and lower effect on TBARS development than the combination, as shown in Fig. 3 [106].

References

1. Eriksson, C.E. (1987) in Autoxidation of Unsaturated Lipids (Chan, H.W.S., ed.), pp. 207–231, Academic Press, London
2. Halliwell, B. and Gutteridge, J.M.C. (1985) in Free Radicals in Biology and Medicine, pp. 20–64, Clarendon Press, Oxford
3. Kaur, H. and Perkins, M.I. (1991) in Free Radicals and Food Additives (Aruoma, O.I. and Halliwell, B., eds.), pp. 37–57, Taylor & Francis, London
4. Löliger, J. (1991) in Free Radicals and Food Additives (Aruoma, O.I. and Halliwell, B., eds.), pp. 121–150, Taylor & Francis, London
5. Gordon, M.H. (1990) in Food Antioxidants (Hudson, B.J.F., ed.), pp. 1–18, Elsevier Applied Science, London
6. Khayat, A. and Schwall, D. (1983) Food Technol. **37**, 130–140
7. Kappus, H. (1991) in Free Radicals and Food Additives (Aruoma, O.I. and Halliwell, B., eds.), pp. 59–76, Taylor & Francis, London
8. NaWar, W.W. (1985) in Food Chemistry (Fennema, O.R., ed.), pp. 245–370, Marcel Dekker, New York
9. Pearson, A.M., Gray, J.I., Wolzak, A.M. and Horenstein, N.A. (1983) Food Technol. **37**, 121–129
10. Decker, E.A. and Hultin, H.O. (1990) J. Food Sci. **55**, 947–953

11. Pike, O.A. and Peng, I.C. (1988) J. Food Sci. **53**, 1245–1246
12. Dawson, L.E. and Gartner, R. (1983) Food Technol. **37**, 112–116
13. Kanner, J.D. and Fennema, O. (1987) J. Agric. Food Chem. **35**, 71–76
14. Schuler, P. (1990) in Food Antioxidants (Hudson, B.J.F., ed.), pp. 99–170, Elsevier Applied Science, London
15. Beirne, D.O. and Ballantyne, A.B. (1987) Int. J. Food Sci. Technol. **22**, 515–523
16. Hsieh, R.J. and Kinsella, J.E. (1989) Adv. Food Res. **33**, 234–320
17. Lee, S.H. and Min, D.B. (1991) J. Agric. Food Chem. **39**, 642–646
18. Korycka-Dahl, M. and Richardson, T.J. (1980) Dairy Sci. **63**, 1181–1198
19. Almeida-Dominguez, N.G. (1992) J. Food Sci. **57**, 112–117
20. Suarna, C. and Southwell-Keely, P.T. (1991) Lipids **26**, 187–190
21. Yamaoka, M., Carrilo, M.J.H., Nakahara, T. and Komiyama, K. (1991) J. Am. Oil Chem. Soc. **68**, 114–118
22. Cillard, J. and Cillard, P. (1986) J. Am. Oil Chem. Soc. **63**, 1165–1169
23. Shibata, H., Yamane, M., Nagasawa, H. and Ochiai, H. (1991) Agric. Biol. Chem. **55**, 2167–2168
24. Papadopoulos, G. and Boskou, D. (1991) J. Am. Oil Chem. Soc. **68**, 669–671
25. Kikuzaki, H. and Nakatani, N. (1989) Agric. Biol. Chem. **53**, 519–524
26. Hanama, A.A. and Nawar, W.W. (1991) J. Agric. Food Chem. **39**, 1063–1069
27. Kikugawa, K., Kunugi, A. and Kurechi, T. (1990) in Food Antioxidants (Hudson, B.J.F., ed.), pp. 65–98, Elsevier Applied Science, London
28. Empson, K.L., Labuza, T.P. and Graf, E. (1991) J. Food Sci. **56**, 560–563
29. Pokorny, J. (1987) in Autoxidation of Unsaturated Lipids (H.W.S., Chan, ed.), pp. 141–206, Academic Press, London
30. Dziezak, J.D. (1986) Food Technol. **40**, 94–102
31. Kochhar, S.P. and Rossell, J.B. (1990) in Food Antioxidants (Hudson, B.J.F., ed.), pp. 19–64, Elsevier Applied Science, London
32. Warner, K. and Frankel, E.N. (1987) J. Am. Oil Chem. Soc. **64**, 213–218
33. Shibata, H., Kurosaki, C. and Ochiai, H. (1988) Agric. Biol. Chem. **52**, 605–606
34. Lee, S.H. and Min, D.B. (1990) J. Agric. Food Chem. **38**, 1630–1634
35. Sutherland, M.W. and Gebicki, J.M. (1982) Arch. Biochem. Biophys. **214**, 1–11
36. Hicks, C.L. (1980) J. Dairy Sci. **63**, 1199–1204
37. Lingnert, H., Åkesson, G. and Eriksson, C.E. (1989) J. Agric. Food Chem. **37**, 23–28
38. Jørgensen, K. and Skibsted, L.H. (1993) Z. Lebensm. Unters. Forsch. **196**, 423–429
39. Gordon, M.H. and Magos, P. (1983) Food Chem. **10**, 141–147
40. White, P.J. and Armstrong, L.S. (1986) J. Am. Oil Chem. Soc. **63**, 525–529
41. Yan, P.S. and White, P.J. (1990) J. Agric. Food Chem. **38**, 1904–1908
42. Chen, Z.Y. and Nawar, W.W. (1991) J. Am. Oil Chem. Soc. **68**, 938–970
43. Ishikawa, Y., Sugiyama, K. and Kakabayashi, N. (1984) J. Am. Oil Chem. Soc. **61**, 950–954
44. Dziedzic, S.Z. and Hudon, B.J.E. (1984) J. Am. Oil Chem. Soc. **61**, 1042–1045
45. Husain, S.R., Terao, J. and Matsushita, S. (1986) J. Am. Oil Chem. Soc. **63**, 1457–1460
46. Lingnert, H. and Eriksson, C.E. (1981) Prog. Food Nutr. Sci. **5**, 453–466
47. Namiki, M. (1988) Adv. Food Res. **32**, 150–184

48. Mann, T.F., Reagan, J.O., Lillard, D.A., Campion, D.R., Lyon, C.E. and Miller, M.F. (1989) J. Food Sci. **54**, 1431–1437
49. Macku, C. and Shibamoto, T. (1991) J. Agric. Food Chem. **39**, 1990–1993
50. Anon. (1987) A Scientific Status Summary. Food Technol. **9**, 163–168
51. Pratt, D.E., Pietro, C.D., Porter, W.I. and Giffee, J.W. (1981) J. Food Sci. **47**, 24–35
52. Murata, K. (1971) Mem. Osaka City Univ. **18**, 19–23
53. Skibsted, L.H. (1992) in Cured Meat Products and Their Oxidative Stability. The Chemistry of Muscle Based Foods (Ledward, D.A., Johnson, D.E. and Knight, M., eds.), pp. 266–286, Royal Society of Chemistry, London
54. Aoyama, M., Maruyama, T., Niiya, I. and Akatsuka, S. (1987) Nippon Shokuhin Kogyo Gakkaishi **34**, 714–719
55. Bermond, P. (1990) in Food Antioxidants (Hudson, B.J.F., ed.), pp. 193–252, Elsevier Applied Science, London
56. Barlow, S.M. (1990) in Food Antioxidants (Hudson, B.J.F., ed.), pp. 253–308, Elsevier Applied Science, London
57. Warner, C.R., Caniels, D.H., Lin, F.S.D., Joe, F.L. and Fazio, T. (1986) J. Agric. Food Chem. **34**, 1–5
58. Jeremiah, L.E. (1987) J. Food Protection **51**, 105–109
59. Harris, P.L. and Cuppett, S.L. (1991) J. Food Protection **54**, 133–135
60. Ochi, T., Isuchiya, K., Aoyama, M., Maruyama, T. and Niiya, I. (1987) Nippon Shokuhin Kogyo Gakkaishi **34**, 720–724
61. Shibata, H., Kurosaki, C., Kawashima, T. and Ochiai, H. (1987) Agric. Biol. Chem. **51**, 3261–3266
62. Toyosaki, T., Yamamoto, A. and Mineshita, T. (1987) J. Food Sci. **52**, 1377–1380
63. Toyosaki, T., Yamamoto, A. and Mineshita, T. (1987) J. Food Sci. **52**, 88–90
64. Toyosaki, T. and Mineshita, T. (1989) J. Agric. Food Chem. **37**, 286–289
65. Hayes, R.E., Bookwalter, G.N. and Bagley, E.B. (1977) J. Food Sci. **42**, 1527–1532
66. Laakso, S. and Lilius, E.M. (1982) J. Agric. Food Chem. **30**, 913–916
67. Wang, J.Y., Miyazawa, T. and Fujimoto, K. (1991) Agric. Biol. Chem. **55**, 1531–1536
68. Wang, J.J., Fujimoto, K., Miyazawa, T. and Endo, Y. (1991) J. Agric. Food Chem. **39**, 351–355
69. Iwami, K., Hattori, M. and Ibuki, F. (1987) J. Agric. Food Chem. **35**, 628–631
70. Taguchi, K., Iwami, K., Kawabata, M. and Ibuki, F. (1988) Agric. Biol. Chem. **52**, 539–545
71. Faraji, H. and Decker, E.A. (1991) J. Food Sci. **56**, 1038–1041
72. Wayner, D.D.M., Burton, G.W., Ingold, K.U., Barclay, L.R.C. and Locke, S.J. (1987) Biochim. Biophys. Acta **924**, 408–419
73. Yamamoto, Y., Sogo, N., Iwao, R. and Miyamoto, T. (1990) Agric. Biol. Chem. **54**, 3099–3104
74. Yamamoto, Y., Omori, M. and Miyamoto, T. (1991) Agric. Biol. Chem. **55**, 2403–2404
75. Riisom, T., Sims, R.J. and Fioriti, J.A. (1980) J. Am. Oil Chem. Soc. **57**, 354–359

76. Taylor, M.J. and Richardson, T. (1981) J. Am. Oil Chem. Soc. 57, 622–626
77. Ahmad, M.M., Hakim, S.A.L. and Shelata, A.A.Y. (1983) J. Am. Oil Chem. Soc. 60, 837–840
78. Pasquel, L.J.D.R. and Babbitt, J.K. (1991) J. Food Sci. 56, 143–145
79. Hudson, B.J.F. and Lewis, J.I. (1983) Food Chemistry 10, 47–55
80. Das, N.P. and Pereira, T.A. (1990) J. Am. Oil Chem. Soc. 67, 255–258
81. Ramanathan, L. and Das, N.P. (1992) J. Agric. Food Chem. 40, 17–21
82. Miura, K. and Nakatani, N. (1989) Agric. Biol. Chem. 53, 3043–3045
83. Soliman, M.A., El-Sawy, A.A.A., Fadel, H.M. and Osmon, F. (1985) J. Agric. Food Chem. 33, 523–528
84. Nagata, M., Osawa, T., Namiki, M., Fukuda, Y. and Ozaki, T. (1987) Agric. Biol. Chem. 51, 1285–1289
85. Smith, R.C. and Lawing, L. (1983) Arch. Biochem. Biophys. 223, 166–172
86. Farr, D.K., Löliger, J. and Savoy, M.-C. (1986) J. Sci. Food Agric. 37, 804–810
87. Kuchiba, M., Mitsutomi, E., Matoba, T. and Hasegawa, K. (1989) Agric. Biol. Chem. 53, 3187–3191
88. Nakatani, N. and Kikuzaki, H. (1987) Agric. Biol. Chem. 51, 2727–2732
89. Ramarathnam, N., Osawa, T., Namiki, M. and Kawakishi, S. (1988) J. Agric. Food Chem. 36, 732–737
90. Onyeneho, S.N. and Hettiarachchy, N.S. (1991) J. Agric. Food Chem. 39, 1701–1704
91. Osawa, T. and Namiki, M. (1985) J. Agric. Food Chem. 33, 777–780
92. Matsuzaki, T. and Koiwai, A. (1988) Agric. Biol. Chem. 52, 2341–2342
93. Igarashi, K., Itoh, M. and Harada, T. (1990) Agric. Biol. Chem. 54, 1053–1055
94. Zhang, K.-Q., Bao, Y., Wu, P., Rosen, R.T. and Ho, C.-T. (1990) J. Agric. Food Chem. 38, 1194–1197
95. Chang, S.S., Matijasevic, B.O., Hsieh, O.L. and Huong, C.L. (1977) J. Food Sci. 42, 1102–1106
96. Economu, K.D., Oreopoulou, V. and Thomopoulos, C.D. (1991) JAOCS 68, 109–113
97. Bracco, U., Löliger, J. and Viret, J.L. (1981) J. Am. Oil Chem. Soc. 58, 686–690
98. Al-Jalay, B., Blank, G., Mcconnell, B. and Al-Khayat, M. (1987) J. Food Protection 50, 25–27
99. Huisman, M., Lindberg, H., Skibsted, L.H. and Bertelsen, G. (1994) Z. Lebensm. Unters. Forsch. 198, 57–59
100. Finckh, B.F. and Kunert, K.J. (1985) J. Agric. Food Chem. 33, 574–577
101. Wasson, D.H., Reppond, K.D. and Kandianis, K.J. (1991) J. Food Sci. 56, 1564–1566
102. Saito, H. and Takeuchi, M. (1989) Agric. Biol. Chem. 53, 539–540
103. Hildebrand, D.H. (1984) J. Am. Oil Chem. Soc. 61, 552–555
104. Kashima, M., Cha, G.S., Isoda, Y., Hirano, J. and Miyazawa, T. (1991) J. Am. Oil Chem. Soc. 68, 119–122
105. Crackel, R.L., Gray, J.I., Booren, A.M., Pearson, A.M. and Buckley, D.J. (1988) J. Food Sci. 53, 656–657
106. Bruun-Jensen, L., Skovgaard, I.M., Skibsted, L.H. and Bertelsen, G. (1994) Z. Lebensm. Unters. Forsch. 199, 210–213

Biochem. Soc. Symp. **61**, 235–246
Printed in Great Britain

Antioxidants in food packaging: a risk factor?

Gerald Scott

Department of Chemical Engineering and Applied Chemistry, Aston University, Birmingham B4 7ET, U.K.

Abstract

It is current practice to test all new additives for packaging polymers for toxicity before permitting them to be used in food contact applications. However, many antioxidants and stabilizers act sacrificially and are converted to oxidation products in the process of preventing polymer degradation. In most cases, little is known about the toxicity of antioxidant transformation products, and in some cases there is reason to suspect that they may be more toxic than the chemicals from which they are derived.

Two possible solutions are presently showing promise. The first is to chemically react the antioxidant or stabilizer with the polymer, either at the polymer synthesis stage or preferably during processing, so that neither the antioxidant nor its transformation products can be leached into food. The second is to use a biological antioxidant (e.g. α-tocopherol) whose oxidation chemistry and toxicology are known.

Antioxidants and stabilizers in the manufacture of packaging

Oxidation of polymers and the role of antioxidants

All polymers used in the packaging industry are subject to oxidation, and the rate at which this occurs depends on their chemical structure and the conditions to which they are exposed during manufacture and use [1]. The straight-chain paraffinic hydrocarbon polymer, polymethylene (**I**) (Fig. 1), is relatively resistant to both thermo- and photo-oxidation when made in the laboratory by decomposition of diazomethane. However, commercial polyethylene (**II**) is not polymethylene, since it contains appreciable amounts of pendent alkyl groups and, even more importantly, olefinic unsaturation as a result of its method of manufacture. Polypropylene (**III**, R = CH$_3$) and other related poly-α-olefins are even more susceptible to oxidation due to the very high concentrations of tertiary hydrogen atoms.

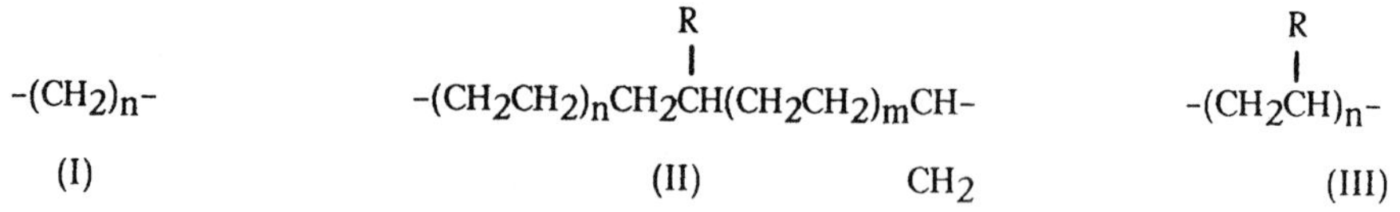

-(CH2)n-
(I)
R
-(CH2CH2)nCH2CH(CH2CH2)mCH-
(II)
CH2
R
-(CH2CH)n-
(III)

Fig. 1. Chemical structure of (I) polymethylene, (II) polyethylene and (III) polypropylene.

However, by far the major cause of environmental instability of the carbon-based polymers is the hydroperoxide group which is introduced during the processing operation [1,2]. To convert polymers into containers or films involves both high temperatures and mechanical action on the polymer in the viscous state. Furthermore, since it is impossible to exclude oxygen during processing, the macroradicals that are produced by shearing of the polymer chains react with oxygen to produce hydroperoxides. This is shown typically for poly(vinyl chloride) (PVC) in Scheme 1 [2], but similar mechano-oxidation occurs with other polymers. Consequently, if the subsequent chain reaction is not inhibited at this stage, extensive oxidation of the polymer will occur. This results, in the case of polypropylene, to molar mass reduction, in polyethylene to cross-linking and in PVC to intense discolouration due to polyconjugation [2]. All these processes are technologically unacceptable since they result in changes in polymer rheology during processing and impairment of polymer performance in service. The hydroperoxidic species, if not destroyed during the manufacturing process, lead to subsequent environmental degradation of the final product, particularly when the artifact is to be exposed to the outdoor environment [3]. Processing stabilizers are therefore added to the polymer before it is extruded or injection-moulded in order to minimize the formation of hydroperoxides which are the primary cause of molecular mass change both during manufacture and use [2].

Cl Cl Cl
-CHCH2CHCH2CHCH2-
PVC
Shear
Cl Cl
-CHCH2CHCH2·
+
Cl
·CHCH2-
O2/PVC
Cl
-CHCH2CH=CH2 + Cl·
Cl
HOOCHCH2-
Cl
-CHCHCH=CH2 + HCl
Cl
O=CCH2-
-CH=CHCH=CH2 + Cl· etc

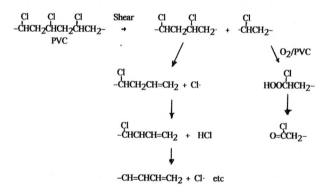

Scheme 1. Mechanodegradation of PVC.

Antioxidant and stabilizer mechanisms

Antioxidants and stabilizers fall into two main classes; those which prevent the formation of free radicals from hydroperoxides and those which interrupt the radical chain reaction, see Scheme 2 [4–6]. Typical examples of chain-breaking and preventive antioxidants are listed in Table 1. By the very nature of their interven-

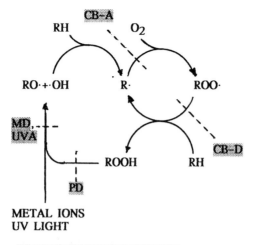

Scheme 2. Mechanisms of antioxidant action.

tion in the removal of free radicals or their precursors from polymers, antioxidants and stabilizers act sacrificially and are partially or wholly transformed to secondary products in exerting their protective effect. These chemical transformations can normally be followed analytically in the polymer during processing. PVC stabilizers act by the preventive mechanism, removing the redox pro-oxidant species (hydrogen chloride and hydroperoxides) produced during processing [2] (see Table 1). One of the most effective 'food approved' PVC stabilizers used in packaging is dibutyl tin maleate (**XVII**; Table 1), and the chemical tranformations occurring during processing in PVC are shown in eqn. (1).

$$\underset{Bu_2Sn}{\overset{O-\overset{O}{\overset{\|}{C}}}{\diagdown}} \overset{CH}{\underset{\|}{\underset{CH}{\|}}} + 2HCl \;\rightarrow\; Bu_2SnCl_2 + O\overset{\overset{O}{\overset{\|}{C}}}{\diagdown}\overset{CH}{\underset{\|}{\underset{CH}{\|}}} + H_2O \quad (1)$$

The end products are the potentially toxic chemicals, maleic anhydride and dibutyl tin chlorides [7]. This reaction is complete within 10 min when PVC is processed at 210 °C [7].

Maleic anhydride itself, although not an antioxidant, is known to undergo a Diels–Alder reaction with polyenic unsaturation, thus effecting the removal of part of the colour [8]. However, this reaction eliminates from the polymer only a small proportion of the free maleic anhydride present (~ 1.5 g/100 g) as a result of eqn. (1) [7].

Table 1. Antioxidant classification.

Mechanism	Code/name	Examples
A. Chain breaking (CB) 1. Electron donors (CB-D) $ROO^{\cdot} + AH \rightarrow ROOH + A^{\cdot}$		Hindered phenols

	IVa, BHT	$R = CH_3$
	IVb, 1076	$R = CH_2CH_2COOC_{18}H_{37}$
	IVc, 1010	$R = (-CH_2CH_2COOCH_2)_4C$
		Aromatic amines

	V, IPPD	$R = iso\text{-}Pr$
2. Electron acceptors (CB-A) $R^{\cdot} + A^{\cdot} \rightarrow RH(C{=}C) + AH$		'Stable' phenoxyls/semiquinones
	VI, G$^{\cdot}$	

| | VII, BQH$^{\cdot}$ | |

| | VIII, SQH$^{\cdot}$ | |

		'Stable' nitroxyls
$R^{\cdot} + A^{\cdot} \rightarrow RA$	IX, 770	
$RA \xrightarrow{\text{Oxidation}} A^{\cdot}$		

		'Spin traps'
	X, MNP	$tBuN{=}O$
	XI, MHPBN	

Table 1 (contd.)

Mechanism	Code/name	Examples
3. Catalytic (CB-A/CB-D)		
$A^{\cdot} + R^{\cdot} \rightarrow [AR]$		where A is $>N-O^{\cdot}$, $G^{\cdot}$,
$[AR] \rightarrow AH + RH(=C)$		BQ or $BQH^{\cdot}$
$AH + ROO^{\cdot} \rightarrow A^{\cdot} + ROOH$		and AH is $>N-OH$, GH,
		$BQH^{\cdot}$ or HQ

B. Preventive
1. Hydroperoxide decomposers
   (PD)

	Code/name	Examples
1.1. Catalytic (PD-C)	XII, DLTP	$(C_{12}H_{25}OCOCH_2)_2S$
	XIII, ZnDC	$(R_2NCSS)_2Zn$
	XIV, ZnDP	$[(RO)_2PSS]_2Zn$
1.2. Stoichiometric (PD-S)	XV, TPP	$P(OPh)_3$
2. Metal deactivators (MD)	XVI	

3. Hydrogen chloride scavenger   XVII, DBTM
   and dienophile

4. Hydrogen chloride scavenger   XVIII, DOTG $Oct_2Sn(SCH_2COOOct)_2$
   and peroxide decomposer

5. UV absorbers   XIX, HOBP

Many CB antioxidant transformation products are able to redox-cycle during processing through reduction by macroalkyl radicals in the polymer. The hindered phenols (**IV**; Table 1) are widely used as processing stabilizers (mechanoantioxidants) for hydrocarbon polymers. The main products formed when butylated hydroxytoluene (BHT; **IVa**) is oxidized are electron (hydrogen) acceptors, **VI–VIII** (see Table 1). These are much more effective than BHT itself as processing stabilizers [9,10], and this has been shown to be due to the cycling of the oxidized and reduced forms of the transformation products in the reducing environment of the processing operation. This catalytic antioxidant mechanism cannot occur efficiently at ambient oxygen pressures, since it requires an appreciable alkyl radical concentration to reduce back the phenoxyl radical to the parent phenol, and alkyl radicals react extremely rapidly with oxygen. Thus peroxyl formation competes with the CB-A reaction and peroxyl radicals are removed by the reduced form of the antioxidant, completing the redox antioxidant cycle. Detailed studies have shown that during high temperature processing of polymers the high shearing forces acting on the polymer in the viscoelastic state, coupled with the low concentrations of oxygen in the system, leads to the rapid regeneration of the CB-D antioxidant during the early stages of the reaction. The chemistry of the 'redox antioxidant' process has been discussed in detail elsewhere [2], but it should be noted here that, because it is a catalytic process, **VI–IX** (Table 1) are highly efficient processing stabilizers.

Designing 'safe' antioxidants for food packaging

Most low-molar-mass additives are able to diffuse relatively rapidly through polymeric substrates and in contact with fats and oils and are readily removed from the package [11–13]. Consequently, there are strict regulations in most countries about allowed additives in packaging [14,15]. Antioxidants and stabilizers have to undergo a rigorous toxicity testing regime before they are licenced as food contact additives. However, in commercial practice, the potentially toxic derived transformation products formed in the package during its manufacture have generally not been tested at all.

In view of the immense amount of work that would be involved in evaluating the toxicity of all the possible transformation products that might be formed from commercial 'approved' antioxidants, recent research has looked in different directions to find a solution to this problem. The first approach is to attach antioxidants and stabilizers to polymers through covalent bonds, so that they cannot be lost from the polymer matrix either during the processing operation or during subsequent service. The second is to use, in packaging materials, only antioxidants that are normally present in the human body or are approved foodstuffs additives whose transformation chemistry has already been studied. The former include the tocopherols and the ubiquinones and the latter the organo-soluble ascorbyl esters and the flavanoids, many of which are accepted for foodstuffs use. Some of these are also available commercially and relatively cheaply because of their increasing use as dietary supplements.

Polymer-bound antioxidants and stabilizers

A great deal of work has been done in both academic and industrial laboratories to chemically attach antioxidants to polymers through covalent bonds [16]. Two main ways of reacting antioxidants with polymers are known: (a) co-polymerization of vinyl monomers containing antioxidant groups during the conventional manufacture of polymers and (b) grafting of an antioxidant containing a polymer-reactive group to a commercial commodity polymer by reactive processing.

Both the above processes are used commercially, but the first is costly and is only used for high-value engineering products, where stability cannot be achieved in any other way. Consequently, it cannot be envisaged as a commercial solution for packaging plastics, where cost is of the essence. The second procedure is much more versatile, since it does not require the production of a new speciality polymer for each application and the stabilizer-modified polymer can be 'tailor-made' during polymer conversion into the fabricated product.

Reactive processing of polymers utilizes internal mixers and extruders as chemical reactors. One of the earliest applications of the technique was to attach thiol antioxidants (ASH) to polyunsaturated rubbers by using the free macro-radicals formed by shearing of the polymer chain (see section entitled Oxidation of polymers and the role of antioxidants) to initiate the Kharasch addition of thiols to double bonds in the polymer chain [17,18], see eqn. (2);

$$ASH \; + \; R'CH{=}CHR'' \longrightarrow ASCHCH_2R'' \overset{R'}{|} \qquad (2)$$

where A is an antioxidant or stabilizer group.

This process, although very useful in rubber-modified polymers, has limited application in saturated polymers due to the very low concentrations of olefinic unsaturation normally present. It can, however, be used in PVC, since unsaturation is the primary product of its mechanodegradation (see Scheme 1). Total attachment of thiol antioxidants (e.g. BHBM, **XX**)

to PVC has been observed during processing [19].

A different solution has been found for the saturated polyolefins [17,18,20–22]. This involves the grafting of unsaturated esters to the hydrocarbon chain by reactive processing. Two modifications of this procedure have been developed.

(a) The first utilizes a symmetrical diester of maleic acid (**XXI**), where A is an antioxidant or stabilizer group and PH is a polymer. Symmetrical maleate esters, unlike vinyl monomers, do not readily homopolymerize, but in the presence of a peroxide radical generator (ROOR), they form adducts, **XXII**, on the polymer backbone in very high yield [see eqn. (3)].

(b) A second method involves the grafting of vinyl antioxidants, **XXIII**, in the presence of a radical generator and a co-agent [21,22] [see eqn. (4)].

$$CH_2=CHCOOA + PH \xrightarrow{\quad ROOR \quad} PCH_2CHCOOA \xrightarrow{\quad\quad} GRAFT \qquad (4)$$

$$\overset{\displaystyle CH_2\dot{C}HCOOA}{\underset{}{|}}$$

XXIII   Co-ag   XXIV

It has been shown that widely used commercial antioxidant structures when covalently attached to polyolefins by the above techniques cannot subsequently be removed by the physical processes involved in the normal food contact applications of packaging materials [16,18].

α-Tocopherol and its oxidation products as processing stabilizers for polyolefins

At first sight there would seem to be an obvious benefit from using the antioxidant constituents of foodstuffs as processing stabilizers for packaging plastics. The foodstuffs additive industry has a long history [4,23] and consequently there is a wide range of non-toxic products potentially available. However, as was indicated above, the non-toxicity of the chemical initially incorporated into the polymer does not guarantee that its derived oxidation products formed during processing will also be innocuous.

We chose to study α-DL-tocopherol in some detail because it is readily available commercially and there is a good deal of information on its oxidation products [24,24a]. The major oxidation products formed from α-tocopherol are α-tocopheryl-*p*-quinone (α-Toc-q), the dehydrodimer (α-Toc-dhd) and the oxidized spirodimer (α-Toc-sd) (see Scheme 3) and these are all found in animal tissues and in edible oils [25]. The dimers are excreted as such, and the *p*-quinone as the hydroquinone.

Initial studies had shown that α-tocopherol was a more effective processing stabilizer for polypropylene (PP) than any of the commercial synthetic antioxidants (e.g. Irganox 1010, **IVc**) currently in use [26]. It was not a very effective heat (air oven) or light stabilizer for PP, but as was seen above, this is not a serious disadvantage and could be a positive advantage in packaging which is used once and then disposed of. The major species identified as transformation products of α-Toc-OH when used as a processing stabilizer for PP are α-Toc-sd, α-Toc-st, α-Toc-q and aldehydes formed by methyl group oxidation are minor products (S. Issenhuth, S. Al-Malaika and G. Scott, unpublished work). α-Toc-q is an effective mechanoantioxidant due to its ability to redox cycle by the catalytic CB-A/CB-D mechanism outlined in Table 1 (Z.-A. Lin, S. Al-Malaika and G. Scott, unpublished work). This is particularly interesting in the light of its close structural relationship to the ubiquinones which are known to redox-cycle synergistically with α-Toc-OH *in vivo* [27]. α-Toc-q is the major product formed under photo-oxidative conditions (T. König, S. Al-Malaika and G. Scott, unpublished work) and this is consistent with the poor photostability of polyolefins stabilized with α-Toc-OH.

It was seen earlier that commercial phenolic antioxidants are transformed during processing to quinonoid products and that these are generally more

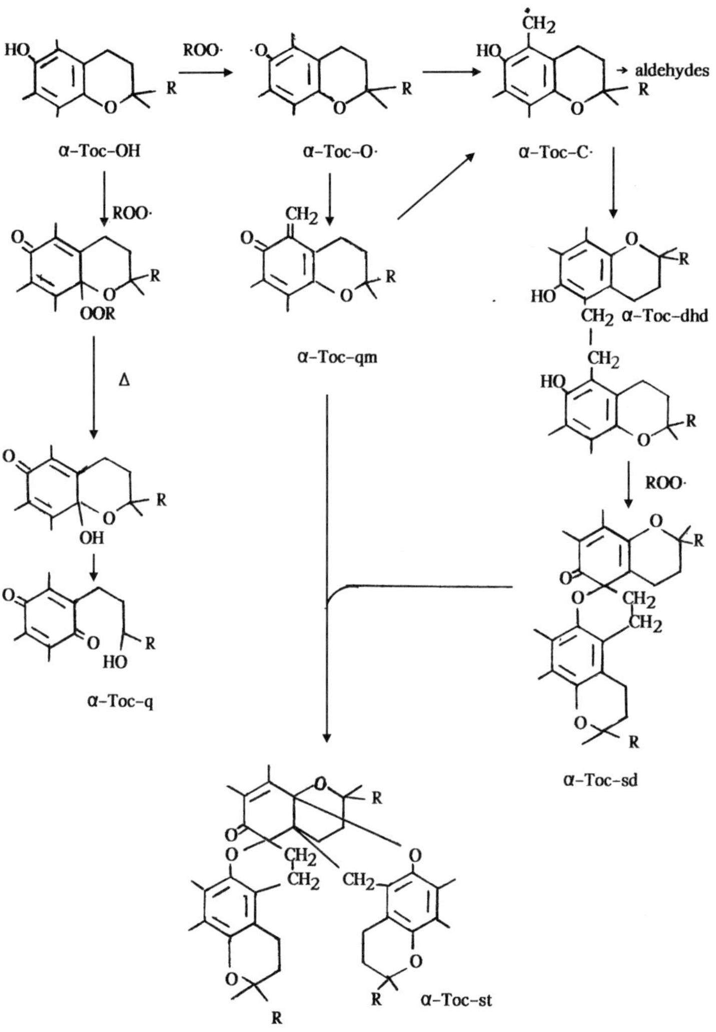

Scheme 3. Oxidation of α-tocopherol.

effective processing stabilizers than the phenols from which they were derived. Since all the oxidation products of α-Toc-OH are quinonoid (see Scheme 3), it seemed possible that the same reversible (redox) antioxidant mechanism might operate with the oxidation products of α-Toc-OH. It has been found (S. Issenhuth, S. Al-Malaika and G. Scott, unpublished work) that all the quinones derived from α-Toc-OH are effective processing stabilizers and that the oxidation sequence outlined in Scheme 3 is partly reversed under the strongly reducing conditions (presence of macroalkyl radicals) in a screw extruder. α-Toc-sd can also be readily reduced by mild reducing agents to α-Toc-dhd, which is itself an effective processing stabilizer. Even α-Toc-OH reduces α-Toc-sd to α-Toc-dhd in refluxing xylene [28]. However, α-Toc-dhd, like α-Toc-q, cannot be reduced back

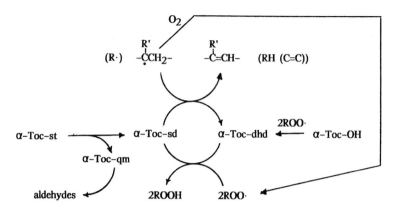

Scheme 4. Redox (catalytic) antioxidant activity of α-tocopherol spiro-dimer (α-Toc-sd).

to α-Toc-OH. It appears then that α-Toc-sd and α-Toc-dhd can redox-cycle reversibly, removing both alkyl and alkylperoxyl radicals (see Scheme 4), almost certainly through the semiquinone in the same way as for other quinones/hydroquinones.

Finally, it is known that *in vivo* α-Toc-O˙ can also redox cycle with α-Toc-OH in the presence of reducing agents. If this could be achieved in the polyolefins during processing then this would extend the period of activity of α-Toc-OH and delay the formation of inactive end-products. Initial attempts to recycle α-Toc-O˙ with ascorbyl esters have not proved successful due to the instability of the ascorbyl moiety under processing conditions (Z. Lin, S. Al-Malaika and G. Scott, unpublished work). Other non-toxic naturally occurring reducing agents are being examined.

Conclusions

Commercial antioxidants and stabilizers undergo chemical transformations during the manufacture of packaging to give products of unknown toxicity. It seems inevitable in the light of the known physical chemistry of the migration of additives from polymers into contacting foodstuffs that these end up, at least in part, in the food chain.

Two possible strategies are discussed to prevent the contamination of foodstuffs by the oxidation products of processing stabilizers. These are: (a) covalent attachment of antioxidants to polymers during synthesis or during polymer conversion to fabricated products; (b) the use of antioxidants which are found already in the human body or which are normal constituents of foodstuffs. Experience with α-tocopherol and its oxidation products suggest that these may be candidates for the latter approach and that the mechanism of their action is related to that occurring *in vivo*.

I am grateful to many co-workers who have contributed to the studies reported and particularly to my colleague Sahar Al-Malaika and to Zau-an Lin, Thomas König, and Silvie Issenhuth for their contributions to the α-tocopherol studies not so far published. We are also grateful to F. Hoffman-La Roche for supporting these studies and to Drs. A. Liniger, F. Nabholz, M. Gmunder and D. Burdick of F. Hoffman-La Roche for helpful discussions and samples of research chemicals.

References

1. Grassie, N. and Scott, G. (1985) Polymer Degradation and Stabilisation, chapt. 4, Cambridge University Press
2. Scott, G. (1993) in Atmospheric Oxidation and Antioxidants (Scott, G., ed.), vol. II, chapt. 3, Elsevier Sci. Publisher
3. Scott, G. (1993) in Atmospheric Oxidation and Antioxidants (Scott, G., ed.), vol. II, chapt. 8, Elsevier Sci. Publisher
4. Scott, G. (1965) in Atmospheric Oxidation and Antioxidants, first edn., chapts. 5 and 6
5. Scott, G. (1993) in Atmospheric Oxidation and Antioxidants (Scott, G., ed.), Vol. I, chapt. 4, Elsevier Sci. Publisher
6. Al-Malaika, S. (1993) in Atmospheric Oxidation and Antioxidants (Scott, G., ed.), Vol. I, chapt. 5, Elsevier Sci. Publisher
7. Scott, G., Tahan, M. and Vyvoda, J. (1978) Eur. Polym. J. **14**, 913
8. Scott, G. (1965) in Atmospheric Oxidation and Antioxidants, first edn., p. 317 et seq.
9. Henman, T.J. (1979) in Developments in Polymer Stabilisation-1 (Scott, G., ed.), p. 39, App. Sci. Pub.
10. Bagheri, R., Chakraborty, K. and Scott, G. (1983) Polym. Deg. Stab. **5**, 145
11. Scott, G. (1988) Food Additives Contaminants **5**, Suppl. No. 1, 421
12. Billingham, N.C. and Calvert, P.D. (1980) in Developments in Polymer Stabilization-3 (Scott, G., ed.), p. 139
13. Billingham, N.C. (1993) in Atmospheric Oxidation and Antioxidants (Scott, G., ed.), chapt. 4, Elsevier Sci. Publisher
14. Crompton, T.R. (1979) Additive Migration from Plastics into Food, Pergamon Press
15. McGuinness, J.D. (1986) Food Additives Contaminants **3**, 95
16. Scott, G. (1993) in Atmospheric Oxidation and Antioxidants (Scott, G., ed.), Vol. II, p. 288 et seq.
17. Scott, G. (1987) in Developments in Polymer Stabilisation-8 (Scott, G., ed.), chapt. 5, Elsevier App. Sci.
18. Scott, G. (1989) in Makromol. Chem., Macromol. Symp. **28**, 59
19. Cooray, B.B. and Scott, G. (1981) Eur. Polym. J. **17**, 385
20. Rekers, J. and Scott, G. (1988) US Patent, 4,743,657
21. Scott, G., Al-Malaika, S. and Ibrahim, A. (1990) US Patent 4,959,410
22. Scott, G. and Al-Malaika, S. (1989) PCT/GB/00909
23. Kochhar, S.P. (1993) in Atmospheric Oxidation and Antioxidants (Scott, G., ed.), Vol. II, Chapter 2
24. Schudel, P., Mayer, H., Metzger, J., Ruegg, R. and Isler, O. (1968) Helv. Chim. Acta **46**, 636

24a. Nilsson, J.L.G., Daves, C.D. and Folkers, K. (1968) Acta Chem. Scand. **22**, 207

25.   Draper, H.H. (1993) in Atmospheric Oxidation and Antioxidants (Scott, G., ed.), Vol. III, p. 272

26.   Laermer, S.F. and Nabholz, F. (1990) Plast. Rubb. Proc. App. **14**, 235

27.   Kagan, V.E., Stoyanovsky, D.A. and Quinn, P.J. (1994) Free Radicals in the Evironment, Medicine and Toxicology (Nohl, H., Esterbauer, H. and Rice-Evans, C., eds.), p. 221, Richelieu Press

28.   Skinner, W.A. and Aloupovic, P. (1963) Science **140**, 803

Biochem. Soc. Symp. **61**, 247–258
Printed in Great Britain

Free radicals and food irradiation

N.J.F. Dodd

CRC Department of Biophysics, Paterson Institute for Cancer Research,
Christie Hospital NHS Trust, Manchester M20 9BX, U.K.

Abstract

Ionizing radiation can be used to control insect and microbial infestation of foodstuffs, inhibit sprouting, delay ripening and reduce the dangers from food-poisoning bacteria. Irradiation produces free radicals, most of which decay rapidly, although some are more persistent. These latter radicals can be detected and characterized by electron spin resonance (ESR). In bone and other calcified tissues, the radiation-induced radicals are distinguishable from naturally occurring radicals, and their stability makes them ideal for radiation dosimetry. The radicals induced in plant material, such as seeds and dried spices, are generally indistinguishable from the endogenous radicals and decay over a period of days or weeks. However, in many of these materials, a radiation-specific radical can be detected at low concentration, thereby permitting identification of irradiated samples, although precluding accurate dosimetry. ESR, although not universally applicable, currently provides the most specific method for the detection of irradiated food.

Introduction

It has been established that exposure of certain foodstuffs to ionizing radiation can (i) prolong shelf life, (ii) control insect and microbial infestation, (iii) inhibit sprouting, (iv) delay ripening and (v) reduce the dangers from food-poisoning bacteria. The method has not gained universal acceptance, but is now permitted for certain specified types of food in more than 30 countries and became legal in the United Kingdom in 1991. Radiation produces very little chemical change in the food — far less than that produced by other methods of food processing, in particular cooking — and the changes that are detected are generally minor changes in the concentration of compounds already present.

The main constituent of most foods is water, irradiation of water leading to the production of a number of highly reactive radicals:

$$H_2O \rightarrow e_{aq}^-, HO^\bullet, H^\bullet \ (H_2, H_2O_2, H_3O^+)$$

These radicals are known to be damaging if produced in close proximity to biologically important molecules such as DNA. In irradiated food, these radicals decay almost instantaneously and are unlikely to constitute a hazard to the subsequent consumer.

On the other hand, some radicals, produced in rigid structures such as bone or cellulose, persist long enough to be ingested. Some radicals undergo rapid decay when exposed to moisture, while others can withstand extreme treatment such as boiling. However, there is no evidence that any of these radicals constitute a hazard to health.

ESR detection of radicals

The presence of radiation-induced radicals in certain foodstuffs provides the possibility of using electron spin resonance (ESR) as a means of monitoring such foodstuffs for the purpose of control and enforcement of the regulations. However, since the nature of the radiation-induced radicals varies greatly from one type of food to another, their stability and ESR characteristics are best considered separately.

Fruit, nuts and spices

The fleshy parts of fruit contain too high a concentration of water for radiation-induced radicals to have sufficient lifetime to be detectable by ESR. Consequently, ESR signals are found only in the seeds or stones and in hard structures such as the stalk. In the case of nuts, it is the shell which is the most likely source of radiation-induced radicals. Many seeds and spices show a broad, non-specific endogenous signal, often associated with pigmentation. On irradiation, this signal increases and, although detectable for days or even months, it decays with a rate that is dependent on storage conditions, in particular humidity and temperature [1–3]. Since many plant tissues exhibit a six-line signal from traces of manganese (Mn^{2+}) ions [4,5], which appears to be unaffected by radiation, it is possible that this signal could be used as an internal standard for quantification of the free radical signal, for example in the case of strawberries (Fig. 1). However, the magnitude of the endogenous free radical signal is probably dependent on the ripeness of the fruit. Hepburn *et al.* [6] have shown that sunlight-induced pigments give ESR signals similar to those produced by ionizing radiation. Storage of paprika at 50 °C in the dark or under artificial light at room temperature is also reported to increase the endogenous signal [7]. Further studies on irradiated strawberries [8] demonstrated the formation of a signal on either side of the main radical signal that was specific for ionizing radiation. This signal was later assigned to radicals in cellulosic constituents of the fruit [9], the two lines separated by about 60 G (6 mT) being the outer lines of a triplet with a ≈ 30 G (3 mT). These authors showed that the radical was formed in the seeds or stones of many types of fruit. Subsequently, the 'cellulose' signal has been reported in the seeds and stems of many different irradiated fruit [8,10–13], in irradiated spices [7,12] and in the shells of irradiated nuts [12]. Complex radiation-induced signals have been observed in mango seeds, a singlet, a doublet with a ≈ 15 G (1.5 mT) and a 'cellulose' signal with a ≈ 55 G (5.5 mT) [5]. It is interesting to note that the latter signal was primarily located in the kernel rather

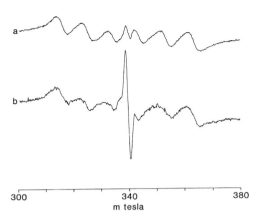

Fig. 1. ESR spectra of strawberry achenes (a) before and (b) after irradiation with a dose of 10 kGy.

than the seed coat, whereas in irradiated black pepper, the 'cellulose' signal is detectable only in the black coat (N.J.F. Dodd, unpublished work) (Fig. 2). The stones of irradiated dates also give complex signals [10,14] which have been shown by Raffi to consist of the 'cellulose' and a 'sugar' signal. This has recently been confirmed by work in Manchester (M.A. Ghelawi, J.S. Moore and N.J.F. Dodd, unpublished work).

Dried fruit and vegetables

The dry outer skin of onions, garlic and shallots give a singlet at $g = 2.00$ which is increased on irradiation and decays only slowly [5]. Similarly, irradiated dried vegetables give simple broad singlets which are similar in shape to those in the unirradiated samples, although of higher intensity, while the single line spectrum of unirradiated dried mushrooms is replaced, on irradiation, by a complex spectrum [10], possibly containing components from cellulose and sugar or other carbohydrate radicals. Irradiation of sultanas, which show no endogenous signal, gives rise to a complex signal that has a surprisingly high stability. Dried papaya [15–18] and banana (Fig. 3) also give a similar signal on irradiation, and comparison of this radiation-induced signal with that from irradiated sugars suggests that it is produced in small crystals of sugar, formed during drying. Consequently, it is probable that many other dried fruits, that are likely to contain microcrystalline sugar, will give similar results.

Bone and shell

Radiation-induced radicals in bone were first reported about 40 years ago [19] and their stability led to the development of an ESR method of archaeological dating [20]. ESR was proposed for dosimetry of irradiated bone grafts [21,22], as a dosimeter in radiotherapy [23] and for dosimetry in cases of accidental exposure to radiation [24]. However, although some attempts were made to use ESR in the detection of irradiated food [1,25–27], the method was largely unknown or ignored until re-examined by the group in Manchester [4]. Since then, the method

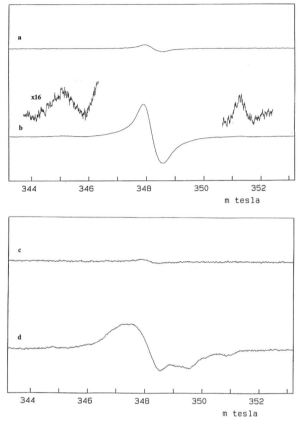

Fig. 2. ESR spectra (a,b) of the black coat and (c,d) of the central 'white' fraction of black pepper, before (a,c) and after (b,d) irradiated to a dose of 10 kGy. Spectrum (b) shows the 'cellulose' signal in the wings, amplified by a factor of 16. Spectrometer gain for spectra (c) and (d) is 4 × that for (a) and (b).

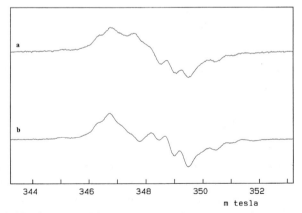

Fig. 3. ESR spectra of (a) dried banana and (b) sucrose irradiated to a dose of 2 kGy.

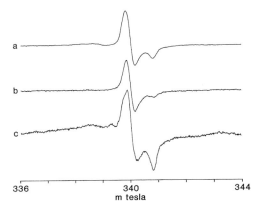

Fig. 4. ESR spectra of (a) chicken bone, (b) fish bone and (c) prawn cuticle irradiated to a dose of 10 kGy. Relative gains are 1, 3 and 6 respectively.

has been widely examined by many groups and recently validated by a collaborative trial involving laboratories in six European countries and one EFTA country [18].

Unirradiated bone gives a broad, weak, ESR signal that may be enhanced slightly by excessive grinding or heating. On irradiation, an asymmetric signal is observed (Fig. 4), that is characteristic of exposure to ionizing radiation and has, so far, not been produced by other treatments, including exposure to UV light or ultrasound. The signal is probably due to several different radicals, the major contribution being from CO_2^- [28]. The most extensive studies have been carried out using chicken bone, in particular the tibiotarsi, although qualitatively identical signals have been observed with bones of other poultry [29], beef and pork [13,30,31] as well as frog [31,32]. A small proportion of the radiation-induced radicals decay within days of irradiation, but the remaining radicals are stable indefinitely [33,34]. In the case of chicken tibiotarsi, cooking produced no more than 10–15% reduction in the signal of the irradiated bones [29,33]. Quantitatively, the harder, more calcified bones give a greater signal for a given radiation dose. This applies even within different bones of the same animal; for example, in chicken there is a 2-fold difference in dose response between the softer bones such as sternum and rib and the harder femur, tibiotarsus, humerus, radius and ulna [33]. Fish bones also show the same characteristic stable signal after irradiation [4,30,31,35,36], although, as expected, this is much weaker than that in the harder bones, and in some cases other, broader signals are also observed. It has also been shown that the fins and scales of irradiated fish show weak but characteristic signals, some of which appear to be the same as that in bone, while others have different characteristics. In the case of irradiated cuticle of prawns and shrimps, some reports indicate the formation of CO_2^- radicals [4], while others suggest radicals from chitin [35]. There appear to be marked differences in the composition of the cuticle of different varieties [37]. The cuticle of scampi (Norway lobster, *Nephrops norvegicus*) shows a characteristic singlet at $g = 2.0009$ in

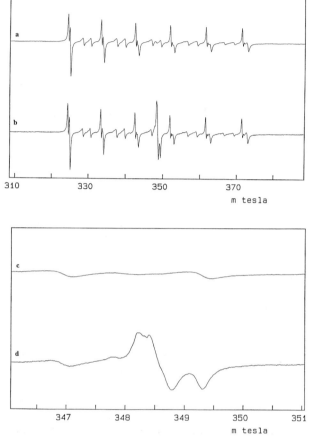

Fig. 5. Mussel shell, (a,c) before and (b,d) after irradiation with a dose of 2 kGy. Spectra (a) and (b) have a sweep width of 80 mT and (c) and (d) a sweep width of 5 mT.

addition to a strong Mn^{2+} signal, present also in the unirradiated material [38,39]. The Mn^{2+} signal is also prominent in unirradiated crab and mussel shells. However, in the latter, the Mn^{2+} signal is complex (Fig. 5), and when a single fragment is examined, it shows marked orientational effects. On irradiation, both shells show the CO_2^- radical signal, at much higher intensity than that in irradiated bone. The linewidth of this signal in mussel shell is narrower than that in crab shell or bone and also appears to be aligned within the matrix.

Quantification

While irradiation frequently produces an enhancement of the endogenous radical signal, this cannot be used as proof of irradiation, since many factors may influence the magnitude of the endogenous signal. Even where large increases are produced by radiation it would be necessary to make accurate quantitative measurements and to know the rate of decay of the signal. Consequently, one requires an ESR signal that is stable and specific for radiation. Three different radiation-specific signals have been detected in the various foodstuffs examined: the 'cellulose' signal, produced in many seeds, spices and the shells of nuts; the 'sugar' signal in dried fruit; the CO_2^- radical signal produced in calcified tissues, such as bone of all types and mollusc shells. The 'cellulose' signal decays, at a rate dependent on storage conditions, in particular moisture, although in date stones and the shells of pistachio nuts the signal has been observed 12 months after irradiation. Consequently, while the presence of this signal is proof of irradiation, it is difficult to estimate the radiation dose. Moreover, the absence of the signal cannot be taken as evidence that the substance has not been irradiated. The 'sugar' signal in dried fruit is stable, but can be removed by rehydration. Therefore, its presence can be taken as proof of irradiation, although its absence is only an indication that there has been no radiation exposure. Quantification of the radiation dose from the magnitude of the signal is unlikely to be accurate, since the concentration of microcrystalline sugars may vary from sample to sample. On the other hand, it may be possible to estimate the original dose by re-irradiation. The stability of the radiation signal in calcified tissues makes it suitable for both qualitative and quantitative determinations [18,34,40,41].

Semi-quantitative methods

The stable radiation-induced signal in calcified tissues initially increases linearly with radiation dose, but at higher doses a saturation effect is observed. The slope of the dose–effect curve and the dose at which saturation occurs both appear to be dependent on the degree of calcification and crystallinity [42–44] of the tissue. Thus the harder meat bones give a larger, less readily saturated signal than the softer fish bones [30,31,45] (Fig. 6). In the case of poultry and fish, the saturation effects occur above the maximum U.K. permitted doses (poultry, 7 kGy; fish, 3 kGy) [46]. Absolute determination of radical concentration by ESR

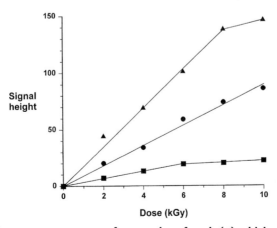

Fig. 6. Dose–response curves for samples of pork (▲), chicken (●) and cod (■) bones.

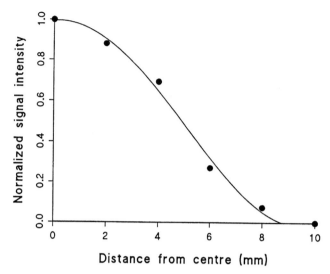

Fig. 7. Graph showing the decrease in signal intensity with distance, on the vertical axis, from the centre of an H_{012} rectangular microwave cavity.

requires precise calibration and measurement of many different parameters [47]. Consequently, in most cases relative measurements are made, comparing changes in the magnitude of the ESR signal and calibrating these against a standard sample of known radical concentration. However, these measurements are still influenced by changes in dielectric constant, which can be produced by differences in moisture content, and by the shape, size and position of the sample, since the response of a standard microwave cavity decreases rapidly as a small sample is moved away from the centre of the cavity (Fig. 7). This latter problem can be minimized in one of two ways. The samples can be powdered and packed into precision bore sample tubes, to fill a depth greater than the depth of the cavity and corrections made for differences in packing density. Alternatively, single fragments of known weight can be carefully positioned at the centre of the cavity, within the region of uniformity, the signals being adjusted to unit weight. In this way, comparison of unknown samples with samples of similar tissue, irradiated to a known dose, can quickly provide a reasonable estimate of dose. However, care must be taken to select the correct tissue as standard, due to the large variation in dose response of different calcified tissues (Fig. 8). The minimum detectable dose for beef or chicken bones is about 50 Gy, while for mussel shell it is as low as 5 Gy [31], but for fish bones is about 500 Gy.

Quantitative methods

It has been shown that samples of the same type of bone taken from different animals [29] or different types of bone from the same animal [33,48] have different dose responses. In particular, the age of the animal or bird [49] has a significant effect. Consequently, accurate radiation dosimetry requires a knowledge

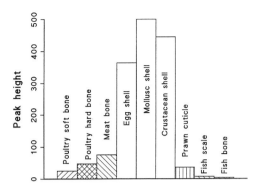

Fig. 8. Histogram showing the variation in height of the CO_2^- radical signal in various calcified tissues, irradiated to 2 kGy.

of the radiation response of each individual sample. This can be determined by re-irradiating the sample several times with a known dose and measuring the ESR signal after each irradiation. The original dose is then found by extrapolation to zero signal [30,31]. In most cases, ESR measurements are made soon after each additional dose of radiation, without allowing time for the initial, rapid, radical decay to occur. The errors introduced by this procedure are probably small, but have not been investigated. Other sources of error are also present, since, in a sample of unknown origin, the original conditions of irradiation may not be reproduced. Several factors that might influence radiation response have been examined using chicken bones [33]. The dose rate and type of irradiation, e.g. low-dose-rate γ-rays or high-dose-rate electrons, appear to have very little influence, but temperature during irradiation has a significant effect. The radical concentration in samples irradiated at $-21\,°C$ is 25% lower than that in samples irradiated at room temperature. Some foods are packed under CO_2, to reduce the growth of micro-organisms. This greatly increases the yield of CO_2^- radicals in powdered bone, but may have no effect in intact bone surrounded by flesh. Cooking irradiated bone causes only a small (10–15%) loss in radiation-induced radicals, but irradiation of cooked bone produces about twice the number of radicals that are produced in uncooked bone. This appears to be due to the change in structure of the bone, in particular loss of collagen and consequent relative increase in calcium content.

Summary

ESR provides a quick and simple method of detecting a wide variety of irradiated foods, due to the appearance of certain radiation-specific signals. In many cases these signals decay within the lifetime of the food and at a rate that is highly dependent on storage conditions, particularly moisture content. Consequently, in such samples, dosimetry is impossible and the absence of a radiation-induced signal cannot be taken as proof that the food has not been irradiated. However, in the case of calcified tissues such as bone or shell the signal remains indefinitely and is unequivocal proof of irradiation. In such cases a qualitative test requires as little as 10 mg of material, which need not be completely dry or free of all traces of flesh or marrow, and the test can be completed within about 5 min. An approximate estimate of radiation dose can be obtained by comparison of the signal height per unit weight with that of an irradiated standard of a similar tissue, provided that the saturation point has not been reached. Accurate dosimetry requires re-irradiation and repeated ESR measurement of the sample, a long and expensive process. Moreover in the case of a cooked bone, it is essential to know whether the initial irradiation was carried out before or after cooking. However, under commercial conditions of irradiation, there will be a significant variation in dose within a batch, and it is only necessary to ensure that the food has been irradiated within certain limits of dose, in order to comply with the regulations. Thus the semi-quantitative ESR method will normally suffice.

References

1. Beczner, J., Farkas, J., Watterich, A., Buda, B. and Kiss, I. (1973) in Proc. Int. Colloquium, The Identification of Irradiated Foodstuffs, pp. 255–267, Commission of European Communities, EUR 5126
2. Beczner, J., Farkas, J., Watterich, A., Mailáth, P.F. and Kiss, I. (1988) in Report of WHO Working Group, Health Impact, Identification and Dosimetry of Irradiated Foods (Bögl, K.W., Regulla, D.F. and Seuss, M.J., eds.), pp. 162–171, Institut für Strahlen Hygiene, ISH-Heft 125
3. Yang, G.C., Mossoba, M.M., Merin, U. and Rosenthal, I. (1987) J. Food Quality 10, 287–294
4. Dodd, N.J.F., Swallow, A.J. and Ley, F.J. (1985) Radiat. Phys. Chem. 26, 451–453
5. Desrosiers, M.F. and McLaughlin, W.L. (1989) Radiat. Phys. Chem. 34, 895–898
6. Hepburn, H.A., Goodman, B.A., McPhail, D.B., Matthews, S. and Powell, A.A. (1986) J. Exp. Bot. 37, 1675–1684
7. Wieser, A. and Regulla, D.F. (1988) in Report of WHO Working Group, Health Impact, Identification and Dosimetry of Irradiated Foods (Bögl, K.W., Regulla, D.F. and Seuss, M.J., eds.), pp. 155–161, Institut für Strahlen Hygiene, ISH-Heft 125
8. Raffi, J.J., Agnel, J.-P.L., Buscarlet, L.A. and Martin, C.C. (1988) J. Chem. Soc. (Faraday Trans. 1) 84, 3359–3362
9. Raffi, J.J. and Agnel, J.-P.L. (1989) Radiat. Phys. Chem. 34, 891–894
10. Stachowicz, W., Strzelczak-Burlinska, G., Michalik, J., Wojtowicz, A., Dziedzic-Goclawska, A. and Ostrowski, K. (1992) J. Sci. Food Agric. 58, 407–415
11. Helle, N., Linke, B., Bögl, K.W. and Schreiber, G.A. (1992) Zeit. Lebensmittel-Unterschung Forschung 195, 129–132
12. Helle, N., Linke, B., Mager, M., Schreiber, G.A. and Bögl, K.W. (1992) Zeit. Ernährungswissenschaft 31, 205–218
13. Goodman, B.A., McPhail, D.B. and Duthie, D.M.L. (1989) J. Sci. Food Agric. 47, 101–111
14. Raffi, J.J., Agnel, J.-P. and Ahmed, S.H. (1991) FoodTec 26–30
15. Helle, N. and Bögl, K.W. (1990) FoodTec 24–39

16. Helle, N., Wiesend, B., Bögl, K.W. and Schreiber, G.A. (1991) Bundesgesundheitsblatt **34**, 317–321

17. Schreiber, G.A., Guggenberger, R., Helle, N., Heide, L., Spiegelberg, A., Holstein, A., Leffke, A., Mayer, M., Wagner, M., Wiesend, B. and Bögl, K.W. (1991) in New Developments in Fundamental and Applied Radiobiology (Seymour, C.B. and Mothersill, C., eds.), pp. 443–448, Taylor and Francis, London

18. Raffi, J.J. (1992) Report, Electron Spin Resonance Intercomparison Studies on Irradiated Foodstuffs, Commission of European Communities, EUR 13630

19. Gordy, W., Ard, W.B. and Shields, H. (1955) Proc. Natl. Acad. Sci. U.S.A. **41**, 983–996

20. Ikeya, M. and Miki, T. (1980) Science **207**, 977–979

21. Stachowicz, W., Michalik, J., Dziedzic-Goclawska, A. and Ostrowski, K. (1970) Nukleonika **17**, 425–431

22. Ostrowski, K., Dziedzic-Goclawska, A., Michalik, J. and Stachowicz, W. (1970) Experientia **26**, 822–823

23. Stachowicz, W., Michalik, J., Dziedzic-Goclawska, A. and Ostrowski, K. (1974) Nukleonika **19**, 845–850

24. Caracelli, I., Terrile, M.C. and Mascarenhas, S. (1986) Health Phys. **50**, 259–263

25. Onderdelinden, D. and Strackee, L. (1970) in Proc. Colloquium, The Identification of Irradiated Foodstuffs (Smeets, J., ed.), pp. 87–95, Commission of European Communities, EUR 4695

26. Onderdelinden, D. and Strackee, L. (1973) in Proc. Colloquium, Identification of Irradiated Foodstuffs, pp. 127–140, Commission of European Communities, EUR 5126

27. Tjaberg, T.B., Underal, B. and Lunde, G. (1972) J. Appl. Bacteriol. **35**, 473–478

28. Geoffroy, M. and Tochon-Danguy, H.J. (1985) Int. J. Radiat. Biol. **48**, 621–633

29. Lea, J.S., Dodd, N.J.F. and Swallow, A.J. (1988) Int. J. Food Sci. Technol. **23**, 625–632

30. Dodd, N.J.F., Lea, J.S. and Swallow, A.J. (1988) Nature (London) **334**, 387

31. Dodd, N.J.F., Lea, J.S. and Swallow, A.J. (1989) Appl. Radiat. Isot. **40**, 1211–1214

32. Raffi, J., Evans, J.C., Agnel, J.-P., Rowlands, C.C. and Lesgards, G. (1989) Appl. Radiat. Isot. **40**, 1215–1218

33. Dodd, N.J.F., Jia, H., Lea, J.S. and Swallow, A.J. (1992) Int. J. Food Sci. Technol. **27**, 371–383

34. Desrosiers, M.F. and Le, F.G. (1993) Appl. Radiat. Isot. **44**, 439–442

35. Desrosiers, M.F. (1989) J. Agric. Food Chem. **37**, 96–100

36. Stewart, E.M., Stevenson, H.M. and Gray, R. (1991) J. Sci. Food Agric. **55**, 653–660

37. Morehouse, K.M. and Desrosiers, M.F. (1993) Appl. Radiat. Isot. **44**, 429–432

38. Stewart, E.M., Stevenson, H.M. and Gray, R. (1992) Int. J. Food Sci. Technol. **27**, 125–132

39. Stewart, E.M., Stevenson, H.M. and Gray, R. (1993) Appl. Radiat. Isot. **44**, 433–437

40. Raffi, J., Belliardo, J.-J., Agnel, J.-P. and Vincent, P. (1993) Appl. Radiat. Isot. **44**, 407–412

41. Desrosiers, M.F., McLaughlin, W.L., Sheahen, L.A., Dodd, N.J.F., Lea, J.S., Evans, J.C., Rowlands, C.C., Raffi, J.J. and Agnel, J.-P.L. (1990) Int. J. Food Sci. Technol. **25**, 682–691

42. Dziedzic-Goclawska, A., Wlodarski, K., Stachowicz, W., Michalik, J. and Ostrowski, K. (1971) Experientia **27**, 1405–1406

43. Ostrowski, K., Dziedzic-Goclawska, A., Stachowicz, W. and Michalik, J. (1972) Histochemie **32**, 343–351

44. Dziedzic-Goclawska, A., Emerich, J., Grzesik, W., Stachowicz, W., Michalik, J. and Ostrowski, K. (1988) J. Bone Mineral Res. **3**, 533–539

45. Bordi, F., Fattibene, P., Onori, S. and Pantaloni, M. (1993) Appl. Radiat. Isot. **44**, 443–447

46. Anon (1990) The Food (Control of Irradiation) Regulations, HMSO, London. Statutory Instrument, 1990 No. 2490

47. Ten Bosch, J.J. (1967) in Ph.D. Thesis, University of Utrecht, Radiation Effects in Collagen: a Quantitative Electron Spin Resonance Study, pp. 56–80, Bronder-Offset, Rotterdam

48. Gray, R. and Stevenson, M.H. (1990) Int. J. Food Sci. Technol. **25**, 506–511

49. Gray, R., Stevenson, M.H. and Kilpatrick, D.J. (1990) Radiat. Phys. Chem. **35**, 284–287

Biochem. Soc. Symp. **61**, 259–271
Printed in Great Britain

Atherogenic and anti-atherogenic factors in the human diet

P.B. Addis*, T.P. Carr*, C.A. Hassel*, Z.Z.Huang† and G.J. Warner‡

*Department of Food Science and Nutrition, 1334 Eckles Avenue,
University of Minnesota, St. Paul, MN 55108, U.S.A., †Department of Family
Practice and Community Health, University of Minnesota, 201 Washington
Avenue, S. E. Minneapolis, MN 55455, U.S.A. and ‡Department of Biochemistry,
Medical College of Pennsylvania, 2900 Queen Lane, Philadelphia, PA 19129,
U.S.A.

Abstract

New atherosclerosis causative factors and preventive modalities have been identified. Atherogenic factors include lipid oxidation products, such as cholesterol oxidation products, malonaldehyde and other aldehydes; *trans*-fatty acids; some saturated fatty acids (lauric, myristic and possibly palmitic acids); and myristic acid plus cholesterol. Lipid oxidation products are well suited to induce arterial damage, based on their known cytotoxic effects; evidence also indicates the possibility of plaque promotion and stimulation of thrombogenesis. Anti-atherogenic factors include antioxidants, fish oils and other polyunsaturates (if protected from oxidation), fibre and trace minerals such as copper, manganese, selenium and zinc. Iron is unique, being considered as both a potential promoter of atherosclerosis (component of ferritin, conceivably inducing lipid oxidation) and a possible anti-atherogenic component (of antioxidant enzyme catalase). It is apparent that an entire new series of research challenges has been uncovered.

Introduction

Coronary heart disease (CHD) and cancer continue to be the greatest causes of morbidity and mortality among developed nations. CHD has always been a controversial disease with respect to its multifactorial etiology and, in view of the latest recommendations to the public on what dietary factors are causative or preventive of CHD, great sums of money have been gained or lost. For this discussion, we have grouped those dietary factors which promote the forerunner to CHD, namely atherosclerosis, as being atherogenic; these are contrasted with those factors believed to be anti-atherogenic, i.e. those which reduce the prevalence or slow the progression of CHD. The fact that many of the factors listed in either grouping are unfamiliar to the reader may reflect the fact that significant new findings are being discovered at a rapid pace and that the original, very popular lipid hypothesis, i.e. the basic idea of how dietary factors (saturated fat and cholesterol) affected CHD, has been undergoing modification for several years. Two examples will be given: (1) saturated fat has long been considered to be cholesterolaemic (and therefore atherogenic) but based on research in the area of low-density lipoprotein (LDL) peroxidation it can be argued that consumption of a polyunsaturated-rich diet could be deleterious because LDL is more susceptible to peroxidation when polyunsaturates are a prominent part of the dietary fat; and (2) hydrogenated vegetable oil shortenings have long been recommended as replacements for animal fats such as butter, lard and tallow; nevertheless, the wisdom of this recommendation is now being questioned in view of several studies linking the consumption of vegetable shortenings to hypercholesterolaemia and CHD. The active principles in the hydrogenated shortenings include the saturated fats along with *trans* isomers formed in the hydrogenation process. These and other equally surprising new findings will be discussed.

In choosing the terms 'atherogenic' and 'anti-atherogenic' we have attempted to simplify the conceptual framework of this review. Therefore, dietary factors that are hypercholesterolaemic are grouped with truly atherogenic (cytotoxic) factors in spite of the fact that hypercholesterolaemia is not exactly the same as atherogenicity. To illustrate, most cases of CHD occur among persons with normal serum cholesterol levels, and many people with hypercholesterolaemia do not exhibit symptoms of CHD. Nevertheless, the risk of CHD rises as serum cholesterol, and more specifically, as serum LDL rises. The exceptions to the latter relationship provide much stimulation for antioxidant/lipid oxidation products (LOPS)/cholesterol oxidation products (COPS) research, because it is possible that elevated serum lipids are less damaging if LOPS/COPS are kept low by a high antioxidant intake.

Atherogenic factors in the human diet

CHD is a multifactorial disease in which diet is only one of many factors involved. Nevertheless, that diet is somewhat easily altered and has enormous economic ramifications, and since Western societies tend to rapidly identify 'scapegoats', large sums of money for research on the lipid hypothesis have been available and there has been, until recently, a tendency to exclude alternative hypotheses regarding diet and CHD. Fortunately, some changes are occurring and many newer areas of CHD research have developed rapidly in the past decade. Based on this newly available data we cite the following as atherogenic factors in the human diet: COPS, LOPS, *trans*-fatty acids and saturated fats (limited to myristic, lauric and possibly palmitic acids), and possibly dietary cholesterol, in combination with high levels of the cholesterolaemic saturated fatty acids. These are summarized in Table 1. Finally, some recent work has identified stored iron (serum ferritin) and therefore dietary iron as a CHD risk factor, but many studies

Table I. Atherogenic factors in the human diet.

Lipid oxidation products
   Cholesterol oxidation products
   Hydroperoxydienes (as precursors to) n-alkanals, *trans*-alkenals, *trans,trans*-
      and *cis,trans*-alka-2,4-dienals, 4-hydroxy-*trans*-2-alkenals
trans-Fatty acids
Some saturated fatty acids
Cholesterol + myristic acid
Iron (ferrous)?

have disputed this finding and there are scientific grounds on which to argue the reverse hypothesis. Therefore, iron will be discussed under both the atherogenic and anti-atherogenic categories.

COPS have been intensively studied for the past two decades and research in this area has received extensive review [1–3]. A synopsis of the research on COPS indicates clearly that cytotoxicity is a common characteristic of a wide variety of COPS. It is also well established that loss of endothelial cells is one of the earliest stages of atherosclerosis, as revealed by studies of monkeys fed high-saturated-fat high-cholesterol diets [4]. Interestingly, powdered eggs were the major source of cholesterol in this study and is a foodstuff known to contain high levels of COPS [5,6]. Several previous studies, involving simultaneous comparisons of purified (by methanolic extraction) cholesterol with the more polar COPS, have consistently demonstrated COPS to be cytotoxic, cholesterol to be free of cytotoxicity, and COPS exhibiting several properties consistent with angiotoxicity [7–9]. These data are summarized in Table 2.

Angiotoxicity is related to the first step of the process leading to clinical CHD — namely, endothelial cell death and endothelial damage. Atherosclerotic lesions of plaque, representing the second step, are found in the intimal layer of cells, causing thickening and eventual occlusion, or at least conditions favouring myocardial infarction. The final stage of CHD is myocardial infarction, frequently the result of thrombosis or arterial spasm. Evidence available suggests a role for COPS in all three stages [1,2].

Some epidemiological data have implicated COPS in CHD. Two populations of immigrants moving from India to London and the West Indies displayed high morbidity and mortality from atherosclerosis without common major risk factors {i.e. high serum LDL, low plasma high-density-lipoprotein (HDL), hypertension, diabetes, or smoking [10,11]}. An important component of Indian cooking is ghee, a clarified butter product. Ghee contains significant levels of COPS (12% of sterols) and could explain the high prevalence of CHD among these populations, especially in the absence of cholesterolaemia [12].

There is also some evidence suggesting that dietary COPS may be atherogenic via their effects on lipoprotein metabolism. Rabbits fed cholesterol containing 5% (w/w) COPS displayed a 5-fold increase in plasma total cholesterol concentration when compared with rabbits fed purified cholesterol [13], data suggesting that the

Table 2. Biological properties of cholesterol oxidation products.

Cytotoxicity
Angiotoxicity
Atherogenicity
Inhibition of hydroxymethylglutaryl-coenzyme A reductase
Inhibition of endothelial cell prostacyclin synthesis
Inhibition of cholesterol 7α-hydroxylase
Inhibition of cholesterol-5,6-epoxide hydrolase
Inhibition of methylsterol oxidases
Stimulation of cholesterol esterification
Increase low-density lipoprotein
Hypercholesterolaemic
Reduction of membrane fluidity
Reduction in cholesterol/phospholipid ratio of membranes
Inhibition of hexose transport by membranes
Modification of membrane calcium flux
Increase osmotic fragility of cells
Mutagenicity

increased plasma cholesterol concentration was attributable to increased very-low-density lipoprotein (VLDL) by the liver. Other studies using HepG2 cells [14] and primary hepatocytes [15] have shown that COPS can stimulate cellular cholesteryl ester synthesis and secretion in lipoproteins. Another potential mechanism by which COPS can increase the atherogenicity of plasma lipoproteins is by increasing LDL cholesteryl ester content, i.e. increasing the cholesteryl ester/apolipoprotein B (apoB) ratio of LDL particles. Carr and co-workers [16] have shown that cholesteryl ester enrichment of plasma LDL is strongly correlated with atherosclerosis development in primates, and that production of cholesteryl ester-enriched LDL is regulated largely by the secretion of apoB-containing lipoproteins by the liver [17]. Recent research in our laboratory has demonstrated that the addition of dietary COPS to HepG2 cells results in the secretion of apoB-containing lipoproteins enriched with cholesteryl esters [18]. These findings could have serious clinical implications, and further research is required to determine the precise role of COPS in the assembly and secretion of hepatic lipoproteins.

The case implicating COPS would be strengthened by linking them to the final step in CHD, thrombosis. Prostacyclin produced by endothelial cells slows the adhesion of platelets to the vessel wall, thereby reducing the risk of loss of integrity, a factor which if left unchecked could result in thrombosis. COPS have been shown to be far more inhibitory of endothelial prostacyclin production than cholesterol [19]. Because platelets secrete platelet-derived growth factor, which in turn stimulates hyperplasia of such cells destined to become foam cells, stage two of CHD can also be accelerated by COPS. A summary of the detrimental properties of COPS is presented in Table 2.

COPS have also been shown to occur in the lipoproteins of fasted humans [20] and to be absorbed post-prandially by chylomicrons and other mechanisms after a meal rich in fat and COPS [21]. The level of COPS peaked about 3 h post-prandial and was, in those subjects that exhibited a sharp increase in plasma COPS, quickly cleared from the circulation in a manner that appeared to represent classic detoxification. In research on the hamster, dietary COPS predominantly appear in the liver [22]. Moreover, lymphatic absorption of COPS in rats has been recently demonstrated [23].

The significance of plasma levels, lipoprotein distribution and absorption of COPS is unknown, but should provide the focus of intense study in the immediate future. This is especially true given new research on the potential role of antioxidants in the prevention of CHD by retarding the peroxidative changes in LDL. We have made informal observations that humans consuming high levels of fruit, vegetables and whole grain cereals tend to experience low levels of circulating plasma COPS. How does the level of COPS caused by *in vivo* lipid oxidation compare with those caused by post-prandial absorption of a meal rich in COPS? This is a crucial question with regard to elucidating the potential role of *in vivo* oxidation and/or dietary COPS in CHD.

COPS are not the LOPS of importance to CHD. Biological oxidations of LDL are now believed to be a necessary step in foam-cell formation [24,25], and involve extensive loss of polyunsaturated fatty acids and the appearance of a number of aldehydic breakdown products [24]; the cytotoxicity of these species is well-established [25]. Therefore, the situation for LOPS and COPS is much the same, as many aspects of CHD are adversely affected by both types of degradation products. The occurrence of LOPS in rancid foods has long been recognized as a quality problem in foodstuffs and the potential for adverse health effects has been previously hypothesized [1,2]. As was the case for COPS, research into these intriguing questions has been stymied by methodology. The traditional methods for measuring rancidity in foods, peroxide value and thiobarbituric acid reagent, were good for assessing potential organoleptic problems but did nothing to monitor the accumulation of individual fatty acid degradation products. Recently, an important advance in this area has been reported [26]. High-field ^{1}H nuclear magnetic resonance spectroscopy has been used to identify numerous aldehydes, many known to be cytotoxic, from heated culinary oils. Logically, the more polyunsaturated oils exhibited the greatest accumulation of detrimental fatty acid breakdown products; saturates were more resistant [26]. Methods now exist for the determination of individual COPS and LOPS in foods, plasma, plasma lipoproteins, and tissues. It is therefore possible for the first time to answer some critical questions regarding the relative importance of both dietary and biologically generated COPS and LOPS and the importance of antioxidants.

The other atherogenic lipids in the human diet include saturated fats, cholesterol and *trans*-fatty acids. Of these, the relationship between dietary saturated fatty acids and plasma cholesterol levels has received the most attention. Early human studies demonstrated that fatty acid chain length and degree of unsaturation were important determinants of cholesterolaemic response [27,28]. Additional studies served as a basis for the development of regression equations [29,30] that have been useful in prediction for groups of subjects' cholesterolaemic responses to short-term modifications in dietary fatty acid consumption. Generally, these equations predict that saturated fatty acids are approximately twice as potent in raising plasma cholesterol levels as are polyunsaturated fatty acids in lowering them. 'Potency' is often expressed as the cholesterolaemic response (in mg/dl) induced per unit of total dietary energy consumed in the form of a given fatty acid. Both Keys and Hegsted documented the negligible influence of stearic acid ($C_{18:0}$) and acknowledged [29,30] the earlier work of Hashim *et al.* [31] and Grande [32] demonstrating that saturated fatty acids less than 12 carbon atoms in length did not significantly influence plasma total cholesterol concentrations. Therefore, as early as 1965, it was generally agreed that almost all of the hyper-cholesterolaemic effects attributed to dietary saturated fatty acids were accounted for by three individual fatty acids: lauric ($C_{12:0}$), myristic ($C_{14:0}$) and palmitic ($C_{16:0}$) acids.

Keys and Hegsted disagreed in their interpretation of the relative cholesterolaemic effects of lauric, myristic and palmitic acids [29,30]. Keys interpreted these three saturated fatty acids to be essentially equivalent on a percent energy basis; Hegsted believed myristic acid to be the most potent saturated fatty acid. In both cases the authors were inferring independent fatty acid effects from multiple regression equations fitted to data compiled from a large number of dietary trials. Limitations of such inferences were duly noted by both authors, in part because of the inter-dependence of these individual dietary fatty acids within the experimental diets used. Characterization of cholesterolaemic effects for specific fatty acids is further complicated by the fact that commonly consumed dietary triacylglycerols are comprised of fatty acids that may also vary in their degree of unsaturation, isomeric orientation of double bonds and position within the triacylglycerol molecule.

In 1970, McGandy attempted to address the independent cholesterolaemic effects of lauric, myristic, palmitic and stearic acids while minimizing some of the limitations posed above [33]. Subjects were fed a semi-synthetic diet in which specific saturated fatty acids were varied independently of one another in a diet containing 300 mg of cholesterol/day and ranging widely in linoleic acid abundance. Results showed a less potent effect for myristic acid and a more potent effect for lauric and stearic acids when expressed relative to the natural fats fed in the earlier study [29]. It was concluded that myristic and palmitic acids were approximately equivalent in hypercholesterolaemic properties and that positional specificity of stearic acid within the triacyglycerol molecule may influence its cholesterolaemic response.

Subsequent to the McGandy study, almost 20 years elapsed before the public policy of heart disease prevention began to drive renewed interest in this area for the purpose of changing the composition of the food supply [34,35]. Bonanome and Grundy [36] fed subjects liquid-formula diets and confirmed earlier findings [27,29,30] that stearic acid was hypocholesterolaemic relative to palmitic acid. Additional work found that lauric acid was also hypocholesterolaemic relative to palmitic acid [37]. However, Hayes and co-workers provided evidence that, under certain conditions, palmitic acid can be approximately equivalent in cholesterolaemic response to oleic acid ($C_{18:10}$, long regarded as neutral [38–40]). These conclusions include the absence or near absence of dietary cholesterol and a low LDL concentration in human subjects or animals. In addition, Hayes provided data in monkeys and gerbils suggesting that, under the conditions described above, myristic and linoleic acids are the only dietary fatty acids with consequential (and opposing) cholesterolaemic effects [41,42]. Dietschy and co-workers demonstrated hypercholesterolaemic responses for lauric, myristic and palmitic acids, relative to all others tested [43,44]. No significant differential effects among these three fatty acids were detected.

Recently, Katan and co-workers [45] attempted an approach similar to McGandy's [33]. Subjects were fed semi-synthetic margarines enriched in either myristic, palmitic or oleic acid such that each fatty acid accounted for at least 10% of total energy. Myristic acid was found to be the most hypercholesterolaemic, followed by palmitic and then oleic. It is interesting and perhaps significant that HDL cholesterol also increased for both men and women on the myristic acid diet.

The *trans*-fatty acid issue is yet another controversial one in CHD research. For decades, the 'authorities' in the U.S. have recommended that the public use vegetable oils and shortenings in place of animal fats such as lard and tallow. However, a recent study of 85000 nurses has suggested a strong relationship between consumption of the *trans* isomer and CHD, either non-fatal myocardial infarction or sudden death from CHD [46]. An 8 year follow-up revealed 431 cases of CHD and a relative risk ratio of 1.5 ($P<0.001$). That the major rise in CHD in this century coincides with increased intake of *trans* isomers and the more recent decline in CHD appears to coincide with the use of more lightly hydrogenated oils was reviewed [46]. In an interesting hypothesis paper, Simopoulos [47] has reviewed literature related to the potential role of *trans*-fatty acids in insulin resistance, a risk factor for CHD. Increasing consumption of *trans* isomers, saturated fat and linoleic acid (provided by the significant increases in vegetable oil consumption and hydrogenated vegetable shortenings) and decreases in linolenic acid consumption could lead to insulin resistance [47]. Other factors involved in insulin resistance include increases in body weight, alcohol intake, and decreases in physical activity and decreases in the consumption of arachidonic, eicosapentaenoic and docosahexaenoic acids. The ability of *trans* isomers to inhibit enzymes involved in elongation and desaturation of fatty acids may exacerbate the situation [48]. Other evidence concerning deleterious *trans* isomer effects include modest elevations of Lp[a] [49], some variants of which are highly atherogenic.

The potential chemical modifications related to the formation of *trans* isomers, the oxidation of *trans* isomers in heated oils and the potential for toxic effects has only begun to be evaluated. In a study of four heated oils, Greek and Italian olive oils, and sunflower and safflower oils, it was noted that a rapid transformation of the *cis* isomer into *trans* isomers occurred as they were heated [50]. Oils with about 0.5% (w/w) *trans* isomer were found after only 7 h of heating at 180 °C to contain as much as 13.5% *trans* fats, with Greek olive oil exhibiting the greatest resistance to change. Most oils are used for far longer periods in restaurants, although some oil is carried out on the food and is replaced with fresh oil.

Iron is the last potentially atherogenic dietary component to be discussed. Although iron is an essential nutrient, an extensive epidemiological study implicated stored iron (plasma ferritin) in CHD in Eastern Finnish men [51]. Iron is well known to initiate tissue oxidative damage. In a study where the function of liver storage iron as a potential risk factor for CHD was evaluated independently and in combination with various lipoprotein indices using the CHD data from 11 countries, along with available data on liver iron stores, CHD mortality rates were found to be best correlated with the liver iron-serum cholesterol product in both men ($r = 0.72$) and, more importantly, in both genders combined ($r = 0.74$). However, the correlation coefficient (r) for the relationship between liver iron and CHD mortality was only 0.23 in men and 0.49 in women, and r for that between iron–cholesterol product and mortality was 0.38 in women [52].

A survey in a total of 82 healthy Dutch volunteers revealed a significant negative association (partial regression coefficient -0.0010, $P \leq 0.05$) between erythrocyte selenium and serum ferritin levels, possibly connected with the mechanism of decreasing glutathione peroxidase activity in erythrocytes following exposure to iron-mediated oxidative stress [53].

The primary research that ignited a controversy on the possible heart–iron relationship was the study conducted by Salonen and co-workers [51]. This study of 1931 randomly selected Eastern Finnish men over a 5-year (1984–1989) period showed that men possessing 200 μg/l ferritin had a 2.2-fold greater (95% confidence interval, 1.2–4.0; $P < 0.01$) risk factor-adjusted risk of acute myocardial infarction when expressed relative to those of men with lower serum ferritin, and the association was stronger in men with serum LDL higher than 5.0 mmol/l (193 mg/dl) than in those with lower LDL levels. The strongest determinants of serum ferritin concentration in the study were the intakes of alcohol and meat. Therefore, the high stored iron level, as assessed by elevated serum ferritin, was suggested as a risk factor in CHD [51]. However, lack of information concerning fruit, vegetable, cereal and antioxidant consumption limits the usefulness of the study.

In a study in West Germany by Oster *et al.* [54], serum iron levels were found not to be associated with the presence of CHD or its severity. There was a moderately positive correlation between the serum ferritin levels and iron concentrations in heart tissue from patients during bypass surgery, whereas serum concentrations of iron and some other trace elements were not correlated with those in the heart tissue. Aronow [55] reported that serum ferritin is not a CHD risk factor in men and women 62 years of age or older. Serum ferritin levels were determined in 577 elderly people after a 14-h fast. CHD was present in 74 of 171 men and in 172 of 406 women. Increased serum ferritin levels were not seen in men or women with documented heart disease and, in fact, 10% of women without CHD displayed elevated ferritin levels, whereas in only 7% of women with CHD these levels were elevated.

On balance, there would appear to no clear consensus regarding the potential role of iron in CHD.

Anti-atherogenic factors in the diet

The studies of anti-atherogenic factors (Table 3) in the human diet are relatively new compared with the traditional studies on atherogenic factors. Nevertheless, the addition or enhancement of anti-atherogenic factors have

Table 3. Anti-atherogenic factors in the human diet.

Antioxidants
Fish oils, protected
Polyunsaturates, protected
Trace minerals: Fe, Cu, Mn, Se, Zn
Fibre

potential to reduce CHD to a greater degree than does the restriction of athero-genic factors. It is easier to add than to prohibit dietary components, especially if prohibition involves foods of high culinary value. Such anti-atherogenic factors include antioxidants, fish oils, polyunsaturates, fibre, and the trace minerals iron, copper and selenium. All can be added to the diet without serious sensory problems, assuming the polyunsaturates, including fish oils, are adequately protected against oxidative deterioration.

The antioxidants are very prominent members of the anti-atherogenic agents in the diet and the chronicle of their discovery supplies a fascinating source of reading material. Early work had clearly established the risk associated with elevated serum LDL, but the laboratory evidence was lacking. In an attempt to learn more about how LDL can load cholesterol ester into arterial cells to produce foam cells, Goldstein and Brown [56] incubated LDL with macrophages. This led to the discovery of receptor-mediated endocytosis by which cholesterol enters the cell [56]. However, the native receptor was, of course, down-regulated, indicating that as cholesterol requirements of the cell were met the process slows; this presented difficulties with hypotheses concerning how foam cells could be formed. Subsequent research demonstrated the existence of the scavenger receptor, one that binds to a modified form of LDL, including oxidized LDL, and one that is not down-regulated [57]. These findings provided the explanation for the produc-tion of foam cells and stimulated interest in preventing oxidation of the lipidic components of LDL, and antioxidants were the obvious choice of weapon.

A recent review by Jialal [58] summarized the strong evidence supporting the concept that antioxidants are potentially a new modality in the prevention of CHD. It is tempting to speculate that the combined effects of increased antioxidant intake and lowering of plasma LDL may have a synergistic beneficial effect on the risk status of CHD. Numerous antioxidants have been studied, including dietary supplements such as α-tocopherol, β-carotene and ascorbic acid; food additives such as butylated hydroxyanisole; and numerous other naturally occurring antioxidants such as the catechins of red wine [59] and green tea [60].

Epidemiological evidence also strongly supports the contention that dietary antioxidants have a protective effect against the free radical reactions that appear to play a key role in CHD [61]. The evidence for these protective effects is strong in part in view of the variety of epidemiological studies that support this hypo-thesis, including cross-sectional comparisons between countries, prospective studies and case-control studies of individuals. Prospective studies have supplied data based on both dietary intake and plasma antioxidant levels [61].

Another group of anti-atherogenic factors is the various plant fibre components of the human diet which function by lowering plasma cholesterol. This area has been recently reviewed by Ripsin and Keenan [62]. Generally, soluble fibre is thought to be more effective as a hypocholesterolaemic agent than insoluble fibre.

Fish oils and other polyunsaturates have long been associated with a decreased risk of CHD [63]. Most of this effect may be ascribable to their ability to lower platelet activity. It is beyond the scope of this review to summarize the extensive, although sometime inconsistent, data concerning the possible protective effect of highly unsaturated oils. It is, however, possible to postulate that these oils, although possible protective in the native state, can become quite toxic if lipid oxidation has occurred extensively [26]. The many potential interrelationships occurring among dietary COPS, LOPS, antioxidants and polyunsaturates, and *in vivo* platelet effects, endothelial injury and amplification or diminution of antioxidant effects and lipid oxidation are complex but potentially very important.

Finally, in spite of the hypothesis concerning iron, ferritin and CHD, and in agreement with the significant and mounting evidence against the 'ferritin hypothesis', the growing evidence suggests that many trace minerals, including iron, have important antioxidant functions and protect biological tissue against free-radical-induced damage. A recent review by Johnson and Fischer [64] summarized data on copper, zinc and manganese, which are components of superoxide dismutases; selenium, a component of glutathione peroxidase; iron, a component of catalase; and copper, as a component of ceruloplasmin. The latter protein oxidizes iron to the ferric state for binding by ferritin. In this manner, free iron is kept in a bound form and is not able to catalyse free-radical reactions.

Summary

This review has focused on the emerging area of dietary lipid oxidation products, antioxidants and *trans*-fatty acids as potential factors influencing CHD. An extensive review of the newer data on saturated fats, a sometimes confusing but often oversimplified area, was presented. It is our opinion that the new areas of antioxidants, lipid oxidation products and *trans*-fatty acids require vigorous research study, since these agents are among the most promising, consistent, logical, and applicable findings that have been reported for many years. It is apparent that an entire new series of research challenges has been uncovered.

Published as paper no. 21885 of the Scientific Journal Series of the Minnesota Agricultural Experiment Station Project 18–23H. We wish to thank Dr. Martin C. Grootveld and Dr. F. Guardiola for technical advice.

References
1. Addis, P.B. (1986) Food Chem. Tox. **24**, 1021–1030
2. Addis, P.B. and Warner, G.J. (1991) in Free Radicals and Food Additives (Aruoma, O.I. and Halliwell, B., eds.), pp. 77–119, Taylor and Francis, London

3. Smith, L.L. (1992) in Biological Effects of Cholesterol Oxides (Peng, S.-K. and Moran, R.J., eds.), pp. 7–32, CRC Press, Boca Raton
4. Faggiotto, A. and Ross, R. (1984) Arteriosclerosis **4**, 341–356
5. Nourooz-Zadeh, J. and Appelqvist, L.-A. (1987) J. Food Sci. **52**, 57–62
6. Sander, B.D., Addis, P.B., Park, S.W. and Smith, D.E. (1989) J. Food Protection **52**, 109–114
7. Peng, S.-K., Taylor, C.B., Tham, P., Werthessen, N.T. and Mikkelson, B. (1978) Arch. Pathol. Lab. Med. **102**, 57–64
8. Peng, S.-K., Sevanian, A. and Morin, R.A. (1992) in Biological Effects of Cholesterol Oxides (Peng, S.-K. and Moran, R.J., eds.), pp. 147–166, CRC Press, Boca Raton
9. Smith, L.L. (1981) in Cholesterol Autoxidation, pp. 361–452, Plenum Press, New York
10. McKeigue, P.M., Adelstein, A.M., Shipley, M.J., Reimersma, R.A., Marmot, M.G., Hunt, S.P., Butler, S.M. and Turner, P.R. (1985) Lancet **2**, 1086–1090
11. Beckles, G.L.A., Kirkwood, B.R., Carson, D.C., Miller, G.J., Alexis, S.D. and Byam, N.T.A. (1986) Lancet **1**, 1298–1301
12. Jacobson, M.S. (1987) Lancet **2**, 656–658
13. Kosykh, V.A., Lankin, V.Z., Podres, E.A., Novikov, D.K., Volgushev, S.A., Victorov, A.V., Repin, V.S. and Smirnov, V.N. (1989) Lipids **24**, 109–115
14. Dashti, N. (1992) J. Biol. Chem. **267**, 7160–7169
15. Drevon, C.A., Engelhorn, S.C. and Steinberg, D. (1980) J. Lipid Res. **21**, 1065–1071
16. Carr, T.P., Parks, J.S. and Rudel, L.L. (1992) Arteriosclerosis Thromb. **12**, 1274–1283
17. Carr, T.P., Hamilton, R.L., Jr. and Rudel, L.L. (1995) J. Lipid Res. **34**, 25–36
18. Warner, G.J. (1994) Ph.D. Thesis, University of Minnesota, St. Paul
19. Peng, S.-K., Hu, B., Peng, A.Y. and Moran, R.J. (1993) Artery **20**, 122–134
20. Addis, P.B., Emanuel, H.A., Bergmann, S.D. and Zavoral, J.H. (1989) Free Radical Biol. Med. **7**, 179–182
21. Emanuel, H.A., Hassel, C.A., Addis, P.B., Bergmann, S.D. and Zavoral, J.H. (1991) J. Food Sci. **56**, 843–847
22. Xiaohong, J. (1992) M.Sc. Thesis, University of Minnesota, St. Paul
23. Osada, K., Sasaki, E. and Sugano, M. (1994) Lipids **29**, 555–559
24. Steinberg, D., Parthasarathy, S., Carew, T.E., Khoo, J.C. and Witzum, J.L. (1989) N. Engl. J. Med. **320**, 915–923
25. Esterbauer, H. and Zollner, H. (1989) Free Radical Biol. Med. **7**, 197–204
26. Claxson, A.W.D., Hawkes, G.E., Richardson, D.P., Naughton, D.P., Haywood, R.M., Chander, C.L., Atherton, M., Lynch, E.J. and Grootveld, M.C. (1994) FEBS Lett. **335**, 81–90
27. Ahrens, E.H., Insull, W., Blomstrand, R., Hirsch, J., Tsaltas, T.T. and Peterson, M.L. (1957) Lancet **1**, 943–953
28. Keys, A., Anderson, J.T. and Grande, F. (1957) Lancet **ii**, 959
29. Keys, A., Anderson, J.T. and Grande, F. (1965) Metabolism **14**, 776–787
30. Hegsted, D.M., McGandy, R.B., Myers, M.L. and Stare, F.J. (1965) Am. J. Clin. Nutr. **17**, 281–295
31. Hashim, S.A., Artega, A. and Van Itallie, T.B. (1960) Lancet **1**, 1105–1112

32. Grande, F. (1962) J. Nutr. **76**, 55–62
33. McGandy, R.B., Hegsted, D.M. and Myers, M.L. (1970) Am. J. Clin. Nutr. **23**, 1288–1298
34. Diet and Health (1989) Implications for Reducing Chronic Disease Risk. National Academy of Sciences Press, Washington, D. C.
35. NCEP (1990) Report of the Expert Panel on Population Strategies for Blood Cholesterol Reduction. U.S. Department of Health and Human Services. NIH Publication No. 90–3046
36. Bonanome, A. and Grundy, S.M. (1988) N. Engl. J. Med. **318**, 1244–1248
37. Dende, M.A. and Grundy, S.M. (1992) Am. J. Clin. Nutr. **56**, 895–898
38. Hayes, K.C., Pronczuk, A., Lindsey, S. and Diersen-Sschade, D. (1991) Am. J. Clin. Nutr. **53**, 491–498
39. Khosla, P. and Hayes, K.C. (1992) Am. J. Clin. Nutr. **55**, 51–62
40. Ng, T.K.W., Hayes, K.C., de Witt, G.F., Jegathesan, M., Satsunasingham, N., Ong, A.S. and Tan, D.T.S. (1992) J. Am. Coll. Nutr. **11**, 383–390
41. Hayes, K.C. and Khosla, P. (1992) FASEB J. **6**, 2600–2607
42. Pronczuk, A., Khosla, P. and Hayes, K.C. (1994) FASEB J. **8**, 1191–1200
43. Woollett, L.A., Spady, D.K. and Dietschy, J.M. (1989) J. Clin. Invest. **84**, 119–128
44. Woollett, L.A., Spady, D.K. and Dietschy, J.M. (1992) J. Clin. Invest. **89**, 1133–1141
45. Zock, P.L., de Vries, H.M. and Katan, M.B. (1994) Arterioscler. Thromb. **14**, 567–575
46. Willett, W.C., Stampfer, M.J., Manson, J.E., Colditz, G.A., Speizer, F.E., Rosner, B.A., Sampson, L.A. and Hennekens, C.H. (1993) Lancet **341**, 581–585
47. Simopoulos, A.P. (1994) Free Radical Biol. Med. **17**, 367–372
48. Koletzko, B. (1992) Acta Paediatr. **81**, 302–306
49. Nestel, P., Noakes, M., Belling, B., McArthur, R., Clifton, P., Janus, E. and Abbey, M. (1992) J. Lipid Res. **33**, 1029–1036
50. Kiritsakis, A., Aspris, P. and Markakis, P. (1989) in Flavors and Off-flavors, (Charalambous, G., ed.), Elsevier Science Publishers B.V., Amsterdam
51. Salonen, J.T., Nyyssönen, K., Korpela, H., Tuomilehto, J., Seppnen, R. and Salonen, R. (1992) Circulation **86**, 803–811
52. Lauffer, R.B. (1990) Med. Hypotheses **35**, 96–102
53. Bukkens, S.G.F., de Vos, N., Kok, F.J., Schouten, E.G., de Bruijn, A.M. and Hofman, A. (1990) J. Am. Coll. Nutr. **9**, 128–135
54. Oster, O., Dahm, M., Oelert, H. and Preilwitz, W. (1989) Clin. Chem. **35**, 851
55. Aronow, W.S. (1993) Am. J. Cardiol. **72**, 347–348
56. Brown, M.S. and Goldstein, J.L. (1976) Science **191**, 150–154
57. Goldstein, J.L., Ho, Y.K., Basu, S.K. and Brown, M.S. (1979) Proc. Natl. Acad. Sci. U.S.A. **76**, 333–337
58. Jialal, I. (1993) Can. J. Cardiol. **9** (Suppl. B), 11B–13B
59. Frankel, E.N., Waterhouse, A.L. and Teissedre, P.L. (1995) J. Agric. Food Chem. **43**, 890–894
60. Namiki, M., Yamashita, K. and Osawa, T. (1993) in Active Oxygens, Lipid Peroxides and Antioxidants (Yagi, K., ed.), pp. 319–332, Japan Scientific Societies Press, Tokyo; CRC Press, Boca Raton

61. Stampfer, M.J. and Rimm, E.B. (1993) Can. J. Cardiol. **9** (Suppl. B), 14B–18B
62. Ripsin, C.M. and Keenan, J.M. (1992) J. Am. Med. Assoc. **267**, 3317–3325
63. Glomset, J.A. (1985) N. Engl. J. Med. **312**, 1253–1254
64. Johnson, M.A. and Fischer, J.G. (1994) Food Tech. **48**, 112–120

Subject index

ABTS [see 2,2'-Azinobis-(3-ethyl
    benzthiazoline-6-sulphonic acid]
Acetaminophen (*see* Paracetamol)
Activated neutrophil, 197
Adaptive response, 51
Adriamycin, 21
Air pollution, 140, 153
Aldehydic breakdown product, 263
Alkoxyl radical, 106, 110
Allergen, 154
ALS (*see* Amyotrophic lateral
    sclerosis)
Alzheimer's disease, 2, 20, 169
Aminopyrine, 166, 167, 168
Amodiaquine, 168
5-Aminosalicylic acid, 166, 169
Amyotrophic lateral sclerosis, 19, 20
Angiotoxicity, 261
Anti-atherogenic factor, 259, 260,
    266–268
Anti-oestrogen, 217
Antioxidant
    cardioprotective action, 217
    chain-breaking, 103
    characterization, 73–93, 224
    commercial application, 227
    defence, 7–11
    in diet, 47, 104, 117–124
    in plasma, 140, 141
    in respiratory tract lining fluid, 140
    mechanism of action, 223
    plant-derived, 2
    use in food packaging, 235–244
Apolipoprotein B, 111, 213, 262
Arterial thrombosis, 210
Arthritis, 18, 19, 22, 93, 195
Arylamine, 166
Asbestos fibre, 156
Ascorbic acid, 140, 142, 143, 227, 230
Atherogenic factor, 259–266
Atherosclerosis, 209, 214
Autoxidation, 4, 5, 66, 222, 223
2,2'-Azinobis-(3-ethyl benzthiazoline-
    6-sulphonic acid), 108

Bioreductive drug, 171
Bone, 249, 251
Breast cancer, 209–211, 215

Caeruloplasmin, 8, 74
Cancer, 117, 209–211, 215
Canthaxanthin, 118, 119
Carbon-centred radical, 70
Carbonyl, 147
Cardioprotection, 210, 216
Cardiovascular disease, 117
Carotenoid, 117–124
β-Carotene, 8, 74, 79, 117–124, 103,
    112
Carotenoid antioxidant, 225
Catalase, 9, 10
Catalytic antioxidant, 244
Cataract, 82
Catechin, 103, 104, 106–110, 112, 113
Catechin/gallate ester, 103, 104,
    107–109, 112, 113
CB-A (*see* Chain-breaking acceptor)
CB-D (*see* Chain-breaking donor)
Chain-breaking acceptor, 237–239
Chain-breaking donor, 237–239
CHD (*see* Coronary heart disease)
Cholesterolaemic response, 264
Cholesterol oxidation product,
    260–263
Cigarette smoke, 21, 74, 124, 140, 141
Clozapine, 163, 165, 168
Coal combustion, 154, 156
COPS (*see* Cholesterol oxidation
    product)
Coronary heart disease, 105, 209–212,
    259–263, 265–268
Cuticle, 251
Cyclization, 67
Cytochrome *c*, 202

Damage removal, 12
Dapsone, 165, 168, 169
Deoxyribose, 185
Detoxification, 10